ME~~~~ SO-AFH-036

ABBREVIATIONS:

12,000 Conveniences at the Expense of Communications and Safety

Eighth Edition

Neil M. Davis, MS, PharmD, FASHP
Professor Emeritus, Temple University
  School of Pharmacy, Philadelphia, PA,
Editor-in-Chief, Hospital Pharmacy
President, Safe Medication Practices
Consulting, Inc.

published by

Neil M. Davis Associates
1143 Wright Drive
Huntingdon Valley, PA 19006-2721

Phone (215) 947-1752
FAX (215) 938-1937
http://www.neilmdavis.com
E-mail med@neilmdavis.com

Contents

Chapter 1
Introduction

L isted are 12,000 current acronyms, symbols, and other abbreviations and 18,000 of their possible meanings. This list has been compiled to assist individuals in reading and transcribing medical records, medically-related communications, and prescriptions. The list, although current and comprehensive, represents a portion of abbreviations in use and their many possible meanings as new ones are being coined every day.

WARNING

Abbreviations are a convenience, a time saver, a space saver, and a way of avoiding the possibility of misspelling words. However, a price can be paid for their use. Abbreviations are sometimes not understood, misread, or are interpreted incorrectly. Their use lengthens the time needed to train individuals in the health fields, wastes the time of healthcare workers in tracking down their meaning, at times delays the patient's care, and occasionally results in patient harm.

The publication of this list of abbreviations is not an endorsement of their legitimacy. It is not a guarantee that the intended meaning has been correctly captured, or an indication that they are in common use. Where uncertainty exists, the one who wrote the abbreviation must be contacted for clarification.

There are many variations in how an abbreviation can be expressed. Anterior-posterior has been written as AP, A.P., ap, and A/P. Since there are few standards and those who use abbreviations do not necessarily follow these standards, this book only shows anterior-posterior as AP. This is done to make it easier to find the meaning of an abbreviation as all the meanings of AP are listed together. This elimination of unnecessary duplication also keeps the book at a convenient size thus enabling it to be sold at a reasonable price. Lower case letters are used when firm custom dictates as in Ag, Na, mCi, etc. The first letter of trademarks are capitalized, whereas nonproprietary names appear in lower case.

The abbreviation AP, is listed as meaning doxorubicin and cisplatin. The reason for this apparent disparity is that the official generic names (United States Adopted Names) are shown rather than the trade names Adriamycin® and Platinol®. In the case of LSD, the official name, lysergide, is given, rather than the chemical name, lysergic acid diethylamide. The Latin derivations for older medical and pharmaceutical abbreviations, (TID, *ter in die,* three times daily) may be found in *Remington.*[1]

Healthcare organizations are wisely advised by the Joint Commission on Accreditation of Healthcare Organizations to formulate an approved list of abbreviations. Every attempt should be made to restrict this list to common abbreviations that are understood by all health professionals who must work with medical records. There are certain dangerous abbreviations that should not be approved, and a warning should be issued about their use (see Table 1 as well as notes in the text). A second list should be published containing dangerous abbreviations which were purposely omitted from the approved list. The reasons for their omission should be stated.

Many inherent problems associated with abbreviations contribute to or cause errors. Reports of such errors have been published routinely.[2-5]

Abbreviations and symbols can also easily be misread or interpreted in a unintended manner. For example:

(1) "HCT250 mg" was intended to mean hydrocortisone 250 mg but was interpreted as hydrochlorothiazide 50 mg (HCTZ50 mg).

(2) Flucytosine was improperly abbreviated as 5 FU causing it to be read as fluorouracil. Flucytosine is abbreviated 5 FC and fluorouracil is 5 FU.

(3) Floxuridine was improperly abbreviated as 5 FU causing it to be read as fluorouracil. Floxuridine is abbreviated FUDR and fluorouracil is 5 FU.

Table 1. Examples of dangerous abbreviations

Problem term	Reason	Suggested term
O.D. for once daily	Interpreted as right eye	Write "once daily"
q.o.d. for every other day	Interpreted as meaning every once a day or read as q.i.d.	Write "every other day"
q.d. for once daily	Read or interpreted as q.i.d.	Write "once daily"
q.n. for every night	Read as every hour	Write "every night," "H.S." or nightly
q hs for every night	Read as every hour	Use "HS" or "at bedtime"
U for Unit	Read as 0, 4, 6 or cc	Write "unit"
O.J. for orange juice	Read as OD or OS	Write "orange juice"
µg (microgram)	When handwritten, misread as mg	Write "mcg"
sq or sub q for subcutaneous	The q is read as every	Use "subcut"
Chemical symbols	Not understood or misunderstood	Write full name
Lettered abbreviations for drug names or drug protocols	Not understood or misunderstood	Use generic or trade name(s)
Apothecary symbols or terms	Not understood or misunderstood	Use metric system
per os for by mouth	OS read as left eye	Use "by mouth," "orally," or "P.O."
D/C for discharge	Interpreted as discontinue (orders for discharge medications result in premature discontinuance of current medication)	Write "discharge"
T̄/d for one per day	Read as T.I.D.	Use "once daily"
/ (a slash mark) for with, and, or per	read as a one	use, "and," "with," or "per"

3

(4) MTX was thought to be mustargen. MTX is methotrexate and mustargen is abbreviated HN_2.

(5) **The abbreviation "U" for unit is the most dangerous one in the book, having caused numerous tenfold insulin overdoses. The word unit should never be abbreviated.** The handwritten U for unit has been mistaken for a zero, causing tenfold errors. The handwritten U has also been read as the number four, six, and as "cc."

(6) OD meant to signify once daily has caused Lugol's solution to be given in the right eye.

(7) OJ meant to signify orange juice, looked like OS and caused Saturated Solution of Potassium Iodide to be given in the left eye.

(8) IVP meant to signify intravenous push (Lasix 20 mg IVP) caused a patient to be given an intravenous pyelogram which is the usual meaning of this abbreviation.

(9) Na Warfarin (Sodium Warfarin) was read as "No Warfarin."

(10) The abbreviation "$\bar{s}$" for without has been thought to mean "with" ($\bar{c}$).

(11) The order for PT, intended to signify a laboratory test order for prothrombin time, resulted in the ordering of a physical therapy consultation.

(12) The abbreviation, "TAB," meant to signify Triple Antibiotic, (a coined name for a hospital sterile topical antibiotic mixture), caused patients to have their wounds irrigated with a diet soda.

(13) A slash mark (/) has been mistaken for a one, causing a patient to receive a 100 unit overdose of NPH insulin when the slash was used to separate an order for two insulin doses:

6 units regular insulin/20 units NPH insulin

(14) Vidarabine, an antiviral agent, was ordered as ara-A, however ara-C which is cytarabine, an antineoplastic agent, was given.

(15) On several occasions, pediatric-strength diphtheria-tetanus toxoids (DT) have been confused with adult-strength tetanus-diphtheria toxoids (Td).

(16) DTP is commonly understood to refer to diphtheria-tetanus-pertussis vaccine. But in some hospitals it is also used as shorthand for a sedative cocktail of Demerol, Thorazine, and Phenergan. Several cases have occurred where a child was vaccinated rather than was given the sedative mixture.

(17) What does the abbreviation MR mean? Some will guess measles-rubella vaccine (M-R-Vax II, Merck), while others will assume mumps-rubella vaccine (Biavax II, Merck).

(18) The abbreviation TIW (three times a week) was thought to mean Tuesday and Wednesday when the I was read as a slash mark. Due to conformation bias (you see what you know) this uncommon abbreviation is seen as the more commonly used TID (three times a day).

(19) PCA meant to be procainamide was interrupted as patient controlled analgesia.

(20) PGE_1 (alprostadil, Caverject) was read P6 E1 (Alcon's ophthalmic pilocarpine and epinephrine solution).

A prescription could be written with directions as follows: "OD OD OD," to mean one drop in the right eye once daily!

Abbreviations should not be used for drug names as they are particularly dangerous. As previously illustrated, there is the possibility that the writer may, through mental error, confuse two abbreviations and use the wrong one. Similarly, the reader may attribute the wrong meaning to an abbreviation. To further confound the problem, some drug name abbreviations have multiple meanings (see CPM, CPZ and PBZ in table 2). The abbreviation AC has been used for three different cancer chemotherapy combinations to mean Adriamycin and either cyclophosphamide, carmustine, or cisplatin.

Beside causing medication errors and incorrect interpretation of medical records, abbreviations can create problems because treatment is delayed while a health professional seeks clarification for the meaning of the abbreviation used. Abbreviations should not be used to designate drugs or combinations of drugs.

Certain abbreviations in the book are followed by a warning, "this is a dangerous abbreviation." This warning

Table 2. Example of abbreviations which have contradictory or ambiguous meanings

BO	=	bowel open; bowel obstruction;
HG	=	Hansen's disease; Hodgkin's disease; Huntington's disease
SDBP	=	seated, standing, or supine diastolic blood pressure
STF	=	special tube feeding; standard tube feeding
CPM	=	cyclophosphamide; chlorpheniramine maleate;
AZT	=	zidovudine; azathioprine
PBZ	=	phenylbutazone; pyribenzamine; phenoxybenzamine
CPZ	=	chlorpromazine; Compazine
DW	=	dextrose in water; distilled water; deionized water
LFD	=	lactose-free diet; low fat diet; and low fiber diet
NBM	=	no bowel movement; normal bowel movement; nothing by mouth;
ESLD	=	end-stage liver disease; end-stage lung disease
MS	=	morphine sulfate; multiple sclerosis; mitral stenosis; musculoskeletal; medical student; minimal support; muscle strength; mental status; milk shake; mitral sound; and morning stiffness
CF	=	cystic fibrosis; Caucasian female; calcium leucovorin (citrovorum factor); complement fixation; cancer-free; cardiac failure; coronary flow; contractile force; cephalothin; Christmas factor; count fingers; and cisplatin and fluorouracil

could be placed after many abbreviations, but was reserved for situations where errors have been published because these abbreviations were used or where the meaning is critical and not likely to be known. Such warning statements should also appear after every abbreviation for a drug or drug combination.

Abbreviations for medical facility names create problems as they are usually not recognized by the readers in other geographic areas. A clue to the fact that one is dealing with such an abbreviation is when it ends with MC, for Medical Center; MH, for Memorial Hospital; CH, for Community Hospital; UH, for University Hospital; and H, for Hospital.

When an abbreviation can not be found in this book or when the listed meaning(s) do not make sense, there is a possibility that the abbreviation has been misread. As an example, a reader could not find the meaning of HHTS. On closer examination it really was +HTS, not HHTS.

Chapter 6 is a table of normal laboratory values. Both the conventional and international values are listed. Each laboratory publishes a list of its normal values. These local lists should be reviewed to see if there are significant differences.

A new section has been added to this edition (chapter 5), a cross-referenced list of 2,100 generic and trademark names. The list contains names of commonly prescribed and new drugs. Trademarks have their first letter capitalized whereas generic names are in lower case. Coded drug names and abbreviations for drug names are found in chapter on abbreviations (chapter 3). This list will enable readers to obtain the generic name for trademark products or trademarks for generic names. It will also serve as a spelling check.

The Council of Biology Editors (CBE), in their 1983 CBE Style Manual listed about 600 abbreviations gathered from 15 internationally recognized authorities and organizations.[6] The majority of these symbols and abbreviations tend to be more scientifically oriented than those which would appear in medical records. In the few situations where the CBE abbreviations differ from what is presented in this book, the CBE abbreviation has been placed in parenthesis after the meaning. As is the practice in the United States, mL has been used rather than ml and the spelling of liter, meter, etc. is used rather than litre and metre, even though ml, litre, and metre are listed in the *CBE Style Manual*. A new edition of the CBE was published in 1995.[7] Again, in this edition, emphasis is placed on scientific abbreviations.

An examination of the 12,000 abbreviations and their 18,000 meanings is a testimonial to the problems and dangers associated with most undefined abbreviations.

The assistance of Ann Sandt Kishbaugh, Merchantville, NJ and Evelyn Canizares and all the others that helped is gratefully acknowledged.

References

1. Gennaro AR, ed. Remington's Pharmaceutical Sciences, 19th ed. Easton, PA: Mack Publishing Co, 1995.

2. Davis NM, Cohen MR. Medication errors: causes and prevention. Huntingdon Valley, PA: Neil M. Davis Associates; 1983.

3. Cohen MR. Medication error reports. Hosp Pharm (appears monthly from 1975 to the present).

4. Cohen MR. Medication errors. Nursing 97 (appears monthly, starting in Nursing 77, to the present).

5. Davis NM. Med Errors. Am J Nursing (appears monthly from 1994 to 1995).

6. CBE Style Manual, 5th ed. Bethesda, MD: Council of Biology Editors; 1983.

7. Scientific Style and Format: The CBE Manual for Authors, Editors, and Publishers, 6th Ed. Council of Biological Editors-Cambridge University Press. Cambridge UK, New York, Victoria Australia: 1995.

Chapter 2

A Healthcare Controlled Vocabulary

Presently there are no standards for physician's orders, consultations, written prescriptions, standing orders, computer order sets, nurse's medication administration records, pharmacy profiles, hospital formularies, etc. Because in the healthcare field everyone does their own thing, there are many variations. These variations in the way abbreviations are expressed are not always understood and at times are misinterpreted. They cause delays in initiating therapy, cause accidents, waste time for everyone in clarifying these documents, lengthen the time it takes to train those working in the healthcare field, lengthen hospital stays, and waste money.

A controlled vocabulary similar to what is used in the aviation industry is needed. Everyone in the aviation industry "follows the book," and uses a controlled vocabulary. All pilots and air traffic controllers say, "alpha", "bravo", "charley." They do not go off on their own and say "adam", "beef", "candy!" They say "one three," not thirteen, because thirteen sounds like thirty. Radio transmission in the aviation industry is not easy to decipher, yet because precision is critical everything possible is done to eliminate error. To prevent errors all radio transmissions are given only in English, every transmission is given in the same order, and must be immediately repeated by the receiver to make sure it was heard correctly. Written and oral communication in the medical professions are just as critical and are also not easy to decipher, so establishing a controlled vocabulary is also necessary in this industry.

Listed below are three organizations that have ongoing projects related to standardizing medical terminology:

Computer-Based Patient Record Institute, Inc.
1000 East Woodfield Rd. Suite 102
Schuamburg, IL 60173

The United States Pharmacopeial Convention, Inc.
12601 Twinbrook Parkway
Rockville, MD, 20852

National Library of Medicine
Unified Medical Language System
8600 Rockville Pike
Bethesda, MD, 20894

Listed below is the start of a Healthcare Controlled Vocabulary. The basis for this controlled vocabulary is established standard terminology and the result of 30 years of studying medication errors by this author.

It is anticipated that a Healthcare Controlled Vocabulary, with professional organizations' input and backing, will grow and some day evolve into an "official standard." Your suggestions and comments are vital to this growth and eventual recognition. It is always safest to avoid the use of abbreviations unless a standard has been established and is well publicized in your work environment.

Standard	What not to use or do	Comments
100 mg (100 space mg)	100mg (100 no space mg)	A USP* standard way of expressing a strength is to leave a space between the number and its units. Leaving this space makes it easier to read the number as can be seen below. 1mg 1 mg 10mg 10 mg 100mg 100 mg
1 mg	1.0 mg	This is a USP standard. When a trailing zero is used, the decimal point is sometimes not seen thus causing a tenfold overdose. These overdoses have caused injury and death.
0.1 mL	.1 mL	When the decimal point is not seen, this is read as 1 mL, causing a ten fold overdose.
once daily (Do not abbreviate.)	The abbreviation OD The abbreviation QD	The classic meaning for OD is right eye. Liquids intended to be given once daily are mistakenly given in the right eye. When the Q is dotted too aggressively it looks like Q.I.D. and the medication is given four times daily. When a lower case q is used, the tail of the q has come up between the q and the d to make it look like qid. In the United Kingdom, Q.D. means four times daily
unit (Do not abbreviate. Write "unit" using a lower-case u)	The abbreviation U	The handwritten U is mistaken for a zero when poorly written causing a 10 fold overdose (i.e. 6 U regular insulin is read as 60). The poorly written U has also been read as a 4, 6, and cc. Write "unit", leaving a space between the number and the word unit.

(continued)

Standard	What not to use or do	Comments
mg (Lower case mg with no period)	mg., Mg., Mg, MG, mgm, mgs	The USP standard expression is the mg
mL (lower case m with a capital L, no period)	mL., ml, ml., mls, mLs, cc	The USP standard expression is the mL
Use generic names or trademarks	Do not abbreviate drug names or combinations of drugs, such as CPZ, PBZ, NTG, MS, 5FC, MTX, 6MP, MOPP, ASA, HCTZ, etc. Do not use shortened names or chemical names	Abbreviated drug names and acronyms are not always known to the reader, at times they have more than one possible meaning, or are thought to be another drug. When the chemical name "6 mercaptopurine" has been used, six doses of mercaptopurine have been mistakenly administered. The generic name, mercaptopurine, should be used. When an unofficial shortened version of the name norfloxacin, norflox was used, Norflex was mistakenly given. An order for Aredia was read as Adriamycin, as some professionals abbreviated the name Adriamycin as "Adria" which looks like Aredia.
The metric system	The apothecary system (grains, drams, minims, ounces, etc.)	The Apothecary system is so rarely used it is not recognized or understood. The symbol for minim (♏︎) is read as mL; the symbol for one dram (♌︎) is read as 3 tablespoons, and gr (grain) is read as gram.
Use properly placed commas for numbers above 999, as in 10,000, or 5,000,000	5000000	Many people have difficulty in reading large numbers such as 5000000. The use of commas helps the reader to read these numbers correctly.

Standard	What not to use or do	Comments
600 mg When possible, do not use decimal expressions.	0.6 g	A USP standard. The elimination of decimals lessens the chance for error.
25 mcg	0.025 mg	Mistakes are made when reading numbers less than 1 with decimals.
Do not use the term "bolus" in conjunction with the administration of potassium chloride injection. Use specific concentrations and the time in which the drug should be administered.		Some physicians will erroneously indicate that potassium chloride injection should be "bolused" or be given "IV push," vaguely meaning that it should not be dripped in slowly. Many deaths have been reported when prescribers have been taken literally and the potassium chloride was given by bolus or IV push. Orders should be specific such as, "20 mEq of potassium chloride in 50 mL of 5% dextrose to run over 30 minutes."
use "and"	Do not use a slash mark or the symbol "&"	A slash mark looks like a one. An order written "6 units regular insulin/20 units NPH insulin," was read as 120 units of NPH insulin. The symbol "&" has been read as a 4.
Orally transmitted medical orders should be read back as heard for verification.	Do not assume that one has spoken or heard correctly.	During oral communications, speakers misspeak and/or transcribers mishear. To minimize these errors, the transmitter must speak clearly and slowly, the transcriber must repeat what was transcribed, and the transmitter must listen attentively when this is being done. This is less likely to occur when the prescription is complete.

(continued)

Standard	What not to use or do	Comments
When prescriptions are written or orally transmitted they must be complete. • dosage form must be specified • strength must be specified • directions must be specified • included in the directions must be the purpose or indication.	Incomplete orders	Prescribers on occasion think of one drug and mistakenly order another. Nurses and pharmacists on occasion misread prescriptions because of error, poor handwriting or poor oral communications, or look alike or sound alike drugs.[1] When the prescription is complete and the purpose or indication is included, these errors are less likely to occur. Listing the purpose or indication on the prescription label will assist in increasing patient compliance.
Written communications must be legible.	Illegible handwriting	Prescribers who cannot or will not write legibly must either print (if this would be legible), type, use a computer, or have an employee write for them and then immediately verify and sign the document.
Prescribe specific doses.	Do not prescribe 2 ampuls or 2 vials	There are often more than one size or concentration of drug available. Failing to be specific will lead to unintended doses being administered.
Establish a list of approved abbreviations with no abbreviation having more than one possible meaning within a context.	Everyone using their own abbreviations.	To understand the scope of this problem examine the contents of this book for abbreviations that have many meanings and for obscure abbreviations which would not generally be recognized.
Use h or hr for hour	°	An order written as q 4° has been read as q 40 or the symbol ° has not been understood.

*USP = United States Pharmacopeia
1. Davis NM, Cohen MR, Teplitsky BS. Look-alike and sound alike drug names: The problem and the solution. Hosp Pharm 1992:27:95–110

Chapter 3

Lettered Abbreviations and Acronyms

Where an abbreviation contains numbers, they are not considered during alphabetizing.

The letter-by-letter (dictionary) system of alphabetizing is used.

Trademarks (proprietary names) have their first letter capitalized, whereas nonproprietary (generic) names are in lower case letters. See WARNING in chapter 1.

A

A	accommodation
	Acinetobacter
	adenine
	age
	alive
	ambulatory
	angioplasty
	anterior
	anxiety
	apical
	arterial
	artery
	Asian
	assessment
A′	ankle
@	at
(a)	axillary temperature
$\bar{a}$	before
A_1	aortic first heart sound

A_2	aortic second sound
A250	5% albumin 250 mL
A1000	5% albumin 1000 mL
A II	angiotensin II
AA	acetic acid
	achievement age
	active assistive
	acute asthma
	African-American
	Alcoholics Anonymous
	alcohol abuse
	alopecia areata
	alveolar-arterial gradient
	amino acid
	anaplastic astrocytomas
	anti-aerobic
	antiarrhythmic agent
	aortic aneurysm
	aplastic anemia
	arm ankle (pulse ratio)
	ascending aorta
	audiologic assessment
	Australia antigen
	authorized absence
	automobile accident

	cytarabine (ara-C) and doxorubicin (Adriamycin)	AAN	AIDS-associated neutropenia analgesic abuse nephropathy analgesic-associated nephropathy attending's admission notes
aa	of each		
A&A	aid and attendance arthroscopy and arthrotomy awake and aware		
A-a	alveolar arterial (gradient)	AAO	alert, awake, & oriented
a/A	arterial-alveolar (gradient)	AAO × 3	awake and oriented to time, place, and person
AAA	abdominal aortic aneurysmectomy (aneurysm) acute anxiety attack aromatic amino acids	AAOC	antacid of choice
		AAP	assessment adjustment pass
A&AA	active and active assistive	AAPC	antibiotic-associated pseudomembranous colitis
AAAE	amino acid activating enzyme		
AAC	Adrenalin, atropine, and cocaine antimicrobial agent-associated colitis	AAPMC	antibiotic-associated pseudomembranous colitis
		a/ApO₂	arterial-alveolar oxygen tension ratio
AACG	acute angle closure glaucoma	AAPSA	age-adjusted prostate-specific antigen
AAD	acid-ash diet antibiotic-associated diarrhea	AAR	antigen-antiglobulin reaction
AADA	Abbreviated Antibiotic Drug Application	AAROM	active-assistive range of motion
[A-a]Do₂	alveolar-arterial oxygen tension gradient	AAS	acute abdominal series androgenic-anabolic steroid aortic arch syndrome atlantoaxis subluxation atypical absence seizure
AAE	active assistance exercise acute allergic encephalitis		
AAECS	amino acid enriched cardioplegic solution		
A/AEX	active assistive exercise	AASCRN	amino acid screen
AAF	African American female	AAT	activity as tolerated alpha-antitrypsin at all times atypical antibody titer
AAFB	alcohol acid-fast bacilli		
AAG	alpha-1-acid glycoprotein	A₁AT	alpha₁-antitrypsin
AAH	acute alcoholic hepatitis	A₁AT-Pᵢ	alpha₁-antitrypsin (phenotyping)
AAI	arm-ankle indices		
AAL	anterior axillary line	AAU	acute anterior uveitis
AAM	African American male amino acid mixture	AAV	adeno-associated vector adeno-associated virus
AAMI	age associated memory impairment	AAVV	accumulated alveolar ventilatory volume
AAMS	acute aseptic meningitis syndrome	AB	abortion Ace® bandage

	antibiotic	ABD PL	abductor pollicis longus
	antibody	ABE	acute bacterial endocarditis
	Aphasia Battery		adult basic education
	apical beat		botulism equine trivalent antitoxin
	armboard		
	products meeting bioequivalence requirements for generic pharmaceuticals	ABEP	auditory brain stem-evoked potentials
		ABF	aortobifemoral (bypass)
A/B	acid-base ratio	ABG	air/bone gap
	apnea/bradycardia		aortoiliac bypass graft
A > B	air greater than bone (conduction)		arterial blood gases
			axiobuccogingival
A & B	apnea and bradycardia	ABH	Ativan, Benadryl, and Haldol
	assault and battery		
ABC	abbreviated blood count	ABI	ankle brachial index (ankle-to-arm systolic blood pressure ratio)
	absolute band counts		
	absolute basophil count		atherothrombotic brain infarction
	advanced breast cancer		
	airway, breathing, and circulation	ABID	antibody identification
		A Big	atrial bigeminy
	all but code (resuscitation order)	ABK	aphakic bullous keratopathy
	aneurysmal bone cyst	ABL	abetalipoproteinemia
	antigen binding capacity		allograft bound lymphocytes
	apnea, bradycardia, and cyanosis		axiobuccolingual
	applesauce, bananas, and cereal (diet)	ABLB	alternate binaural loudness balance
	argon beam coagulator	ABLC	amphotericin B lipid complex
	aspiration, biopsy and cytology	A/B Mods	apnea/bradycardia moderate stimulation
	artificial beta cells		
	avidin-biotin complex	ABMS	autologous bone marrow support
ABCD	amphotericin B colloid dispersion	A/B MS	apnea/bradycardia mild stimulation
ABCDE	botulism toxoid pentavalent	ABMT	autologous bone marrow transplantation
ABD	after bronchodilator	ABN	abnormality(ies)
ABd	plain gauze dressing, type of	abnl bld	abnormal bleeding
Abd	abdomen	A.B.N.M.	American Board of Nuclear Medicine
	abdominal	abnor.	abnormal
	abductor	ABO	absent bed occupant
ABDCT	atrial bolus dynamic computer tomography		blood group system (A, AB, B, and O)
ABD GR	abdominal girth	ABP	ambulatory blood pressure
ABD PB	abductor pollicis brevis		

	androgen binding protein		acyclovir
	arterial blood pressure		adenocarcinoma
ABPA	allergic bronchopulmo-		against clinical advice
	nary aspergillosis		aminocaproic acid
ABPM	allergic bronchopulmo-		anterior cerebral artery
	nary mycosis		anterior communicating
	ambulatory blood pressure		artery
	monitoring		anticanalicular antibodies
ABR	absolute bed rest	AC/A	accommodation
	auditory brain (evoked)		convergence–accommoda-
	responses		tion (ratio)
ABS	absent	ACAT	acyl coenzyme A:
	absorbed		cholesterol
	absorption		acyltransferase
	Accuchek® blood sugar	ACB	alveolar-capillary block
	acute brain syndrome		antibody-coated bacteria
	admitting blood sugar		aortocoronary bypass
	antibody screen		before breakfast
	at bedside	AC̄B	assist with bath
A/B SS	apnea/bradycardia self-	AC & BC	air and bone conduction
	stimulation	ACBE	air contrast barium
ABT	aminopyrine breath test		enema
	antibiotic therapy	ACC	acalculous cholecystitis
ABVD	Adriamycin®, bleomycin,		accident
	vinblastine, and		accommodation
	dacarbazine (DTIC)		adenoid cystic carcinomas
ABW	actual body weight		administrative control
ABx	antibiotics		center
AC	abdominal circumference		advanced colorectal
	acetate		cancer
	acromioclavicular		ambulatory care center
	acute		amylase creatinine
	air conditioned		clearance
	air conduction		automated cell count
	anchored catheter	AcCoA	acetyl-coenzyme A
	antecubital	ACCR	amylase creatinine
	anticoagulant		clearance ratio
	assist control	ACCU	acute coronary care unit
	activated charcoal	ACCU✔	Accuchek® (blood
	before meals		glucose monitoring)
	doxorubicin (Adriamycin)	ACD	absolute cardiac dullness
	and cyclophosphamide		acid-citrate-dextrose
A/C	anterior chamber of the		allergic contact dermatitis
	eye		anemia of chronic disease
	assist/control		anterior cervical
5-AC	azacitidine		diskectomy
ACA	acrodermatitis chronica		anterior chamber diameter
	atrophicans		anterior chest diameter

	before dinner	A/CK	Accuchek®
	dactinomycin	ACL	anterior cruciate ligament
AC-DC	bisexual (homo- and	aCL	anticardiolipin (antibody)
	heterosexual	ACLF	adult congregate living
ACDDS	Alcoholism/Chemical		facility
	Dependency	ACLR	anterior cruciate ligament
	Detoxification Service		repair
ACDF	anterior cervical	ACLS	advanced cardiac life
	diskectomy fusion		support
ACDK	acquired cystic disease of	ACM	Arnold-Chiari
	the kidney		malformation
ACDs	anticonvulsant drugs	ACME	aphakic cystoid macular
ACE	adrenocortical extract		edema
	adverse clinical event	ACMV	assist-controlled
	aerosol cloud enhancer		mechanical ventilation
	angiotensin-converting	ACN	acute conditioned neurosis
	enzyme	ACNU	nidran
	doxorubicin (Adriamycin),	ACOA	Adult Children of
	cyclophosphamide, and		Alcoholics
	etoposide	A COMM A	anterior communicating
ACEI	angiotensin-converting		artery
	enzyme inhibitor	ACP	acid phosphatase
ACF	accessory clinical findings		ambulatory care program
	acute care facility	ACPA	anticytoplasmic antibodies
	anterior cervical fusion	AC-PH	acid phosphatase
ACHES	abdominal pain, chest	ACPO	acute colonic pseudo-
	pain, headache, eye		obstruction
	problems, and severe	ACPP	adrenocorticopolypeptide
	leg pains (early danger	ACPPD	average cost per patient day
	signs of oral	ACPP PF	acid phosphatase prostatic
	contraceptive adverse		fluid
	effects)	ACQ	acquired
ACG	angiocardiography	ACR	adenomatosis of the colon
ACH	adrenal cortical hormone		and rectum
	aftercoming head		anterior chamber
	arm girth, chest depth,		reformation
	and hip width		anticonstipation regimen
ACh	acetylcholine	ACS	acute chest syndrome
ACHA	air-conduction hearing aid		acute confusional state
AChE	acetylcholinesterase		American Cancer Society
AC & HS	before meals and at		anodal-closing sound
	bedtime		before supper
ACI	adrenal cortical	ACSL	automatic computerized
	insufficiency		solvent litholysis
	aftercare instructions	ACSVBG	aortocoronary saphenous
AC IOL	anterior chamber		vein bypass graft
	intraocular lens	ACSW	Academy of Certified
ACJ	acromioclavicular joint		Social Workers

ACT	activated clotting time	ADAM	adjustment disorder with anxious mood
	aggressive comfort treatment	ADAS	Alzheimer's Disease Assessment Scale
	allergen challenge test		
	anticoagulant therapy	ADAS COG	Alzheimer's Disease Assessment Scale-Cognitive Subscale
ACT-D	dactinomycin		
Act Ex	active exercise	ADAT	advance diet as tolerated
ACTG	AIDS Clinical Trial Group	ADAU	adolescent drug abuse unit
ACTH	corticotropin (adrenocorticotrophic hormone)	ADB	amorous disinhibited behavior
		ADC	Aid to Dependent Children
ACT-Post	activated clotting time post-filter		AIDS (acquired immune deficiency syndrome) dementia complex
ACT-Pre	activated clotting time pre-filter		anxiety disorder clinic
ACTSEB	anterior chamber tube shunt encircling band		average daily consumption
ACU	ambulatory care unit	ADCC	antibody-dependent cellular cytotoxicity
ACV	acyclovir	ADD	adduction
	amifostine, cisplatin, and vinblastine		attention deficit disorder
	assist control ventilation		average daily dose
	atrial/carotid/ventricular	ADDH	attention deficit disorder with hyperactivity
A-C-V	A wave, C wave, and V wave	ADDL	additional
ACVD	acute cardiovascular disease	ADDM	adjustment disorder with depressed mood
acyl-CoA	acyl coenzyme A	ADDP	adductor pollicis
AD	accident dispensary	ADDs	AIDS (acquired immune deficiency syndrome)-defining diseases
	admitting diagnosis		
	advance directive (living will)	ADDU	alcohol and drug dependence unit
	air dyne	ADE	acute disseminated encephalitis
	alternating days (this is a dangerous abbreviation)		adverse drug event
	Alzheimer's disease	ADEM	acute disseminating encephalomyelitis
	antidepressant		
	atopic dermatitis	ADEPT	antibody-directed enzyme prodrug therapy
	axis deviation		
	right ear	AEDP	assisted end diastolic pressure
A&D	admission and discharge		
	alcohol and drug	ADFU	agar diffusion for fungus
	ascending and descending		
	vitamins A and D	ADG	atrial diastolic gallop
ADA	adenosine deaminase	ADH	antidiuretic hormone
	American Diabetes Association		
	anterior descending artery		

20

	atypical ductal hyperplasia		anticipate discharge tomorrow
ADHD	attention-deficit hyperactivity disorder		Auditory Discrimination Test
ADI	allowable daily intake		
	axiodistoincisal		any damn thing (a placebo)
A-DIC	doxorubicin and dacarbazine	ADTP	Adolescent Day Treatment Program
Adj D/O	adjustment disorder		Alcohol Dependence Treatment Program
ADL	activities of daily living		
ad lib	as desired	A5D5W	alcohol 5%, dextrose 5% in water for injection
	at liberty		
ADM	admission	ADX	audiological diagnostic
	adrenomedullin	AE	above elbow (amputation)
	doxorubicin		accident and emergency (department)
ADME	absorption, distribution, metabolism, and excretion		acute exacerbation
			adaptive equipment
Ad-OAP	doxorubicin, vincristine, cytarabine, and prednisone		adverse event
			air entry
			antiembolitic
ADOL	adolescent		arm ergometer
ADP	arterial demand pacing		aryepiglottic (fold)
	adenosine diphosphate	A&E	accident and emergency (department)
ADPKD	autosomal dominant polycystic kidney disease	AEA	above elbow amputation
			anti-endomysial antibody
ADPV	anomaly of drainage of pulmonary vein	AEB	as evidenced by
			atrial ectopic beat
ADQ	abductor digiti quinti	AEC	at earliest convenience
	adequate	AECB	acute exacerbations of chronic bronchitis
ADR	acute dystonic reaction		
	adverse drug reaction	AED	antiepileptic drug
	alternative dispute resolution		automated external defibrillator
	doxorubicin (Adriamycin)	AEDD	anterior extradural defects
ADRIA	doxorubicin (Adriamycin)	AEDP	automated external defibrillator pacemaker
ADS	admission day surgery	AEEU	admission entrance and evaluation unit
	anatomical dead space	AEG	air encephalogram
	anonymous donor's sperm		Alcohol Education Group
	antibody deficiency syndrome	AEM	active electrode monitor
ADs	advance directives (living wills)		ambulatory electrogram monitor
			antiepileptic medication
ADSU	ambulatory diagnostic surgery unit	AEP	auditory evoked potential
		AEq	age equivalent
ADT	alternate-day therapy	AER	acoustic evoked response

	albumin excretion rate	AFM×2	double aerosol face mask
	auditory evoked response	AFO	ankle fixation orthotic
Aer. M.	aerosol mask		ankle-foot orthosis
AERS	adverse event reporting system	AFOF	anterior fontanel–open and flat
Aer. T.	aerosol tent	AFP	alpha-fetoprotein
AES	adult emergency service		anterior faucial pillar
	anti-embolic stockings		ascending frontal parietal
AEs	adverse events	AFQT	Armed Forces Qualification Test
AET	alternating esotropia		
	atrial ectopic tachycardia	AFRD	acute febrile respiratory disease
AF	acid-fast		
	afebrile	Aft/Dis	aftercare/discharge
	amniotic fluid	AFV	amniotic fluid volume
	anterior fontanel	AFVSS	afebrile, vital signs stable
	antifibrinogen		
	aortofemoral	AFX	air-fluid exchange
	ascitic fluid	AG	abdominal girth
	atrial fibrillation		adrenogenital
AFB	acid-fast bacilli		aminoglycoside
	aorto-femoral bypass		anion gap
	aspirated foreign body		antigen
AFBG	aortofemoral bypass graft		anti-gravity
AFBY	aortofemoral bypass (graft)		atrial gallop
AFC	adult foster care	Ag	silver
	air filled cushions	A/G	albumin to globulin ratio
AFDC	Aid to Family and Dependent Children	AGA	accelerated growth area
			acute gonococcal arthritis
AFE	amniotic fluid embolization		antigliadin antibody
			appropriate for gestational age
AFEB	afebrile		
AFEU	ante partum fetal evaluation unit		average gestational age
		AG/BL	aminoglycoside/beta-lactam
aFGF	acidic fibroblast growth factor		
		AGD	agar gel diffusion
AFI	acute febrile illness	AGE	acute gastroenteritis
	amniotic fluid index		advanced glycation end product
A fib	atrial fibrillation		
AFIP	Armed Forces Institute of Pathology		angle of greatest extension
			anterior gastroenterostomy
AFKO	ankle-foot-knee orthosis		irreversible advanced glycosylation end products
AFL	atrial flutter		
AFLP	acute fatty liver of pregnancy		
A Flu	atrial flutter	AGF	angle of greatest flexion
AFM	atomic force microscopy	AGG	agammaglobulinemia
	doxorubicin (Adriamycin), fluorouracil, and methotrexate	aggl.	agglutination
		AGI	alpha-glucosidase inhibitor

AGL	acute granulocytic leukemia	AHF	antihemophilic factor
A GLAC-TO-LK	alpha galactoside leukocytes	AHF-M	antihemophilic factor (human), method M, (monoclonal purified)
AGN	acute glomerulonephritis	AHFS	American Hospital Formulary Service
AgNO₃	silver nitrate		
α₁-AGP	alpha₁-acid glycoprotein	AHG	antihemophilic globulin
AGPT	agar-gel precipitation test	AHGS	acute herpetic gingival stomatitis
AGS	adrenogenital syndrome		
AG SYND	adrenogenital syndrome	AHHD	arteriosclerotic hypertensive heart disease
AGTT	abnormal glucose tolerance test		
AGU	aspartylglycosaminuria	AHI	apnea/hypopnea index
AGVHD	acute graft-versus-host disease	AHJ	artificial hip joint
		AHL	apparent half-life
AGVI	Ahmed glaucoma valve implantation	AHM	ambulatory Holter monitoring
AH	abdominal hysterectomy	AHMO	anterior horizontal mandibular osteotomy
	amenorrhea and hirsutism		
	amenorrhea-hyperprolac-tinemia	AHN	adenomatous hyperplastic nodule
	antihyaluronidase		Assistant Head Nurse
A&H	accident and health (insurance)	AHP	acute hemorrhagic pancreatitis
AHA	acetohydroxamic acid (Lithostat®)	AHS	adaptive hand skills
			allopurinol hypersensitivity syndrome
	acquired hemolytic anemia		
	autoimmune hemolytic anemia	AHT	alternating hypertropia
			autoantibodies to human thyroglobulin
AHAs	alpha hydroxy acids		
AHase	antihyaluronidase	AHTG	antihuman thymocyte globulin
AHB_c	hepatitis B core antibody		
AHC	acute hemorrhagic conjunctivitis	AI	accidentally incurred
			apical impulse
	acute hemorrhagic cystitis		allergy index
	Adolescent Health Center		aortic insufficiency
AHCA	American Healthcare Association		artificial insemination
			artificial intelligence
AHD	antecedent hematological disorder	A & I	Allergy and Immunology (department)
	arteriosclerotic heart disease	AIA	Accommodation Independence Assessment
	autoimmune hemolytic disease		allergen-induced asthma
AHE	acute hemorrhagic encephalomyelitis		allyl isopropyl acetamide
			anti-insulin antibody
AHEC	Area Health Education Center		aspirin-induced asthma
		AI-Ab	anti-insulin antibody

AIBF	anterior interbody fusion	AIOD	aortoiliac occlusive disease
AICA	anterior inferior cerebellar artery	AION	anterior ischemic optic neuropathy
	anterior inferior communicating artery	AIP	acute infectious polyneuritis
AICD	activation-induced cell death		acute intermittent porphyria
	automatic implantable cardioverter/ defibrillator	AIPC	androgen-independent prostate cancer
AICS	acute ischemic coronary syndromes	AIR	accelerated idioventricular rhythm
AID	acute infectious disease	AIS	Abbreviated Injury Score
	aortoiliac disease		adolescent idiopathic scoliosis
	artificial insemination donor		anti-insulin serum
	automatic implantable defibrillator	AISA	acquired idiopathic sideroblastic anemia
AIDH	artificial insemination donor husband	AIS/ISS	Abbreviated Injury Scale/ Injury Severity Score
AIDKS	acquired immune deficiency syndrome with Kaposi's sarcoma	AITN	acute interstitial tubular nephritis
		AITP	autoimmune thrombocytopenia purpura
AIDS	acquired immune deficiency syndrome		
AIE	acute inclusion body encephalitis	AIU	absolute iodine uptake
		AIVR	accelerated idioventricular rhythm
AIF	aortic-iliac-femoral		
AIH	artificial insemination with husband's sperm	AJ	ankle jerk
		AJCC	American Joint Committee on Cancer
AIHA	autoimmune hemolytic anemia	AJO	apple juice only
		AJR	abnormal jugular reflex
AIHD	acquired immune hemolytic disease	AK	above knee (amputation)
			actinic keratosis
AIIS	anterior inferior iliac spine		artificial kidney
AILD	angioimmunoblastic lymphadenopathy with dysproteinemia	AKA	above-knee amputation
			alcoholic ketoacidosis
			all known allergies
			also known as
AIMS	Abnormal Involuntary Movement Scale	AKS	alcoholic Korsakoff syndrome
	Arthritis Impact Measurement Scales		arthroscopic knee surgery
		AKU	artificial kidney unit
AIN	acute interstitial nephritis	AL	acute leukemia
	anal intraepithelial neoplasia		argon laser
			arterial line
AINS	anti-inflammatory non-steroidal		assisted living
			axial length

	left ear	ALK ISO	alkaline phosphatase isoenzymes
Al	aluminum	ALK-P	alkaline phosphatase
ALA	alpha-linolenic acid (α-linolenic acid)	ALL	acute lymphoblastic leukemia
	aminolevulinic acid		acute lymphocytic leukemia
	anti-lymphocyte antibody		allergy
ALAC	antibiotic-loaded acrylic cement	ALLD	arthroscopic lumbar laser diskectomy
ALAD	abnormal left axis deviation	ALLO	allogeneic
ALARA	as low as reasonably achievable	Allo-BMT	allogenic bone marrow transplantation
ALAT	alanine transaminase (alanine aminotransferase; SGPT)	ALM	acral lentiginous melanoma
			alveolar lining material
ALAX	apical long axis	ALMI	anterolateral myocardial infarction
ALB	albumin	ALN	anterior lower neck
	albuterol		anterior lymph node
	anterior lenticular bevel	ALND	axillary lymph node dissection
ALC	acute lethal catatonia	ALNM	axillary lymph node metastasis
	alcohol		
	alcoholic liver cirrhosis	ALO	axiolinguo-occlusal
	allogeneic lymphocyte cytotoxicity	Al(OH)₃	aluminum hydroxide
	alternate level of care	ALOS	average length of stay
	Alternate Lifestyle Checklist	ALP	alkaline phosphatase
	axiolinguocervical		argon laser photocoagulation
ALCL	anaplastic large-cell lymphoma		Alupent
ALC R	alcohol rub	ARPF	anterior release posterior fusion
ALD	adrenoleukodystrophy	ALTP	argon laser trabeculo-plasty
	alcoholic liver disease		
	aldolase	ALPZ	alprazolam (Xanax)
ALDH	aldehyde dehydrogenase	ALR	adductor leg raise
ALDOST	aldosterone	ALRI	acute lower-respiratory-tract infection
ALF	acute liver failure		anterolateral rotary instability
ALFT	abnormal liver function tests		
ALG	antilymphoblast globulin	ALS	acute lateral sclerosis
	antilymphocyte globulin		advanced life support
ALH	atypical lobular hyperplasia		amyotrophic lateral sclerosis
ALI	argon laser iridotomy	ALT	alanine transaminase (SGPT)
A-line	arterial catheter		
ALK	alkaline		argon laser trabeculo-plasty
	automated lamellar keratoplasty		
ALK ∅	alkaline phosphatase		

	autolymphocyte therapy		arthroscopic
2 alt	every other day (this is a dangerous abbreviation)		microdiskectomy
			axiomesiodistal
ALTB	acute laryngotracheobron-		dactinomycin
	chitis		(actinomycin D)
ALTE	acute (apparent) life threatening event		methyldopa (alpha methyldopa)
alt hor	every other hour (this is a dangerous abbreviation)	AME	agreed medical examination
ALUP	Alupent		anthrax
ALVAD	abdominal left ventricular		meningoencephalitis
	assist device		apparent
ALWMI	anterolateral wall		mineralocorticoid
	myocardial infarct		excess (syndrome)
ALZ	Alzheimer's disease		Aviation Medical
AM	adult male		Examiner
	amalgam	AMegL	acute megokaryoblastic
	anovulatory menstruation		leukemia
	morning (a.m.)	AMES-	American sign language
	myopic astigmatism	LAN	
AMA	against medical advice	AMF	aerobic metabolism
	American Medical		facilitator
	Association		autocrine motility factor
	antimitochondrial	AMG	acoustic myography
	antibody		aminoglycoside
AMAC	adults molested as		axiomesiogingival
	children		Federal Republic of
AMAD	morning admission		German's equivalent to
AM/ADM	morning admission		United States Food,
AMAG	adrenal medullary		Drug, and Cosmetic Act
	autograft	AMI	acute myocardial
AMAL	amalgam		infarction
AMAP	as much as possible		amitriptyline
AMAT	anti-malignant antibody		axiomesioincisal
	test	AML	acute myelogenous
A-MAT	amorphous material		leukemia
AMB	ambulate		angiomyolipoma
	ambulatory		anterior mitral leaflet
	amphotericin B	AMM	agnogenic myeloid
	as manifested by		metaplasia
AMBER	advanced multiple beam	AMML	acute myelomonocytic
	equalization		leukemia
	radiography	AMMOL	acute myelomonoblastic
AMC	arm muscle circumference		leukemia
	arthrogryposis multiplex	AMN	adrenomyeloneuropathy
	congenita	amnio	amniocentesis
AM/CR	amylase to creatinine ratio	AMN SC	amniotic fluid scan
AMD	age-related macular	AMOL	acute monoblastic
	degeneration		leukemia

AMP	adenosine monophosphate	ANA SWAB	anaerobic swab
	ampicillin	ANC	absolute neutrophil count
	ampere	ANCA	antineutrophil cytoplasmic
	ampul		antibody
	amputation	anch	anchored
A-M pr	Austin-Moore prosthesis	ANCN	absolute neutrophil count
AMPT	metyrosine (alphameth-		nadir
	ylpara tyrosine)	ANCOVA	analysis of covariance
AMR	acoustic muscle reflex	AND	anterior nasal discharge
	alternating motion rates	ANDA	Abbreviated New Drug
AMRI	anterior medial rotary		Application
	instability	anes	anesthesia
AMS	acute mountain sickness	ANF	antinuclear factor
	aggravated in military		atrial natriuretic factor
	service	ANG	angiogram
	altered mental status	ANG II	angiotensin II
	amylase	ANGIO	angiogram
	auditory memory span	ANH	acute normovolemic
m-AMSA	amsacrine (acridinyl		hemodilution
	anisidide)		artificial nutrition and
AMSIT	portion of the mental		hydration
	status examination:	ANISO	anisocytosis
	A—appearance,	ANK	ankle
	M—mood,		appointment not kept
	S—sensorium,	ANLL	acute nonlymphoblastic
	I—intelligence,		leukemia
	T—thought process	ANM	Assistant Nurse Manager
AMT	Adolph's Meat Tenderizer	ANN	axillary node–negative
	aminopterin	ANOVA	analysis of variance
	amount	ANP	Adult Nurse Practitioner
AMTS	Abbreviated Mental Test		atrial natriuretic peptide
	Score		(anaritide acetate)
AMU	accessory-muscle use		axillary node–positive
AMV	alveolar minute	ANS	answer
	ventilation		autonomic nervous system
	assisted mechanical	ANSER	Aggregate
	ventilation		Neurobehavioral
AMY	amylase		Student Health and
AMY/CR	amylase/creatinine		Education Review
	ratio	ANT	anterior
AN	amyl nitrate		enheptin (2-amino-5-
	anorexia nervosa		nitrothiazol)
	Associate Nurse	ante	before
	avascular necrosis	ANTI	anti blood group A
ANA	antinuclear antibody	A:AGT	antiglobulin test
ANAD	anorexia nervosa and	Anti bx	antibiotic
	associated disorders	anti-GAD	antibodies to glutamic
ANAG	acute narrow angle		acid decarboxylase
	glaucoma		

27

anti-HBc	antibody to hepatitis B core antigen (HBcAg)	AODA	alcohol and other drug abuse
anti-HBe	antibody to hepatitis B e antigen (HBeAg)	AODM	adult onset diabetes mellitus
anti-HBs	antibody to hepatitis B surface antigen (HBsAg)	A of 1	assistance of one
		A of 2	assistance of two
		AOI	area of induration
ant sag D	anterior sagittal diameter	ao-il	aorta-iliac
ANTU	alpha naphthylthiourea	AOL	augmentation of labor
ANUG	acute necrotizing ulcerative gingivitis	AOLC	acridine-orange leukocyte cytospin
ANV	acute nausea and vomiting	AOLD	automated open lumbar diskectomy
ANX	anxiety anxious	AOM	acute otitis media alternatives of management
AO	Agent Orange		
	anterior oblique	AONAD	alert, oriented, and no acute distress
	aorta		
	aortic opening	AOO	anodal opening odor
	axio-occlusal		continuous arterial asynchronous pacing
	plate, screw (orthopedics)		
	right ear	AOP	anemia of prematurity
A-O	atlanto-occipital (joint)		anodal opening picture
A/O	alert and oriented		aortic pressure
A & O	alert and oriented		apnea of prematurity
A&O × 3	awake and oriented to person, place, and time	AOR	Alvarado Orthopedic Research
A&O × 4	awake and oriented to person, place, time, and object		at own risk
			auditory oculogyric reflex
		AORT REGURG	aortic regurgitation
AOAA	aminooxoacetic acid		
AOAP	as often as possible	AORT STEN	aortic stenosis
AOB	alcohol on breath		
AOBS	acute organic brain syndrome	AOS	ambulatory outpatient surgery
AOC	abridged ocular chart		anode opening sound
	advanced ovarian cancer		antibiotic order sheet
	amoxicillin, omeprazole, and clarithromycin		aortic ostial stenoses
		AOSC	acute obstructive suppurative cholangiotomy
	anode opening contraction		
	antacid of choice	AOSD	adult-onset Still's disease
	area of concern	AOTe	anodal opening tetanus
AOCD	anemia of chronic disease	AP	abdominoperineal
AOCL	anodal opening clonus		acute pancreatitis
AOD	adult onset diabetes		aerosol pentamidine
	alleged onset date		alkaline phosphatase
	arterial occlusive disease		angina pectoris
	Assistant-Officer-of-the-Day		antepartum

	anterior-posterior (x-ray)	APCD	adult polycystic disease
	arterial pressure	APCIs	atrial peptide clearance inhibitors
	apical pulse		
	appendectomy	APCKD	adult polycystic kidney disease
	appendicitis		
	atrial pacing	APD	action potential duration
	attending physician		afferent pupillary defect
	doxorubicin and cisplatin		pamidronate disodium (aminohydroxypropylidene diphosphate)
A&P	active and present		
	anterior and posterior		
	assessment and plans		anterior-posterior diameter
	auscultation and percussion		atrial premature depolarization
A/P	ascites/plasma ratio		automated peritoneal dialysis
$A_2 > P_2$	second aortic sound greater than second pulmonic sound	APDC	Anxiety and Panic Disorder Clinic
APA	antiphospholipid antibody	APDT	acellular pertussis vaccine with diphtheria and tetanus toxoids
APAA	anterior parietal artery aneurysm		
APACHE	Acute Physiology and Chronic Health Evaluation	APE	absolute prediction error
			acute psychotic episode
			acute pulmonary edema
APAD	anterior-posterior abdominal diameter		Adriamycin, cisplatin (Platinol), and etoposide
APAG	antipseudomonal aminoglycosidic penicillin		anterior pituitary extract
		APG	ambulatory patient group
APAP	acetaminophen (N acetyl-para-aminophenol)		Apgar (score)
		APGAR	appearance (color), pulse (heart rate), grimace (reflex irritability), activity (muscle tone), and respiration (score reflecting condition of newborn)
APB	abductor pollicis brevis		
	atrial premature beat		
APC	absolute phagocyte count		
	activated protein C		
	acute pharyngoconjunctiivitis (fever)	APH	adult psychiatric hospital
			alcohol-positive history
			antepartum hemorrhage
	adenoidal-pharyngeal-conjunctival	APHIS	Animal and Plant Health Inspection Service
	adenomatous polyposis of the colon and rectum	APIS	Acute Pain Intensity Scale
	advanced prostate cancer	APIVR	artificial pacemaker-induced ventricular rhythm
	antigen-presenting cell		
	aspirin, phenacetin, and caffeine	APKD	adult polycystic kidney disease
	atrial premature contraction		adult-onset polycystic kidney disease
	autologous packed cells		

29

APL	abductor pollicis longus
	accelerated painless labor
	acute promyelocytic leukemia
	anterior pituitary-like (hormone)
	chorionic gonadotropin
AP & L	anteroposterior and lateral
APLA	anti-phospholipid antibody
APLD	automated percutaneous lumbar diskectomy
APMPPE	acute posterior multifocal placoid pigment epitheliopathy
APMS	acute pain management service
APN	acute pyelonephritis
APO	adverse patient occurrence
	apolipoprotein A-1
	doxorubicin (Adriamycin), prednisone, and vincristine (Oncovin)
APO(a)	apolipoprotein (A)
APOE	apolipoprotein E
APOE-4	apolipoprotein-E (gene)
APOPPS	adjustable postoperative protective prosthetic socket
APP	amyloid precursor protein
APPG	aqueous procaine penicillin G (dangerous terminology; since it is for intramuscular use only, write as penicillin G procaine)
appr.	approximate
appt.	appointment
APPY	appendectomy
APR	abdominoperineal resection
APRT	abdominopelvic radiotherapy
APRV	airway pressure release ventilation
APS	Acute Physiology Scoring (system)
	adult protective services
	Adult Psychiatric Service
	antiphospholipid syndrome
APSAC	anistreplase (anisoylated plasminogen streptokinase activator complex)
APSD	Alzheimer's presenile dementia
APSP	assisted peak systolic pressure
aPTT	activated partial thromboplastin time
APU	ambulatory procedure unit
	antepartum unit
APUD	amine precursor uptake and decarboxylation
APVC	partial anomalous pulmonary venous connection
APVR	aortic pulmonary valve replacement
APW	aortopulmonary window
aq	water
AQ	accomplishment quotient
aq dest	distilled water
A quad	atrial quadrageminy
AR	Achilles reflex
	acoustic reflex
	active resistance
	airway resistance
	alcohol related
	ankle reflex
	aortic regurgitation
	Argyll Robertson (pupil)
	assisted respiration
	at risk
	aural rehabilitation
	autorefractor
Ar	argon
A&R	adenoidectomy with radium
	advised and released
A-R	apical-radial (pulses)
ARA	adenosine regulating agent
ara-A	vidarabine
ara-AC	fazarabine
ara-C	cytarabine

ARAS	ascending reticular activating system	ARN	acute retinal necrosis
ARB	any reliable brand	AROM	active range of motion artifical rupture of membranes
ARBOR	arthropod-borne virus		
ARBOW	artificial rupture of bag of water	ARP	absolute refractory period
ARC	abnormal retinal correspondence		alcohol rehabilitation program
	Alcohol Rehabilitation Center	ARPKS	autosomal recessive polycystic kidney disease
	anomalous retinal correspondence	arr	arrive
	AIDS related complex	ARROM	active resistive range of motion
	American Red Cross		
ARCBS	American Red Cross Blood Services	ARRT	American Registry of Radiologic Technologists
ARD	acute respiratory disease		
	adult respiratory distress	ARS	antirabies serum
	antibiotic removal device	ART	Accredited Record Technician
	antibiotic retrieval device		
	aphakic retinal detachment		Achilles (tendon) reflex test
ARDMS	American Registry of Diagnostic Medical Sonographers		acoustic reflex threshold(s)
			assessment, review, and treatment
ARDS	adult respiratory distress syndrome		arterial
ARE	active-resistive exercises		automated reagin test (for syphilis)
ARF	acute renal failure		
	acute respiratory failure	ARTIC	articulation
	acute rheumatic fever	Art T	art therapy
ARG	alkaline reflux gastritis	ARU	alcohol rehabilitation unit
	arginine	ARV	AIDS related virus
ARHL	age-related hearing loss	ARW	Accredited Rehabilitation Worker
ARHNC	advanced resected head and neck cancer		
		ARWY	airway
ARI	acute renal insufficiency	AS	activated sleep
	aldose reductase inhibitor		anabolic steroid
ARL	average remaining lifetime		anal sphincter
			androgen suppression
ARLD	alcohol related liver disease		ankylosing spondylitis
			anterior synechia
ARM	anxiety reaction, mild		aortic stenosis
	artificial rupture of membranes		atherosclerosis
			doctor called through answering service
ARMD	age-related macular degeneration		atropine sulfate
			AutoSuture®
ARMS	amplification refractory mutation system		left ear

ASA	American Society of Anesthesiologists	ASB	anesthesia standby
	argininosuccinate		asymptomatic bacteriuria
	aspirin (acetylsalicylic acid)	ASBO	adhesive small-bowel obstruction
	atrial septal aneurysm	ASC	altered state of consciousness
ASA I	American Society of anesthesiologists' classification		ambulatory surgery center
	Healthy patient with localized pathological process		anterior subcapsular cataract
			antimony sulfur colloid
			apocrine skin carcinoma
			ascorbic acid
ASA II	A patient with mild to moderate systemic disease	ASCAD	atherosclerotic coronary artery disease
ASA III	A patient with severe systemic disease limiting activity but not incapacitating	ASCCC	advanced squamous cell cervical carcinoma
		ASCI	acute spinal cord injury
		ASCO	American Society of Clinical Oncology
ASA IV	A patient with incapacitating systemic disease	ASCR	autologous stem cell rescue
ASA V	Moribund patient not expected to live. (These are American Society of Anesthesiologists' patient classifications. Emergency operations are designated by "E" after the classification.)	ASCT	autologous stem cell transplantation
		ASCUS	atypical squamous cell of undetermined significance
		ASCVD	arteriosclerotic cardiovascular disease
		ASCVR	arteriosclerotic cardiovascular renal disease
5-ASA	mesalamine (5-aminosalicylic acid) (this is a dangerous abbreviation as it is mistaken for five aspirin tablets)	ASD	atrial septal defect
			aldosterone secretion defect
		ASD I	atrial septal defect, primum
		ASD II	atrial septal defect, secundum
ASAA	acquired severe aplastic anemia	ASDH	acute subdural hematoma
ASACL	American Society of Anesthesiologists Classification	ASE	acute stress erosion
		ASF	anterior spinal fusion
AS/AI	aortic stenosis/aortic insufficiency	ASFR	age-specific fertility rate
		ASH	asymmetric septal hypertrophy
A's and B's	apnea and bradycardia	AsH	hypermetropic astigmatism
ASAP	as soon as possible		
ASAT	aspartate transaminase (aspartate aminotransferase) (SGOT)	ASHD	arteriosclerotic heart disease
		ASI	Anxiety Status Inventory

ASIH	absent, sick in hospital		ASTZ	antistreptozyme test
ASIMC	absent, sick in medical center		ASU	acute stroke unit ambulatory surgical unit
ASIS	anterior superior iliac spine		ASV	antisnake venom
			ASVD	arteriosclerotic vessel disease
ASK	antistreptokinase		ASYM	asymmetric (al)
ASKase	antistreptokinase		ASX	asymptomatic
ASL	American Sign Language antistreptolysin (titer)		AT	activity therapy (therapist) Addiction Therapist
ASLO	antistreptolysin-O			antithrombin
ASLV	avian sarcoma and leukosis virus (Rous virus)			applanation tonometry ataxia-telangiectasia atrial tachycardia
AsM	myopic astigmatism			atraumatic
ASMA	anti-smooth muscle antibody		AT 10	dihydrotachysterol
			ATB	antibiotic
ASMI	anteroseptal myocardial infarction			atypical tuberculosis
			ATC	aerosol treatment chamber
ASO	aldicarb sulfoxide			alcoholism therapy classes
	allele-specific oligodeoxynucleotide (probes)			all-terrain cycle antituberculous chemoprophylaxis
	antistreptolysin-O titer			around the clock
	arteriosclerosis obliterans			Arthritis Treatment Center
	automatic stop order		ATCC	American Type Culture Collection
ASOT	antistreptolysin-O titer			
ASP	acute suppurative parotitis		ATD	antithyroid drug(s)
	acute symmetric polyarthritis			asphyxiating thoracic dystrophy
	asparaginase			anticipated time of discharge
	aspartic acid			autoimmune thyroid
ASPVD	arteriosclerotic peripheral vascular disease			disease
ASR	aldosterone secretion rate		ATE	adipose tissue extraction
	automatic speech recognition		ATEM	analytical transmission electron microscopy
ASS	anterior superior supine assessment		At Fib	atrial fibrillation
			AT III FUN	antithrombin III functional
asst	assistant			
AST	Aphasia Screening Test		ATG	antithymocyte globulin
	aspartate transaminase (SGOT)		ATHR	angina threshold heart rate
	astemizole		ATI	Abdominal Trauma Index
	astigmatism		ATL	Achilles tendon lengthening
ASTH	asthenopia			adult T-cell leukemia
ASTI	acute soft tissue injury			anterior tricuspid leaflet
AS TOL	as tolerated			atypical lymphocytes
ASTIG	astigmatism			
ASTRO	astrocytoma			

ATLL	adult T-cell leukemia lymphoma	AUC	area under the curve
ATLS	acute tumor lysis syndrome	AUC_t	area under the curve to last time point
	advanced trauma life support	AUD	arthritis of unknown diagnosis
ATM	acute transverse myelitis		auditory
	atmosphere	AUD COMP	auditory comprehension
At ma	atrial milliamp	AUG	acute ulcerative gingivitis
ATN	acute tubular necrosis	AUGIB	acute upper gastrointestinal bleeding
ATNC	atraumatic normocephalic		
aTNM	autopsy staging of cancer		
ATNR	asymmetrical tonic neck reflex	AUIC	area under the inhibitory curve
ATP	addiction treatment program	AUL	acute undifferentiated leukemia
	adenosine triphosphate	AUR	acute urinary retention
	anterior tonsillar pillar	AUS	acute urethral syndrome
	autoimmune thrombo-cytopenia purpura		artificial urinary sphincter
			auscultation
ATPase	adenosine triphosphatase	AUTO SP	automatic speech
ATPS	ambient temperature & pressure, saturated with water vapor	AV	anteverted
			anticipatory vomiting
			arteriovenous
ATR	Achilles tendon reflex		atrioventricular
	atrial		auditory visual
	atropine		auriculoventricular
ATRA	all-*trans* retinoic acid (tretinoin-Vesanoid®)	A:V	arterial-venous (ratio in fundi)
atr fib	atrial fibrillation	AVA	aortic valve atresia
ATRO	atropine		arteriovenous anastomosis
ATU	alcohol treatment unit	AVB	atrioventricular block
ATV	all-terrain vehicle	AVC	acrylic veneer crown
ATS	antitetanic serum (tetanus antitoxin)	AVD	aortic valve disease
			apparent volume of distribution
	anxiety tension state		arteriosclerotic vascular disease
ATSO4	atropine sulfate		
ATT	antitetanus toxoid		
	arginine tolerance test	AVDP	asparaginase, vincristine, daunorubicin, and prednisone
at. wt	atomic weight		
AU	allergenic (allergy) units		avoirdupois
	arbitrary units	$AVDO_2$	arteriovenous oxygen difference
	both ears		
Au	gold	AVE	aortic valve echocardiogram
A/U	at umbilicus		
198_{Au}	radioactive gold	AVF	arteriovenous fistula
AUB	abnormal uterine bleeding		augmented unipolar foot (left leg)
AuBMT	autologous bone marrow transplant		

avg	average		as well as
AVGS	autologous vein graft stent	A waves	atrial contraction wave
		AWB	autologous whole blood
AVGs	ambulatory visit groups	AWDW	assault with a deadly weapon
AVH	acute viral hepatitis		
AVHB	atrioventricular heart block	AWI	anterior wall infarct
		AWMI	anterior wall myocardial infarction
AVJR	atrioventricular junctional rhythm		
		AWO	airway obstruction
AVL	augmented unipolar left (left arm)	AWOL	absent without leave
		AWP	airway pressure
AVLT	auditory verbal learning test		average wholesale price
		AWRU	active wrist rotation unit
AVM	arteriovenous malformation	AWS	alcohol withdrawal syndrome
AVN	arteriovenous nicking		
	atrioventricular node	AWU	alcohol withdrawal unit
	avascular necrosis	ax	axillary
AVNR	atrioventricular nodal re-entry	AXB	axillary block
		AXC	aortic cross clamp
AVNRT	atrioventricular node recovery time	ax-fem.fem.	axilla-femoral-femoral (graft)
	atrioventricular nodal re-entry tachycardia	AXND	axillary node dissection
		AXR	abdomen x-ray
A-VO$_2$	arteriovenous oxygen difference	AXT	alternating exotropia
		AZA	azathioprine (Imuran®)
AVOC	avocation	AZA-CR	azacitidine
AVP	arginine vasopressin	5-AZC	azacitidine
AVR	aortic valve replacement	AzdU	azidouridine
	augmented unipolar right (right arm)	AZE	azelastine hydrochloride
		AZQ	diaziquone
AVRT	atrioventricular reciprocating tachycardia	AZT	zidovudine (azidothymidine)
AVS	atriovenous shunt	A-Z test	Aschheim-Zondek test (diagnostic test for pregnancy)
AVSD	atrioventricular septal defect		
AVSS	afebrile, vital signs stable		
AVT	atrioventricular tachycardia		
	atypical ventricular tachycardia		
AvWS	acquired von Willebrand's syndrome		
AW	abdominal wall		
	abnormal wave		
	airway		
A/W	able to work	B	bacillus
A&W	alive and well		bands
AWA	alcohol withdrawal assessment		bilateral
			black

B

	bloody	BACOP	bleomycin, Adriamycin®, cyclophosphamide, vincristine, and prednisone
	bolus		
	both		
	brother		
	botulism (Vaccine B is botulism toxoid)	BACs	bacterial artificial chromosomes
B_1	thiamine HCl	BACT	bacteria
B I	Billroth I (gastric surgery)		base activated clotting time
B II	Billroth II (gastric surgery)	BAD	dipolar affective disorder
B_2	riboflavin	BaE	barium enema
B_3	nicotinic acid	BAE	bronchial artery embolization
b/4	before		
B_5	pantothenic acid	BAEDP	balloon aortic end diastolic pressure
B_6	pyridoxine HCl		
B_7	biotin	BAEP	brain stem auditory evoked potential
B_8	adenosine phosphate		
B_9	benign	BAERs	brain stem auditory evoked responses
B_{12}	cyanocobalamin		
Ba	barium	BAG	buccoaxiogingival
BA	backache	BAHA	bone-anchored hearing aid
	Baptist	BAL	balance
	benzyl alcohol		blood alcohol level
	bile acid		British antilewisite (dimercaprol)
	biliary atresia		
	blood agar		bronchoalveolar lavage
	blood alcohol	BALB	binaural alternate loudness balance
	bone age		
	Bourns assist	BALF	bronchoalveolar lavage fluid
	branchial artery		
	broken appointment	BaM	barium meal
	bronchial asthma	BAND	band neutrophil (stab)
	buccoaxial	BANS	back, arm, neck and scalp
B > A	bone greater than air	BAO	basal acid output
B < A	bone less than air	BAP	blood agar plate
B & A	brisk and active	BAPT	Baptist
BAAM	Beck airway airflow monitor	Barb	barbiturate
		BARN	bilateral acute retinal necrosis
Bab	Babinski		
BAC	benzalkonium chloride	BAR Troche	Benadryl, Ativan, and Reglan troche
	blood alcohol concentration		
		BAS	bile acid sequestrants
	buccoaxiocervical		boric acid solution
BACI	bovine anti-cryptosporidium immunoglobulin	BaS	barium swallow
		BASA	baby aspirin (81 mg chewable tablets of aspirin)
BACON	bleomycin, doxorubicin, lomustine, vincristine, and mechlorethamine		
		BASIS	Basic Achievement Skills Individual Screener

BASK	basket cells	BBL	bottle blood loss
baso.	basophil	BBM	banked breast milk
BASO STIP	basophilic stippling	BBOW	bulging bag of water
		BBP	butyl benzyl phthalate
BAT	Behavioral Avoidance Test	BBR	bibasilar rales
		BBS	bilateral breath sounds
	brightness acuity tester	BBSE	bilateral breath sounds equal
BATO	boronic acid adduct of technetium oxime		
		BBSI	Brigance Basic Skills Inventory
batt	battery		
BAVP	balloon aortic valvuloplasty	BBT	basal body temperature
		BB to MM	belly button to medial malleolus
BAU	bioequivalent allergy units		
BAV	bicuspid aortic valve	B Bx	breast biopsy
BAW	bronchoalveolar washing	BC	back care
BB	baby boy		battered child
	backboard		bed and chair
	back to back		beta carotene
	bad breath		bicycle
	bed bath		birth control
	bed board		bladder cancer
	beta-blocker		blood culture
	blanket bath		Blue Cross
	blood bank		bone conduction
	blow bottle		Bourn control
	blue bloaters		breast cancer
	body belts		buccocervical
	both bones		buffalo cap (cap for intravenous line)
	breakthrough bleeding		
	breast biopsy	B/C	because
	brush biopsy		blood urea nitrogen/creatinine ratio
	buffer base		
B&B	bismuth and bourbon	B&C	bed and chair
	bowel and bladder		biopsy and curettage
B/B	backward bending		board and care
BBA	born before arrival		breathed and cried
BBB	baseball bat beating	BCA	balloon catheter angioplasty
	blood-brain barrier		
	bundle branch block		basal cell atypia
BBBB	bilateral bundle branch block		brachiocephalic artery
		BCAA	branched-chain amino acids
BBC	Brown-Buerger cystoscope	BC < AC	bone conduction less than air conduction
BBD	baby born dead	BC > AC	bone conduction greater than air conduction
	before bronchodilator		
	benign breast disease	B. cat	*Branhamella catarrhalis*
BBFA	both bones forearm	B-CAVe	bleomycin, lomustine, doxorubicin, and vinblastine
BBFP	blood and body fluid precautions		

BCB	Brilliant cresyl blue (stain)	BCQ	breast central quadrantectomy
BCBR	bilateral carotid body resection	BCR	bulbocavernosus reflex
		BCRS	Brief Cognitive Rate Scale
BC/BS	Blue Cross/Blue Shield		
BCC	basal cell carcinoma birth control clinic	BCRT	breast conservation followed by radiation therapy
BCCa	basal cell carcinoma		
BCD	basal cell dysplasia borderline of cardiac dullness	BCS	battered child syndrome breast conserving surgery Budd-Chiari syndrome
BCDH	bilateral congenital dislocated hip	BCSS	bone cell stimulating substance
BCE	basal cell epithelioma beneficial clinical event	BCT	Bag Carrying Test breast-conserving therapy
B cell	large lymphocyte	BCU	burn care unit
BCF	basic conditioning factor Baylor core formula	BCUG	bilateral cystourethrogram
		BD	band neutrophil base deficit base down behavior disorder Behçet's disease bile duct birth date birth defect blood donor brain dead bronchial drainage bronchodilator buccodistal United Kingdom abbreviation for twice a day
BCG	bacille Calmette-Guérin vaccine bicolor guaiac	
BCH	benign coital headache	
BCHA	bone-conduction hearing aid	
BCL	basic cycle length bio-chemoluminescence	
B/C/L	BUN,(blood urea nitrogen),creatinine, lytes (electrolytes)	
BCLP	bilateral cleft lip and palate	
BCM	below costal margin birth control medication body cell mass	
		BDAE	Boston Diagnostic Aphasia Examination
BCME	bis (chloromethyl) ether	BDBS	Bonnet-Dechaume-Blanc syndrome
BCNP	Board Certified Nuclear Pharmacist		
BCNU	carmustine	BDC	burn-dressing change
BCOC	bowel care of choice bowel cathartic of choice	BDD	bronchodilator drugs
		BDE	bile duct exploration
BCP	biochemical profile birth control pills blood cell profile carmustine, cyclophosphamide, and prednisone	BDF	bilateral distal femoral black divorced female
		BDI	Beck Depression Inventory
		BDI SF	Beck's Depression Inventory-Short Form
		BDL	below detectable limits bile duct ligation
BCPAP	Broun's continuous positive airway pressure	BDM	black divorced male

BDNF	brain-derived neurotrophic factor	BE-PEG	balanced electrolyte with polyethylene glycol
B-DOPA	bleomycin, dacarbazine, vincristine (Oncovin), prednisone, and doxorubicin (Adriamycin)	BEV	billion electron volts bleeding esophageal varices
		BF	black female
			boyfriend
BDP	beclomethasone dipropionate best demonstrated practice		bone fragment breakfast fed breast-feed
BDR	background diabetic retinopathy	B/F	bound-to-free ratio
		BFA	baby for adoption
BDV	Borna disease virus		basilic forearm
BE	bacterial endocarditis		bifemoral arteriogram
	barium enema	BFC	benign febrile convulsion
	Barrett's esophagus	bFGF	basic fibroblast growth factor
	base excess		
	below elbow	BFL	breast firm and lactating
	bread equivalent	BFM	black married female
	breast examination	BFNC	benign familial neonatal convulsions
B↑E	both upper extremities		
B↓E	both lower extremities	BFP	biologic false positive
B & E	brisk and equal	BFR	blood filtration rate
BEA	below elbow amputation		blood flow rate
BEAC	carmustine (BiCNU), etoposide, cytarabine (ara-C), and cyclophosphamide	B. frag	Bacillus fragilis
		BFT	bentonite flocculation test biofeedback training
		BFU_e	erythroid burst-forming unit
BEAM	carmustine (BiCNU), etoposide, cytarabine (ara-C), and melphalan brain electrical activity mapping	BG	baby girl
			basal ganglia
			blood glucose
			bone graft
		B-G	Bender Gestalt (test)
BEAR	Bourn's electronic adult respirator	BGA	Bundesgesundheitsamt (German drug regulatory agency)
BEC	bacterial endocarditis		
BED	biochemical evidence of disease	B-GA-LACTO	beta galactosidase
BEE	basal energy expenditure	BGC	basal-ganglion calcification
BEF	bronchoesophageal fistula		
BEH	benign essential hypertension	BGCT	benign glandular cell tumor
		BGDC	Bartholin gland duct cyst
Beh Sp	behavior specialist	BGDR	background diabetic retinopathy
BEI	butanol-extractable iodine		
BEL	blood ethanol level	BGL	blood glucose level
BEP	bleomycin, etoposide, and cisplatin (Platinol)	BGM	blood glucose monitoring
	brain stem evoked potentials	BGTT	borderline glucose tolerance test

39

BH	breath holding		components (see
	bowel habits		SMA 6)
BHC	benzene hexachloride	BIGEM	bigeminal
bHCG	beta human chorionic	BIH	benign intracranial
	gonadotropin		hypertension
BHD	carmustine, hydroxyurea,		bilateral inguinal hernia
	and dacarbazine	BIL	bilateral
B-HEXOS-	beta hexosaminidase A		brother-in-law
A-LK	leukocytes	BILAT	bilateral short leg case
	brain-heart infusion	SLC	
BHI	biosynthetic human	BILAT	bilateral salpingo-
	insulin	SXO	oophorectomy
	brain-heart infusion	Bili	bilirubin
BHN	bridging hepatic necrosis	BILI-C	conjugated bilirubin
BHR	bronchial hyperrespon-	BIL MRY	bilateral myringotomy
	siveness (hyperactivity)	BIMA	bilateral internal
BHP	boarding home placement		mammary arteries
BHS	beta-hemolytic	BIN	twice a night (this is a
	streptococci		dangerous abbreviation)
	breath-holding spell	BIO	binocular indirect
BHT	breath hydrogen test		ophthalmoscopy
BI	Barthel Index	BIOF	biofeedback
	base in	BIP	bipolar affective disorder
	brain injury		bleomycin, ifosfamide,
	bowel impaction		and cisplatin (Platinol)
Bi	bismuth		brain injury program
BIA	bioelectrical impedance	BiPD	biparietal diameter
	analysis	BIPP	bismuth iodoform paraffin
	biospecific interaction		paste
	analysis	BIR	back internal rotation
BIB	brought in by	BIRB	Biomedical Institutional
BIBA	brought in by ambulance		Review Board
BIC	brain injury center	BIS	Bispectral Index
BICAP	bipolar electrocoagulation	bisp	bispinous diameter
	therapy	BIVAD	bilateral ventricular assist
Bicarb	bicarbonate		device
BiCNU®	carmustine	BIW	twice a week (this is a
BICROS	bilateral contralateral		dangerous abbreviation)
	routing of signals	BIZ-PLT	bizarre platelets
BICU	burn intensive care unit	BJ	Bence Jones (protein)
BID	brought in dead		biceps jerk
	twice daily		body jacket
BIDA	amonafide		bone and joint
BIDS	bedtime insulin, daytime		Bristoljet® syringe
	sulfonylurea	BJE	bone and joint
BIF	bifocal		examination
BIG	botulism immune globulin		bones, joints, and
BIG 6	analysis of 6 serum		extremities

BJI	bone and joint infection	BLM	bleomycin sulfate
BJM	bones, joints, and muscles	BLOBS	bladder obstruction
BJP	Bence Jones protein	BLOC	brief loss of consciousness
BK	below knee (amputation)		
	bradykinin	BLPB	beta-lactamase-producing bacteria
	bullous keratopathy		
BKA	below knee amputation	BLPO	beta-lactamase-producing organism
BKC	blepharokerato-conjunctivitis		
		BLQ	both lower quadrants
bkft	breakfast	BLR	blood flow rate
Bkg	background	BLS	basic life support
BKTT	below knee to toe (cast)	BLT	blood-clot lysis time
BKWC	below knee walking cast		brow left transverse
BKWP	below-knee walking plaster (cast)	B.L. unit	Bessey-Lowry units
		BM	black male
BL	baseline (fetal heart rate)		bone marrow
	bioluminescence		bone metastases
	bland		bowel movement
	blast cells		breast milk
	blood level	BMA	biomedical application
	blood loss		bismuth subsalicylate, metronidazole, and amoxicillin
	bronchial lavage		
	Burkitt's lymphoma		
B/L	brother-in-law		bone marrow aspirate
BLB	Boothby-Lovelace-Bulbulian (oxygen mask)	BMB	bone marrow biopsy
		BMC	bone marrow cells
			bone marrow culture
BLBK	blood bank		bone mineral content
BLBS	bilateral breath sounds	BMD	Becker muscular dystrophy
BL = BS	bilateral equal breath sounds		
			bone marrow depression
bl cult	blood culture		bone mineral density
B-L-D	breakfast, lunch, and dinner	BME	basal medium Eagle (diploid cell culture)
bldg	bleeding		biomedical engineering
bld tm	bleeding time		brief maximal effort
BLE	both lower extremities	BMF	between meal feedings
BLEO	bleomycin sulfate		black married female
BLESS	bath, laxative, enema, shampoo, and shower	BMG	benign monoclonal gammopathy
BLG	bovine beta-lactoglobulin	BMI	body mass index
BLIC	beta-lactamase inhibitor combination	BMJ	bones, muscles, joints
		BMK	birthmark
BLIP	beta-lactamase inhibiting protein	BMM	black married male
		BMMM	bone marrow micrometastases
BLL	bilateral lower lobe		
	brows, lids, and lashes	B-MODE	brightness modulation
BLLS	bilateral leg strength	BMP	behavior management plan

BMR	basal metabolic rate	BOH	bundle of His
	best motor response	BOLD	bleomycin, vincristine
BMT	bilateral myringotomy and		(Oncovin®), lomustine,
	tubes		and dacarbazine
	bismuth subsalicylate,	BOM	benign ovarian mass
	metronidazole, and		bilateral otitis media
	tetracycline	BOMA	bilateral otitis media,
	bone marrow transplant		acute
BMTN	bone marrow transplant	BOME	bilateral otitis media with
	neutropenia		effusion
BMTT	bilateral myringotomy	BoNT/A	Botulinum neurotoxin
	with tympanic tubes		type A
BMTU	bone marrow transplant	BOO	bladder outlet obstruction
	unit	BOOP	bronchitis obliterans with
BMU	basic multicellular unit		organized pneumonia
BN	bladder neck	BOP	bleeding on probing
BNC	binasal cannula	BOR	bowels open regularly
	bladder neck contracture		bronchia-oto-renal
BNCT	boron neutron capture		(syndrome)
	therapy	BOS	base of support
BNF	British National	BOT	base of tongue
	Formulary	BOU	burning on urination
BNI	blind nasal intubation	BOUGIE	bougienage
BNL	below normal limits	BOVR	Bureau of Vocational
	breast needle localization		Rehabilitation
Bn M	bone marrow	BOW	bag of water
BNO	bladder neck obstruction	BOW-I	bag of water-intact
	bowels not open	BOW-R	bag of water-ruptured
BNP	brain natriuretic peptide	BP	bathroom privileges
BNPA	binasal pharyngeal airway		bed pan
BNR	bladder neck retraction		bench press
BNS	benign nephrosclerosis		benzoyl peroxide
BO	base out		bipolar
	because of		birthplace
	behavior objective		blood pressure
	body odor		British Pharmacopeia
	bowel obstruction		bullous pemphigoid
	bowel open		bypass
	bucco-occlusal	BP-200	Bourn's Infant Pressure
B & O	belladonna & opium		Ventilator
	(suppositories)	BPA	birch pollen allergy
BOA	born on arrival	BPAD	bipolar affective disorder
	born out of asepsis	BPb	whole blood lead
BOB	ball on back		concentration
BOC	beats of clonus	BPI	bipolar affective disorder,
BOD	bilateral orbital		Type I
	decompression	BPD	biparietal diameter
Bod Units	Bodansky units		borderline personality
BOE	bilateral otitis externa		disorder

	bronchopulmonary dysplasia		bowel rest
BPd	diastolic blood pressure		breech
BPF	bronchopleural fistula		bridge
BPH	benign prostatic hypertrophy		bright red
			brown
		Br	bromide
BPG	bypass graft		bromine
BPI	bactericidal/permeability increasing (protein)	BRA	bananas, rice (rice cereal), and applesauce (diet)
BPIG	bacterial polysaccharide immune globulin		brain
		BRADY	bradycardia
BPL	benzylpenicilloylpolylysine	BRANCH	branch chain amino acids
BPLA	blood pressure, left arm	BRAO	branch retinal artery occlusion
BPM	beats per minute		
	breaths per minute	BRAT	bananas, rice (rice cereal), applesauce, and toast
BPN	bacitracin, polymyxin B, and neomycin sulfate		Baylor rapid autologous transfuser
BPO	benzoyl peroxide		blunt thoracic abdominal trauma
	bilateral partial oophorectomy		
BPP	biophysical profile	BRATT	bananas, rice (rice cereal), applesauce, tea, and toast
BPPP	bilateral pedal pulses present	BRB	blood-retinal barrier
			bright red blood
BP,P,R,T,	blood pressure, pulse, respiration, and temperature	BRBR	bright red blood per rectum
		BRBPR	bright red blood per rectum
BPPV	benign paroxysmal postural vertigo		
		BRCM	below right costal margin
BPR	blood per rectum	BRex	breathing exercise
	blood pressure recorder	Br Fdg	breast-feeding
BPRS	Brief Psychiatric Rating Scale	BRJ	brachial radialis jerk
		BRM	biological response modifiers
BPS	bilateral partial salpingectomy		
		BRO	brother
	blood pump speed	BROM	back range of motion
BPs	systolic blood pressure	BRONK	bronchoscopy
BPSD	bronchopulmonary segmental drainage	BRP	bathroom privileges
		BR RAO	branch retinal artery occlusion
BPV	benign paroxysmal vertigo		
		BR RVO	branch retinal vein occlusion
	benign positional vertigo		
	bovine papilloma virus	BrS	breath sounds
Bq	becquerel	BRSV	bovine respiratory syncytial virus
BQR	brequinar sodium		
BR	bathroom	BRU	basic remodeling unit (osteon)
	bedrest		
	Benzing retrograde	BRVO	branch retinal vein occlusion
	birthing room		
	blink reflex		

BS	barium swallow	BSN	Bachelor of Science in Nursing
	bedside		
	before sleep		bowel sounds normal
	Bennett seal	BSNA	bowel sounds normal and active
	blood sugar		
	Blue Shield	BSNMT	Bachelor of Science in Nuclear Medicine Technology
	bowel sounds		
	breath sounds		
B & S	Bartholin and Skene (glands)	BSNT	breast soft and nontender
		BSNUTD	baby shots not up to date
	bending and stooping	BSO	bilateral salpingo-oophorectomy
BS×4	bowel sounds in all four quadrants		
			l-buthionine sulfoximine
BSA	body surface area	bSOD	bovine superoxide dismutase
	bowel sounds active		
BSAB	Balthazar Scales of Adaptive Behavior	BSOM	bilateral serous otitis media
BSAb	broad-spectrum antibiotics	BSP	Bromsulphalein®
BSB	bedside bag	BSPA	bowel sounds present and active
	body surface burned		
BSC	bedside care	BSPM	body surface potential mapping
	bedside commode		
	burn scar contracture	BSR	bowels sounds regular
BSCC	bedside commode chair	BSRT (R)	Bachelor of Science in Radiologic Technology (Registered)
	Bjork-Shiley convexoconcave (valves)		
BSD	baby soft diet	BSS	Baltimore Sepsis Scale
	bedside drainage		bedside scale
BSE	bovine spongiform encephalopathy		bismuth subsalicylate
			black silk sutures
	breast self-examination	BSS®	balanced salt solution
BSEC	bedside easy chair	BSSG	sitogluside
BSepF	black separated female	BSSO	bilateral sagittal split osteotomy
BSepM	black separated male		
BSER	brain stem evoked responses	BSSS	benign sporadic sleep spikes
BSF	black single female	BSST	breast self-stimulation test
	busulfan	BST	bedside testing
BSG	Bagolini striated glasses		bovine somatotropin
BSGA	beta streptococcus group A		brief stimulus therapy
		BSU	Bartholin, Skene's, urethra (glands)
BSI	body substance isolation		
	brain stem injury		behavioral science unit
BSL	blood sugar level	BSu	blood sugar
BS L base	breath sounds diminished, left base	BSUTD	baby shots up to date
			Base Service Unit
BSM	black single male	BSW	Bachelor of Social Work
	blood safety module		bedscale weight
		BT	bedtime

	behavioral therapy	BTX	Botulinum toxin
	bituberous	BU	base up (prism)
	bladder tumor		below umbilicus
	Blalock-Taussig (shunt)		Bodansky units
	bleeding time		burn unit
	blood type		busulfan
	blood transfusion	BUA	broadband ultrasound
	brain tumor		attenuation
	breast tumor	BUdR	bromodeoxyuridine
	bowel tones	BUE	both upper extremities
B/T	between	BUFA	baby up for adoption
Bt#	bottle number	BUN	blood urea nitrogen
BTA	below the ankle		bunion
BTB	back to bed	BUR	back-up rate (ventilator)
	beat-to-beat (variability)	Burd	Burdick suction
	break-through bleeding	BUS	Bartholin, urethral, and
BTBV	beat to beat variability		Skene's glands
BTC	bilateral tubal cautery	BUT	break up time
	bladder tumor check	BV	bacterial vaginitis
	by the clock		biological value
BTE	Baltimore Therapeutic		blood volume
	Equipment	BVAD	biventricular assist device
	behind-the-ear (hearing	BVD	bovine viral diarrhea
	aid)	BVE	blood volume expander
BTF	blenderized tube feeding	BVH	biventricular hypertrophy
BTFS	breast tumor frozen	BVL	bilateral vas ligation
	section	BVM	bag valve mask
BTG	beta thromboglobulin	BVMG	Bender Visual-Motor
BTHOOM	beats the hell out of me		Gestalt (test)
	(better stated as	BVO	branch vein occlusion
	"differed diagnosis")	BVR	Bureau of Vocational
BTI	biliary tract infection		Rehabilitation
	bitubal interruption	BVRO	bilateral vertical ramus
BTL	bilateral tubal ligation		osteotomy
BTM	bismuth subcitrate,	BVRT	Benton Visual Retention
	tetracycline, and		Test
	metronidazole	BVT	bilateral ventilation tubes
BTO	bilateral tubal occlusion	BW	birth weight
BTP	bismuth tribromophenate		bite-wing (radiograph)
	breakthrough pain		body water
BTPABA	bentiromide		body weight
BTPS	body temperature pressure	B & W	Black and White (milk of
	saturated		magnesia & aromatic
BTR	bladder tumor recheck		cascara fluidextract)
BTS	Blalock-Taussig shunt	BWA	bed wetter admission
BTSH	bovine thyrotropin	BWCS	bagged white cell study
BTU	behavior therapy unit	BWF	Blackwater fever
BTW	back to work	BWFI	bacteriostatic water for
BTW M	between meals		injection

BWidF	black widowed female
BWidM	black widowed male
BWS	battered woman syndrome
BWs	bite-wing (x-rays)
BWX	bite-wing x-ray
Bx	biopsy
B x B	back to back
BX BS	Blue Cross and Blue Shield
BXM	B cell crossmatch
ΦBZ	phenylbutazone
BZD	benzodiazepine
BZDZ	benzodiazepine

C

C	ascorbic acid
	carbohydrate
	Catholic
	Caucasian
	Celsius
	centigrade
	clubbing
	conjunctiva
	constricted
	cyanosis
	cytosine
	hundred
$\bar{c}$	with
C′	cervical spine
C+	with contrast
C−	without contrast
C_1–C_7	cervical vertebra 1 through 7
C_1–C_8	cervical nerves 1 through 8
C_1 to C_9	precursor molecules of the complement system
C_1 to C_{12}	cranial nerves 1 to 12
C3	complement C3
C4	complement C4
CI-CV	Drug Enforcement Agency scheduled substances class one through five
C_{II}	second cranial nerve
CA	cancelled appointment
	Candida albicans
	carcinoma
	cardiac arrest
	carotid artery
	celiac artery
	cellulose acetate (filter)
	chronologic age
	Cocaine Anonymous
	community-acquired
	compressed air
	continuous aerosol
	coronary angioplasty
	coronary artery
Ca	calcium
CA 125	cancer antigen 125
C&A	Clinitest® and Acetest®
CAA	colo-anal anastamosis
	crystalline amino acids
CAB	catheter-associated bacteriuria
	cellulose acetate butyrate
	coronary artery bypass
CABG	coronary artery bypass graft
CaBI	calcium bone index
CaBP	calcium-binding protein
CABS	coronary artery bypass surgery
CAC	cardioacceleratory center
	Certified Alcohol Counselor
	Community Action Center
CACI	computer-assisted continuous infusion
$CaCl_2$	calcium chloride
$CaCO_3$	calcium carbonate
CACP	cisplatin
CAD	cadaver (kidney donor)
	computer-aided diagnosis
	coronary artery disease
CADAC	Certified Alcohol and Drug Abuse Counselor
CADASIL	cerebral autosomal dominant arteriopathy

	with subcortical infarcts and leukoencephalopathy		you ever taken a drink (eye opener) first thing in the morning?
CADD®	Computerized Ambulatory Drug Delivery (pump)	CAH	chronic active hepatitis
CADP	computer-assisted design of prosthesis		chronic aggressive hepatitis
CADXPL	cadaver transplant		congenital adrenal hyperplasia
CAE	cellulose acetate electrophoresis	CAHB	chronic active hepatitis B
	coronary artery endarterectomy	CAI	carbonic anhydrase inhibitors
	cyclophosphamide, doxorubicin (Adriamycin), and etoposide		carboxyamide aminoimidazoles
		'caid	Medicaid
CAEC	cardiac arrhythmia evaluation center	CAIV	cold-adapted influenza virus vaccine
CaEDTA	calcium disodium edetate	CAL	callus
CAF	chronic atrial fibrillation		calories (cal)
	controlled atrial flutter/fibrillation		chronic airflow limitation
		Calb	albumin clearance
	cyclophosphamide, doxorubicin (Adriamycin), and fluorouracil	cal ct	calorie count
		CALD	chronic active liver disease
CAFF	controlled atrial fibrillation/flutter	CALGB	Cancer and Leukemia Group B
CAFT	Clinitron® air fluidized therapy	CALLA	common acute lymphoblastic leukemia antigen
CAG	chronic atrophic gastritis	CAM	Caucasian adult male
	closed angle glaucoma		cell adhesion molecules
	continuous ambulatory gamma globin (infusion)		child abuse management
			confusion assessment method
	coronary arteriography		cystic adenomatoid malformation
CaG	calcium gluconate	CAMCOG	Cambridge Cognitive Examination
CAGE	a questionnaire for alcoholism evaluation (JAMA 1984; 252: 1905-7) C Have you ever felt the need to cut down on your drinking? A Have you ever felt annoyed by criticism of your drinking? G Have you ever felt guilty about your drinking? E Have	CAMD	computer-aided molecular design
		CAMF	cyclophosphamide, Adriamycin, methotrexate, and fluorouracil
		CAMP	cyclophosphamide, doxorubicin (Adriamycin), methotrexate, and procarbazine
		cAMP	cyclic adenosine monophosphate

CAMs	cell adhesion molecules	C-arm	fluoroscopy image intensifier
CAN	contrast-associated nephropathy	CARN	Certified Addiction Registered Nurse
	cord around neck		
CA/N	child abuse and neglect	CART	classification and regression tree
CANC	cancelled		
c-ANCA	antineutrophil cytoplasmic antibody	CAS	carotid artery stenosis
			cerebral arteriosclerosis
CANDA	computer-assisted new drug application		Chemical Abstract Service
CANP	Certified Adult Nurse Practitioner		Clinical Asthma Score
			combined androgen suppression
CAO	chronic airway (airflow) obstruction		computer-assisted surgery
CaO₂	arterial oxygen concentration	CASA	cancer-associated serum antigen
CAP	capsule		Center on Addiction and Substance Abuse
	chemistry admission profile		computer-assisted semen analysis
	chloramphenicol		
	community-acquired pneumonia	CASHD	coronary arteriosclerotic heart disease
	compound action potentials	CASP	Child Analytic Study Program
	cyclophosphamide, doxorubicin (Adria-mycin), and cisplatin	CASS	computer-aided sleep system
CaP	carcinoma of the prostate	CAST®	color allergy screening test
Ca/P	calcium to phosphorus ratio	CAT	Cardiac Arrest Team
CAPB	central auditory processing battery		carnitine acetyl transferase
			cataract
CAPD	chronic ambulatory peritoneal dialysis		Children's Apperception Test
CAPLA	computer-assisted product license application		coital alignment technique
			computed axial tomography
CAPS	caffeine, alcohol, pepper, and spicy food (dietary restrictions)	CATH	methcatinone
			catheter
CAPWA	computerized arterial pulse waveform analysis		catheterization
			Catholic
		CATS	catecholamines
		CAU	Caucasian
CAR	cardiac ambulation routine	CAV	computer-aided ventilation
CARB	carbohydrate		congenital absence of vagina
CARBO	Carbocaine®		cyclophosphamide, doxorubicin (Adriamycin), and vincristine
	carboplatin		
CARD	Cardiac Automatic Resuscitative Device		

CAV-1	canine adenovirus type 1		Evaluation and
CAVB	complete atrioventricular block		Research
		CBF	cerebral blood flow
CAVC	common artrioventricular canal	CBFS	cerebral blood flow studies
CAVE	cyclophosphamide, doxorubicin, (Adriamycin) vincristine, and etoposide	CBFV	cerebral blood flow velocity
		CBG	capillary blood glucose
		CBI	continuous bladder irrigation
CAVH	continuous atriovenous hemofiltration	CBM	cryopreserved bone marrow
CAVHD	continuous arteriovenous hemodialysis	CBN	chronic benign neutropenia
CAV-P-VP	cyclophosphamide, doxorubicin (Adriamycin), vincristine, cisplatin, and etoposide		collected by nurse
		CBP	chronic benign pain copper-binding protein
		CBPS	coronary bypass surgery
		CBR	carotid bodies resected
CAVR	continuous arteriovenous rewarming		chronic bedrest complete bedrest
CAVU	continuous arteriovenous ultrafiltration	CBRAM	controlled partial rebreathing-anesthesia method
CAX	central axis		
CB	cesarean birth chronic bronchitis code blue	CB RRR s̄ M/R/G	cardiac beat, regular rhythm and rate without murmurs, rubs, or gallops
c/b	complicated by		
C & B	chair and bed crown and bridge	CBS	Charles Bonnet's syndrome chronic brain syndrome coarse breath sounds Cruveilhier-Baumgarten syndrome
CBA	chronic bronchitis and asthma County Board of Assistance		
		CBT	cognitive behavioral therapy
CBAVD	congenital bilateral absence of the vas deferens	CBU	cumulative breath units
		CBV	central blood volume
CBC	carbenicillin complete blood count contralateral breast cancer	CBZ	carbamazepine
		CBZE	carbamazepine epoxide
		CC	cardiac catheterization Catholic cerebral concussion chief complaint chronic complainer circulatory collapse clean catch (urine) comfort care coracoclavicular
CBCDA	carboplatin		
CBCT	community based clinical trials		
CBD	closed bladder drainage common bile duct		
CBDE	common bile duct exploration		
CBE	child birth education		
CBER	Center for Biologics		

	cord compression	CCC-SP	Certificate of Clinical Competence in Speech-Language Pathology
	corpus collosum		
	creatinine clearance		
	critical condition	CCD	charged-coupled device
	cubic centimeter (cc), (mL)		childhood celiac disease
	with correction (with glasses)	CCDC	Certified Chemical Dependency Counselor
C_c	concentration of drug in the central compartment	CCDS	color-coded duplex sonography
C/C	cholecystectomy and operative cholangiogram	CCE	clubbing, cyanosis, and edema
			countercurrent electrophoresis
	complete upper and lower dentures	CCF	cephalin cholesterol flocculation
CCII	Clinical Clerk–2nd year		compound comminuted fracture
C & C	cold and clammy		congestive cardiac failure
CCA	calcium-channel antagonist		crystal-induced chemotactic factor
	circumflex coronary artery	CCFE	cyclophosphamide, cisplatin, fluorouracil, and estramustine
	common carotid artery		
	concentrated care area		
	critical care area	CCG	Children's Cancer Group
CCAC	cysteine-cysteic acid complex	CCH	community care home
CCAP	capsule cartilage articular preservation		Cook County Hospital
		CCHD	complex congenital heart disease
CCAT	common carotid artery thrombosis		cyanotic congenital heart disease
CCB	calcium channel blocker(s)	CCHF	Congo-Crimean hemorrhagic fever
	Community Care Board	CCI	chronic coronary insufficiency
	corn, callus, and bunion		
CCC	Cancer Care Center	CCK	cholecystokinin
	central corneal clouding (Grade 0+ to 4+)	CCK-OP	cholecystokinin octapeptide
	Certificate of Clinical Competency	CCK-PZ	cholecystokinin pancreozymin
	child care clinic	CCL	cardiac catheterization laboratory
	Comprehensive Cancer Center		critical condition list
C/cc	colonies per cubic centimeter	CCl_4	carbon tetrachloride
CC & C	colony count and culture	CCM	calcium citrate malate
CCC-A	Certificate of Clinical Competence in Audiology		cyclophosphamide, lomustine (CCNU; CeeNU), and methotrexate

50

CCMSU	clean catch midstream urine	CCUA	clean catch urinalysis
		CCUP	colpocystourethropexy
CCMU	critical care medicine unit	CCV	Critical Care Ventilator (Ohio)
CCN	continuing care nursery		
CCNS	cell cycle-nonspecific	CCW	childcare worker
CCNU	lomustine		counterclockwise
C-collar	cervical collar	CCWR	counterclockwise rotation
CCP	crystalloid cardioplegia	CCX	complications
CCPD	continuous cycling (cyclical) peritoneal dialysis	CCY	cholecystectomy
		CD	cadaver donor
			candela
CCR	cardiac care reversal		Castleman's disease
	cardiac catheterization recovery		celiac disease
			cervical dystonia
	continuous complete remission		cesarean delivery
			character disorder
	counterclockwise rotation		chemical dependency
C_{cr}	creatinine clearance		childhood disease
CCRC	continuing care residential community		chronic dialysis
			closed drainage
CCRN	Certified Critical Care Registered Nurse		clusters of differentiation
			common duct
			communication disorders
CCRT	combined chemo-radiotherapy		complicated delivery
			conjugate diameter
CCRU	critical care recovery unit		continuous drainage
CCS	cell cycle-specific		convulsive disorder
CC & S	cornea, conjunctiva, and sclera		Crohn's disease
			cyclodextran
			cytarabine and daunorubicin
CCSK	clear cell sarcoma of the kidney		
		Cd	cadmium
CCT	calcitriol		concentration of drug
	carotid compression tomography	C/D	cigarettes per day
			cup to disk ratio
	Certified Cardiographic Technician	CD4	antigenic marker on helper/inducer T cells (also called OKT 4, T4, and Leu3)
	closed cerebral trauma		
	closed cranial trauma		
	congenitally corrected transposition (of the great vessels)		
		CD8	antigenic marker on suppressor/cytotoxic T cells (also called OKT 8, T8, and Leu 8)
	crude coal tar		
CCTGA	congenitally corrected transposition of the great arteries		
		C&D	curettage and desiccation
			cystectomy and diversion
CCT in PET	crude coal tar in petroleum		cytoscopy and dilatation
CCTV	closed circuit television	CDA	Certified Dental Assistant
CCU	coronary care unit		chenodeoxycholic acid (chenodiol)
	critical care unit		

	congenital dyserythro-poietic anemia		color Doppler imaging
2CdA	cladribine (chlorodeoxyadenosine)		Cotrel Duobosset Instrumentation
CDAD	*Clostridium difficile*-associated diarrhea	CDIC	*Clostridium difficile*-induced colitis
CDAI	Crohn's Disease Activity Index	C Dif	*Clostridium difficile*
CDAK	Cordis Dow Artificial Kidney	CDK	climatic droplet keratopathy
CDAP	continuous distended airway pressure	CDKI	cyclin-dependent kinase inhibitor
CDB	cough and deep breath	CDLE	chronic discoid lupus erythematosus
CDC	calculated day of confinement	CdLS	Cornelia de Lange's syndrome
	cancer detection center	CDP	chemical dependence profile
	carboplatin, doxorubicin, and cyclophosphamide		Child Development Program
	Centers for Disease Control and Prevention		crystalline degradation product
	Certified Drug Counselor		cytidine diphosphate
	chenodeoxycholic acid (chenodiol)	CDQ	corrected development quotient
	Clostridium difficile colitis	CDR	Clinical Dementia Rating
CDCA	chenodeoxycholic acid (chenodiol)		continuing disability review
CDD	Certificate of Disability for Discharge	CDRH	Center for Devices and Radiological Health
	Clostridium difficile disease	CDR(H)	cup-to-disk ratio horizontal
CDDP	cisplatin	CDRs	complementary determining regions
CDE	canine distemper encephalitis	CDR(V)	cup-to-disk ratio vertical
	Certified Diabetes Educator	CDS	closed door seclusion
	common duct exploration		color Doppler sonography
CDGP	constitutional delay of growth and puberty	CDSC	Communicable Disease Surveillance Centre (United Kingdom)
CDH	chronic daily headache	CDSPIES	congestive heart failure, drugs, spasm, pneumothorax, infection, embolism, and secretions (differential diagnosis mnemonic)
	congenital diaphragmatic hernia		
	congenital dislocation of hip		
	congenital dysplasia of the hip		
CDI	Children's Depression Inventory	CDT	carbohydrate-deficient transferrin
	clean, dry, and intact		Chemical Dependency Technician

CDU	chemical dependency unit	CEN	Certified (Nurse)–
CDV	canine distemper virus		Emergency Room
	cardiovascular	CENOG	computerized
CDX	chlordiazepoxide		electroneuro-
cdyn	dynamic compliance		ophthalmogram
CE	California encephalitis	CEO	chief executive officer
	capillary electrophoresis	CEP	cardiac enzyme panel
	cardiac enlargement		cognitive evoked potential
	cardiac enzymes		congenital erythropoietic
	cardioesophageal		porphyria
	cataract extraction		countercurrent
	central episiotomy		electrophoresis
	chemoembolization		cyclophosphamide,
	cholesterol ester		etoposide, and cisplatin
	community education		(Platinol)
	consultative examination	CEPH	cephalic
	continuing education		cephalosporin
	contrast echocardiology	CEPH	cephalin flocculation
C&E	consultation and	FLOC	
	examination	CER	conditioned emotional
	cough and exercise		response
	curettage and	CE&R	central episiotomy and
	electrodesiccation		repair
CEA	carcinoembryonic antigen	CERA	cortical evoked response
	carotid endarterectomy		audiometry
CEB	calcium entry blocker	CERD	chronic end-stage renal
	carboplatin, etoposide,		disease
	and bleomycin	CERULO	ceruloplasmin
CEC	Council for Exceptional	CERV	cervical
	Children	CES	cognitive environmental
CECD	congenital endothelial		stimulation
	corneal dystrophy		estrogen, conjugated
CECT	contrast-enhanced		(conjugated estrogen
	computed tomography		substance)
CED	cystoscopy-endoscopy	CESD	Center for Epidemiologic
	dilation		Studies – Depression
CEF	chick embryo fibroblast	CESI	cervical epidural steroid
CEFOT	cefotaxime		injection
CEFOX	cefoxitin	CETP	cholesterol ester transfer
CEFTAZ	ceftazidime		protein
CEFUR	cefuroxime	CEV	cyclophosphamide,
CEI	continuous extravascular		etoposide, and
	infusion		vincristine
	converting enzyme	CF	calcium leucovorin
	inhibitor		(citrovorum factor)
CEL	cardiac exercise		cancer-free
	laboratory		cardiac failure
CEMD	consultative examination		Caucasian female
	by physician		Christmas factor

	cisplatin and fluorouracil	CFT	chronic follicular tonsillitis
	complement fixation		
	contractile force		complement fixation test
	count fingers	CFTR	cystic fibrosis transmembrane (conductance) regulator
	cystic fibrosis		
C&F	cell and flare		
	chills and fever	CFU	colony-forming units
CFA	common femoral artery	CFU-E	colony-forming unit–erythroid
	complete Freund's adjuvant		
		CFU-G	colony-forming unit–granulocyte
	cryptogenic fibrosing alveolitis		
		CFU-G/M	colony-forming unit–granulocyte/macro-phage
	cystic fibrosis anthropathy		
CFAC	complement-fixing antibody consumption		
		CFU-M	colony-forming unit–macrophage
C-factor	cleverness factor		
CFCs	chlorofluorocarbons	CFU-S	colony-forming unit–spleen
CFD	color-flow Doppler		
CFF	critical fusion (flicker) frequency	CG	cardiogreen (dye)
			cholecystogram
			contact guarding
CFFT	critical flicker fusion threshold		contralateral groin
		CGA	comprehensive geriatric assessment
CFI	confrontation fields intact		
CFIDS	chronic fatigue immune dysfunction syndrome		contact guard assist
		CGB	chronic gastrointestinal (tract) bleeding
CFL	cisplatin, fluorouracil, and leucovorin calcium		
		CGD	chronic granulomatous disease
CFLX	ciprofloxacin		
	circumflex	CGI	Clinical Global Impressions (scale)
CFM	close fitting mask		
	craniofacial microsomia	CGIC	Clinical Global Impression of Change
	cyclophosphamide, fluorouracil, and mitoxantrone		
		CGL	chronic granulocytic leukemia
CFNS	chills, fever, and night sweats		with correction/with glasses
CFP	cystic fibrosis protein	CGM	central gray matter
CFPT	cyclophosphamide, fluorouracil, prednisone, and tamoxifen	CGMP	Current Good Manufacturing Practices
		cGMP	cyclic guanine monophosphate
CFR	case-fatality rates	CGN	chronic glomerulonephritis
	Code of Federal Regulations		
		CGRP	calcitonin gene-related peptide
CFS	cancer family syndrome		
	Child and Family Service	CGS	cardiogenic shock
	childhood febrile seizures		catgut suture
	chronic fatigue syndrome		

	centimeter-gram-second system	CCNU	
		cHct	central hematocrit
CGTT	cortisol glucose tolerance test	CHD	center hemodialysis
			changed diaper
cGy	centigray		childhood diseases
CH	chest		chronic hemodialysis
	chief		common hepatic duct
	child (children)		congenital heart disease
	chronic		coordinate home care
	cluster headache	CHE	chronic hepatic encephalopathy
	congenital hypothyroidism		
	convalescent hospital	CHEF	clamped homogeneous electric field
	crown-heal		
C_h	hepatic clearance	CHEM 7	laboratory tests for glucose, blood urea nitrogen, creatinine, potassium, sodium, chloride, and carbon dioxide
ch^1	Christ Church chromosone		
CH_{50}	total hemolytic complement		
C&H	cocaine and heroin		
CHA	compound hypermetropic astigmatism		
		CHEMO	chemotherapy
	congenital hypoplastic anemia	ChemoRx	chemotherapy
		CHESS	chemical shift suppression
CHAI	continuous hepatic artery infusion	CHF	congestive heart failure
			Crimean hemorrhagic fever
CHAM-OCA	cyclophosphamide, hydroxyurea, dactinomycin, methotrexate, vincristine, leucovorin, and doxorubicin	CHFV	combined high frequency of ventilation
		CHG	change
		CHI	closed head injury
			creatinine-height index
		CHIN	community health information network
CHAM-PUS	Civilian Health and Medical Program of the Uniformed Services	CHIP	iproplatin
			comprehensive health insurance plan
CHAP	child health associate practitioner	Chix	chickenpox
		CHL	conductive hearing loss
CHARGE	coloboma (of eyes), hearing deficit, choanal atresia, retardation of growth, genital defects (males only), and endocardial cushion defect	ChloMP	chlorambucil, mitoxantrone, and prednisolone
		ChlVPP	chlorambucil, vinblastine, procarbazine, and prednisone
		CHN	central hemorrhagic necrosis
CHB	complete heart block		community nursing home
CHBHA	congenital Heinz body hemolytic anemia	CHO	carbohydrate
			Chinese hamster ovary
CHC	concentric hypertrophic cardiomyopathy	C_{H_2O}	free-water clearance
CH_{3^-}	semustine	C_2H_5OH	alcohol (ethyl alcohol)

55

chol	cholesterol	CIBD	chronic inflammatory bowel disease
c̄ hold	withhold		
CHOP	cyclophosphamide, doxorubicin, vincristine (Oncovin), prednisone	CIBI	Clinician Interview Based Impression (of change)
		CIBIC	Clinician Interview-Based Impression of Change
CHPB	Canadian Health Protection Branch (the equivalent of the U.S. Food and Drug Administration)	CIBP	chronic intractable benign pain
		CIC	cardioinhibitory center circulating immune complexes clean intermittent catheterization completely in the canal (hearing aid) coronary intensive care
CHPX	chickenpox		
CHR	Cercaria-Hullen reaction chronic		
CHRPE	congenital hypertrophy of the retinal pigment epithelium		
		CICE	combined intracapsular cataract extraction
CHRS	congenital hereditary retinoschisis	CICU	cardiac intensive care unit
CHS	Chediak-Higashi syndrome contact hypersensitivity	CICVC	centrally inserted central venous catheter
CHT	closed head trauma	CID	cervical immobilization device combined immunodeficiency cytomegalic inclusion disease
CHU	closed head unit		
CHUC	Certified Health Unit Coordinator		
CHW	community health workers		
CI	cardiac index cesium implant Clinical Instructor cochlear implant commercial insurance complete iridectomy confidence interval continuous infusion coronary insufficiency	CIDP	chronic inflammatory demyelinating polyradiculoneuropathy
		CIDS	cellular immunodeficiency syndrome continuous insulin delivery system
Ci	curie(s)	CIE	chemotherapy induced emesis congenital ichthyosiform erythroderma counterimmunoelectrophore crossed immunoelectrophoresis
CIA	calcaneal insufficiency avulsion chronic idiopathic anhidrosis		
CIAA	competitive insulin autoantibodies		
CIAED	collagen induced autoimmune ear disease	CIEA	continuous infusion epidural analgesia
CIB	Carnation Instant Breakfast® crying-induced bronchospasm cytomegalic inclusion bodies	CIEP	counterimmunoelectrophore crossed immunoelectrophoresis
		CIG	cigarettes
		CIH	continuous infusion haloperidol

56

CIHD	chronic ischemic heart disease	CITP	capillary isotachophoresis
CII	continuous insulin infusion	CIU	chronic idiopathic urticaria
CIIA	common internal iliac artery	CIV	common iliac vein continuous intravenous (infusion)
CIM	change in menses corticosteroid-induced myopathy	CIVI	continuous intravenous infusion
CIMCU	cardiac intermediate care unit	CIXU	constant infusion excretory urogram
CIN	cervical intraepithelial neoplasia	CIWA-Ar	Clinical Institute Withdrawal Assessment for Alcohol–revised
	chemotherapy induced neutropenia	CJD	Creutzfeldt-Jakob disease
	chronic interstitial nephritis	CJR	centric jaw relation
C_{IN}	insulin clearance	CK	check creatine kinase
CIND	cognitive impairment, no dementia	CK-BB	creatine kinase BB band
		CKC	cold knife conization
CINE	chemotherapy-induced nausea and emesis	CK-ISO	creatine kinase isoenzyme
	cineangiogram	CK-MB	creatine kinase MB band
CIP	Cardiac Injury Panel	CK MM	creatine kinase MM band
	critical illness polyneuropathy	CKW	clockwise
		Cl	chloride
CIPD	chronic intermittent peritoneal dialysis	CL	central line chemoluminescence
Circ	circulation circumcision circumference		clear liquid cleft lip cloudy critical list cycle length lung compliance
circ. & sen.	circulation and sensation	C_L	compliance of the lungs
CIS	continuous interleaved sampling carcinoma *in situ*	CLA	community living arrangements
CI&S	conjunctival irritation and swelling	CLAS	congenital localized absence of skin
CISCA	cisplatin, cyclophospha- mide, and doxorubicin (Adriamycin)	CLASS	computer laser assisted surgical system
Cis-DDP	cisplatin	CLASS I	congestive heart failure with no limitation with ordinary activity, (New York Heart Association Classification)
CIS-R	Clinical Interview Schedule, Revised		
CIT	conventional immunosuppressive therapy	CLASS II	congestive heart failure with slight limitation of physical activity
	conventional insulin therapy	CLASS III	congestive heart failure

	with marked limitation of physical activity	CLS	capillary leak syndrome
			community living skills
CLASS IV	congestive heart failure with inability to engage in any physical activity without symptoms	CLSE	calf lung surfactant extract (Infasurf®)
Clav	clavicle	CLT	chronic lymphocytic thyroiditis
CLB	chlorambucil		complex lymphedema therapy
	coccidian-like body		cool lace tent
CLBBB	complete left bundle branch block	Cl_T	total body clearance
CLBD	cortical Lewy body disease	CLV	cutaneous leukocytoclastic vasculitis
CLBP	chronic low back pain	CL VOID	clean voided specimen
CLC	cork leather and celastic (orthotic)	clysis	hypodermoclysis
CL/CP	cleft lip and cleft palate	cm	centimeter
CLD	chronic liver disease	CM	capreomycin
	chronic lung disease		cardiac monitor
Cl_d	dialysis clearance		case management
CLE	centrilobular emphysema		case manager
	continuous lumbar epidural (anesthetic)		Caucasian male
CLEIA	chemiluminescent enzyme immunoassay		centimeter (cm)
			chondromalacia
CLEP	college level examination program		cochlear microphonics
			common migraine
CLF	cholesterol-lecithin flocculation		continuous microwave
			continuous murmur
CLG	clorgyline		contrast media
CLH	chronic lobular hepatitis		costal margin
Cl_h	hepatic clearance		cow's milk
CLI	clomipramine		culture media
Cl_{int}	intrinsic clearance		cutaneous melanoma
CLL	chronic lymphocytic leukemia		cystic mesothelioma
			tomorrow morning (this is a dangerous abbreviation)
CLLE	columnar-lined lower esophagus	cm1	circumflex marginal 1
cl liq	clear liquid	cm2	circumflex marginal 2
Cl_{nr}	nonrenal clearance	cm^3	cubic centimeter
CLO	Campylobacter-like organism	CMA	Certified Medical Assistant
	close		compound myopic astigmatism
	cod liver oil		cow's milk allergy
CL & P	cleft lip and palate	CMAF	centrifuged microaggregate filter
CL PSY	closed psychiatry	CMAPs	compound muscle action potentials
Cl_r	renal clearance		
CLRO	community leave for reorientation	C_{max}	maximum concentration of drug

58

CMB	carbolic methylene blue	CMID	cytomegalic inclusion disease
CMBBT	cervical mucous basal body temperature	C_{min}	minimum concentration of drug
CMC	carpal metacarpal (joint)	CMIR	cell-mediated immune response
	carboxymethylcellulose	CMJ	carpometacarpal joint
	chloramphenicol	CMK	congenital multicystic kidney
	chronic mucocutaneous candidosis	CML	cell-mediated lympholysis
	closed mitral commissurotomy		chronic myelogenous leukemia
CMD	cytomegalic disease		chronic myeloid leukemia
CMDRH	Center for Medical Devices and Radiological Health (of the Food and Drug Administration)	CMM	Comprehensive Major Medical (insurance)
			cutaneous malignant melanoma
CME	cervicomediastinal exploration (examination)	CMME	chloromethyl methyl ether
		CMML	chronic myelomacrocytic leukemia
	continuing medical education	CMMS	Columbia Mental Maturity Scale
	cystoid macular edema	CMO	Chief Medical Officer
CMER	current medical evidence of record		comfort measures only (resuscitation order)
CMF	cyclophosphamide, methotrexate and fluorouracil		consult made out
		CMP	cardiomyopathy
			chondromalacia patellae
CMFP	cyclophosphamide, methotrexate, fluorouracil, and prednisone		cushion mouthpiece
		CMPF	cow's milk, protein-free
		CMPT	cervical mucous penetration test
CMFT	same as CMF with tamoxifen	CMR	cerebral metabolic rate
CMFVP	cyclophosphamide, methotrexate, fluorouracil, vincristine, and prednisone	CMRNG	chromosomally mediated resistant *Neisseria gonorrhoeae*
		$CMRO_2$	cerebral metabolic rate for oxygen
CMG	cystometrogram	CMS	children's medical services
CMGN	chronic membranous glomerulonephritis		circulation motion sensation
CMH	current medical history		chocolate milkshake
CMHC	community mental health center		constant moderate suction
CMHN	Community Mental Health Nurse	CMSUA	clean midstream urinalysis
CMI	cell-mediated immunity	CMT	carpometatarsal (joint)
	clomipramine		Certified Medical Transcriptionist
	Cornell Medical Index		

	Certified Music Therapist	CNH	central neurogenic hypernea
	cervical motion tenderness		contract nursing home
	Charcot-Marie tooth (disease)	CNHC	chronodermatitis nodularis helicis chronicus
	choline magnesium trisalicylate (Trilisate)		community nursing home care
	continuing medication and treatment	CNL	chemonucleolysis
	cutis marmorata telangiectasia	CNLD	chronic neonatal lung disease
CMTX	chemotherapy treatment	CNM	certified nurse midwife
CMV	cisplatin, methotrexate, and vinblastine	CNMT	Certified Nuclear Medicine Technologist
	controlled mechanical ventilation	CNN	congenital nevocytic nevus
	conventional mechanical ventilation	CNO	Chief Nursing Officer
	cool mist vaporizer	CNOR	Certified Nurse, Operating Room
	cytomegalovirus	CNP	capillary nonprofusion
CMVS	culture midvoid specimen	CNPS	cardiac nuclear probe scan
CN	cranial nerve		
	tomorrow night (this is a dangerous abbreviation)	CNRN	Certified Neurosurgical Registered Nurse
C_n	cyanide	CNS	central nervous system
C/N	contrast-to-noise ratio		Clinical Nurse Specialist
CN II–XII	cranial nerves 2–12		coagulase-negative staphylococci
CNA	Certified Nurse Aide		Crigler-Najjar syndrome
	chart not available	CNSHA	congenital nonspherocytic hemolytic anemia
C_{Na}	sodium clearance	CNT	could not tell
CNAG	chronic narrow angle glaucoma		could not test
CNAP	continuous negative airway pressure	CNTA	combined neurosurgical and transfacial approach
CNC	clinical nurse coordinator	CNTF	ciliary neurotrophic factor
	Community Nursing Center	CNV	choroidal neovascularization
CNCbl	cyanocobalamin	CNVM	choroidal neovascular membrane
CND	canned	CO	carbon monoxide
	cannot determine		cardiac output
CNDC	chronic nonspecific diarrhea of childhood		castor oil
CNE	chronic nervous exhaustion		centric occlusion
	could not establish		Certified Orthoptist
CNF	cyclophosphamide, mitoxantrone (Novatantrone), and fluorouracil		cervical orthosis
			court order
		Co	cobalt
		C/O	check out

60

	complained of
	complaints
	under care of
CO_2	carbon dioxide
CO_3	carbonate
COA	children of alcoholic
	coenzyme A
CoA	coarctation of the aorta
COAD	chronic obstructive airway disease
	chronic obstructive arterial disease
COAG	chronic open angle glaucoma
COAGSC	coagulation screen
COAP	cyclophosphamide, vincristine (Oncovin), cytarabine (ara-C), and prednisone
COAR	coarctation
COARCT	coarctation
COB	cisplatin, vincristine (Oncovin), and bleomycin
COBE	chronic obstructive bullous emphysema
COBS	chronic organic brain syndrome
COBT	chronic obstruction of biliary tract
COC	combination oral contraceptive
	continuity of care
COCCIO	coccidioidomycosis
COCM	congestive cardiomyopathy
COD	cataract, right eye
	cause of death
	codeine
	coefficient of oxygen delivery
	condition on discharge
CODE 99	patient in cardiac or respiratory arrest
COD-MD	cerebro-oculardysplasia muscular dystrophy
CODO	codocytes
COE	court-ordered examination
COEPS	cortically originating

	extrapyramidal symptoms
COFS	cerebro-oculo-facio-skeletal
COG	center of gravity
	Central Oncology Group
	cognitive function tests
COGN	cognition
COGTT	cortisone-primed oral glucose tolerance test
COH	carbohydrate
COHB	carboxyhemoglobin
Coke	Coca-Cola®
	cocaine
COL	colonoscopy
COLD	chronic obstructive lung disease
COLD A	cold agglutin titer
Collyr	eye wash
col/ml	colonies per milliliter
colp	colporrhaphy
COM	chronic otitis media
COMF	comfortable
COMLA	cyclophosphamide, vincristine (Oncovin), methotrexate, calcium leucovorin, and cytarabine
COMP	complications
	composite
	compound
	compress
	cyclophosphamide, vincristine (Oncovin), methotrexate, and prednisone
COMT	catechol-o-methyl transferase
CON	catheter over a needle
	certificate of need
CON A	concanavalin A
conc.	concentrated
CONG	congenital
	gallon
CONPA-DRI I	cyclophosphamide, vincristine, doxorubicin, and melphalan

61

CONPA-DRI II	conpadri I plus high-dose methotrexate		Therapy Assistant
CONPA-DRI III	conpadri I plus intensified doxorubicin	COTE	comprehensive occupational therapy evaluation
cont	continuous	COTT CH	cottage cheese
	contusions	COTX	cast off to x-ray
CONTRAL	contralateral	COU	cardiac observation unit
CONTU	contusion		cataracts, both eyes
CONV	conversation	COWA	controlled oral word association
Conv. ex.	convergence excess		
CO-Ox	Co-oximetry	COWS	cold to the opposite and warm to the same
COP	change of plaster		
	cicatricial ocular pemphigoid	COX	Coxsackie virus cytochrome C oxidase
	colloid osmotic pressure	CP	centric position
	complaint of pain		cerebral palsy
	cycophosphamide, vincristine (Oncovin), and prednisone		Certified Paramedic
			chemical peel
			chemistry profiles
COP 1	copolymer 1		chest pain
COPD	chronic obstructive pulmonary disease		chloroquine-primaquine
			chondromalacia patella
COPE	chronic obstructive pulmonary emphysema		chronic pain
			chronic pancreatitis
COPP	cyclophosphamide, vincristine, procarbazine, and prednisone		cleft palate
			clinical pathway
			closing pressure
COPS	community outpatient service		convenience package
			cor pulmonale
COPT	circumoval precipitin test		creatine phosphokinase
COR	conditioned orientation response		cyclophosphamide and cisplatin (Platinol)
			cystopanendoscopy
	coronary	C_p	concentration of drug plasma
CORA	conditioned orientation reflex audiometry		
			phosphate clearance
CORE	cardiac or respiratory emergency	C&P	compensation and pension
			complete and pushing
CORT	Certified Operating Room Technician		cystoscopy and pyelography
COS	cataract, left eye	CPA	cardiopulmonary arrest
	Chief of Staff		carotid photoangiography
	clinically observed seizure		cerebellar pontine angle
C_{osm}	osmolal clearance		chest pain alert
COSTART	Coding symbols for a thesaurus of adverse reaction terms		conditioned play audiometry
			costophrenic angle
COT	content of thought		cyclophosphamide
COTA	Certified Occupational		

	cyproterone acetate	CPETU	chest pain evaluation and treatment unit
CPAF	chlorpropamide-alcohol flush	CPF	cerebral perfusion pressure
C_{PAH}	para-amino hippurate clearance	CPFT	Certified Pulmonary Function Technologist
CPAP	continuous positive airway pressure	CPG	clinical practice guidelines
CPB	cardiopulmonary bypass	CPG2	carboxypeptidase G2
	competitive protein binding	CPGN	chronic progressive glomerulonephritis
CPBA	competitive protein-binding assay	CPH	chronic persistent hepatitis
CPBP	cardiopulmonary bypass	CPhT	Certified Pharmacy Technician
CPC	cerebral palsy clinic	CPI	constitutionally psychopathia inferior
	chronic passive congestion	CPID	chronic pelvic inflammatory disease
	clinicopathologic conference	CPIP	chronic pulmonary insufficiency of prematurity
	continue plan of care	CPK	creatine phosphokinase (BB, MB, MM are isoenzymes)
CPCR	cardiopulmonary-cerebral resuscitation		
CPCS	clinical pharmacokinetics consulting service	CPK-1	creatine phosphokinase MM fraction
CPD	cephalopelvic disproportion	CPK-2	creatine phosphokinase MB fraction
	chorioretinopathy and pituitary dysfunction	CPK-BB	creatine phosphokinase BB fraction
	chronic peritoneal dialysis	CPKD	childhood polycystic kidney disease
	citrate-phosphate-dextrose	CPK-MB	creatine phosphokinase of muscle band
CPDA-1	citrate-phosphate-dextrose-adenine	CPL	criminal procedure law
CPDD	calcium pyrophosphate deposition disease	CPM	central pontine myelinolysis
CPE	cardiogenic pulmonary edema		chlorpheniramine maleate
	chronic pulmonary emphysema		Clinical Practice Model
	Clinical Pastoral Education		continue present management
	clubbing, pitting, or edema		continuous passive motion
	complete physical examination		counts per minute
CPE-C	cyclopentenylcytosine		cycles per minute
CPER	chest pain emergency room		cyclophosphamide
CPET	cardiopulmonary exercise testing	CPmax	peak serum concentration
		CPMDI	computerized

63

	pharmacokinetic model-driven drug infusion		Chinese paralytic syndrome
CPmin	trough serum concentration		chloroquine-pyrimethamine sulfadoxine
CPMM	constant passive motion machine		clinical performance score
CPN	chronic pyelonephritis		clinical pharmacokinetic service
CPO	continue present orders		coagulase-positive staphylococci
CPP	central precocious puberty		complex partial seizures
	cerebral perfusion pressure		cumulative probability of success
	chronic pelvic pain	CPs	clinical pathways
	cryo-poor plasma	CPS I	carbamyl phosphate synthetase I
CPPB	continuous positive pressure breathing	CPSC	Consumer Product Safety Commission
CPPD	calcium pyrophosphate dihydrate	CPT	camptothecin
	cisplatin		carnitine palmitoyl transferase
CP & PD	chest percussion and postural drainage		chest physiotherapy
			child protection team
CPPV	continuous positive pressure ventilation		chromo-perturbation
			cold pressor test
CPQ	Conner's Parent Questionnaire		Continuous Performance Test
CPR	cardiopulmonary resuscitation		current perception threshold
	computer-based patient records		Current Procedural Terminology (coding system)
	computerized patient record	CPT-11	irinotecan hydrochloride
	tablet (French)	CPTA	Certified Physical Therapy Assistant
CPR-1	all measures except cardiopulmonary resuscitation	CPT/C	current perception threshold, computerized
CPR-2	no extraordinary measures (to resuscitate)	CPTH	chronic post-traumatic headache
CPR-3	comfort measures only	CPUE	chest pain of unknown etiology
CPRAM	controlled partial rebreathing anesthesia method	CPX	complete physical examination
CP/ROMI	chest pain, rule out myocardial infarction	CPZ	chlorpromazine
			Compazine® (CPZ is a dangerous abbreviation as it could be either)
CPRS-OCS	Comprehensive Psychiatric Rating Scale, Obsessive-Compulsive Subscale		
CPS	cardiopulmonary support	CQI	continuous quality improvement
	chest pain syndrome		
	child protective services		

CR	cardiac rehabilitation	CRBP	cellular retinol-binding
	cardiorespiratory		protein
	case reports	CRC	case review committee
	chief resident		Clinical Research
	chorioretinal		Coordinator
	clockwise rotation		child-resistant container
	closed reduction		clinical research center
	colon resection		colorectal cancer
	complete remission	CR & C	closed reduction and cast
	contact record	CrCl	creatinine clearance
	controlled release	CRD	childhood rheumatic
	cosmetic rhinoplasty		disease
	creamed		chronic renal disease
	cycloplegia retinoscopy		chronic respiratory
Cr	chromium		disease
C & R	convalescence and		cone-rod dystrophy
	rehabilitation		congenital rubella
	cystoscopy and retrograde		deafness
CR_1	first cranial nerve		crown-rump distance
CRA	central retinal artery	CREAT	serum creatinine
	chronic rheumatoid	CREP	crepitation
	arthritis	CREST	calcinosis, Raynaud's
	cis-retinoic acid		disease, esophageal
	(isotretinion,		dysmotility,
	Accutane®)		sclerodactyly, and
	Clinical Research		telangiectasia
	Associate	CRF	cardiac risk factors
	colorectal anastomosis		case report form
	corticosteroid-resistant		chronic renal failure
	asthma		corticotropin-releasing
CRABP	cellular retinoic acid		factor
	binding protein	CRFZ	closed reduction of
CRAbs	chelating recombinant		fractured zygoma
	antibodies	CRI	Cardiac Risk Index
CRADA	Cooperative Research and		catheter-related infection
	Development Agree-		chronic renal insufficiency
	ment (with NIH)	CRIB	Clinical Risk Index for
CRAG	cerebral radionuclide		Babies
	angiography	CRIE	crossed radioimmuno-
CrAg	cryptococcal antigen		electrophoresis
CRAMS	circulation, respiration,	CRIF	closed reduction and
	abdomen, motor, and		internal fixation
	speech	CRIMF	closed reduction/
CRAN	craniotomy		intermaxillary fixation
CRAO	central retinal artery	CRIS	controlled-release infusion
	occlusion		system
CRAX	crackers	crit	hematocrit
CRBBB	complete right bundle	CRL	crown rump length
	branch block	CRM	cream

	cross-reacting mutant		capillary refill time
CRM +	cross-reacting material positive		cathode ray tube
			central reaction time
CRMD	children with retarded mental development		Certified Rehabilitation Therapist
CRN	crown		copper reduction test
CRNA	Certified Registered Nurse Anesthetist		cranial radiation therapy
		Cr Tr	crutch training
CRNI	Certified Registered Nurse Intravenous	CRTT	Certified Respiratory Therapy Technician
CRNP	Certified Registered Nurse Practitioner	CRTX	cast removed take x-ray
CRO	cathode ray oscilloscope	CRU	cardiac rehabilitation unit
	contract research organization(s)		clinical research unit
CROM	cervical range of motion	CRV	central retinal vein
CROS	contralateral routing of signals	CRVF	congestive right ventricular failure
CRP	chronic relapsing pancreatitis	CRVO	central retinal vein occlusion
	coronary rehabilitation program	CIIRx	Century II Bicarbonate Dialysis Machine
	C-reactive protein	CRYO	cryoablation
C&RP	curettage and root planning		cryosurgery
CRPA	C-reactive protein agglutinins	CRYST	crystals
		CS	cardioplegia solution
CRPD	chronic restrictive pulmonary disease		cat scratch
			cervical spine
CRPF	chloroquine-resistant *Plasmodium falciparum*		cesarean section
			chest strap
CRQ	Chronic Respiratory (Disease) Questionnaire		cholesterol stone
			cigarette smoker
CRR	community rehabilitation residence		clinical stage
			close supervision
CRS	Carroll Self-Rating Scale		conditionally susceptible
	catheter-related sepsis		congenital syphilis
	Chinese restaurant syndrome		conjunctiva-sclera
	colon-rectal surgery		consciousness
	congenital rubella syndrome		conscious sedation
			consultation
	cryoreductive surgery		consultation service
	cytokine-release syndrome		coronary sinus
CRST	calcification, Raynaud's phenomenom, scleroderma, and telangiectasia		corticosteroid(s)
			Cushing's syndrome
			cycloserine
		C&S	conjunctiva and sclera
			cough and sneeze
			culture and sensitivity
CRT	cadaver renal transplant	C/S	cesarean section
			culture and sensitivity

CSA	compressed spectral activity	CSICU	cardiac surgery intensive care unit
	controlled substance analogue	CSII	continuous subcutaneous insulin infusion
	corticosteroid-sensitive asthma	CS IV	clinical stage 4
CsA	cyclosporin	CSLU	chronic status leg ulcer
CSB	caffeine sodium benzoate	CSM	carotid sinus massage
	Cheyne-Stokes breathing		cerebrospinal meningitis
	Children's Services Board		cervical spondylotic myelopathy
CSB I & II	Chemistry Screening Batteries I and II		circulation, sensation, and movement
CSBF	coronary sinus blood flow		Committee on Safety of Medicines (United Kingdom)
CSBO	complete small bowel obstruction	CSME	cotton spot macular edema
CSC	cornea, sclera, and conjunctiva	CSMN	chronic sensorimotor neuropathy
	cryopreserved stem cells	CSN	cystic suppurative necrosis
CSCI	continuous subcutaneous infusion	CSNRT	corrected sinus node recovery time
CSCR	central serous chorioretinopathy	CSNS	carotid sinus nerve stimulation
CSD	cat scratch disease	CSO	Consumer Safety Officer (FDA)
	celiac sprue disease		copied standing orders
C S&D	cleaned, sutured, and dressed	CSOM	chronic serous otitis media
CSDD	Center for the Study of Drug Development		chronic suppurative otitis media
CSE	combined spinal/epidurals	CSP	cellulose sodium phosphate
	cross-section echocardiography		chiral stationary phase
C sect.	cesarean section	C-spine	cervical spine
CSF	cerebrospinal fluid	CSR	central supply room
	colony-stimulating factors		Cheyne-Strokes respiration
CSFELP	cerebrospinal fluid electrophoresis		corrective septorhinoplasty
CSFP	cerebrospinal fluid pressure	C-S RT	cranio-spinal radiotherapy
CSGIT	continuous-suture graft-inclusion technique	CSS	carotid sinus stimulation
C-Sh	chair shower		Central Sterile Services
CSH	carotid sinus hypersensitivity		chemical sensitivity syndrome
	chronic subdural hematoma		chewing, sucking, and swallowing
CSI	Computerized Severity Index	C_{ss}	concentration of drug at steady-state
	continuous subcutaneous infusion		

CSSD	closed system sterile drainage	CTAP	clear to auscultation and percussion
CST	cardiac stress test		computed tomography during arterial portography
	castration		
	central sensory conducting time	CTB	ceased to breathe
	cerebroside sulfotransferase		cholera toxin B
		CTC	Cancer Treatment Center
	Certified Surgical Technologist		circular tear capsulotomy
	contraction stress test		clinical trial certificate (United Kingdom's equivalent to the Investigational New Drug Application)
	convulsive shock therapy		
	cosyntropin stimulation test		
	static compliance		
C_{STAT}	static lung compliance	CTCL	cutaneous T-cell lymphoma (mycosis fungoides)
CSU	cardiac surgery unit		
	cardiac surveillance unit	CT & DB	cough, turn & deep breath
	cardiovascular surgery unit	CTD	carpal tunnel decompression
	casualty staging unit		chest tube drainage
	catheter specimen of urine		connective tissue disease
CSW	Clinical Social Worker		corneal thickness depth
CT	calcitonin		cumulative trauma disorder
	cardiothoracic		
	carpal tunnel	CTDW	continues to do well
	cellulose triacetate (filter)	CTF	Colorado tick fever
	cervical traction		continuous tube feeding
	chemotherapy	C/TG	cholesterol to triglyceride ratio
	chest tube		
	circulation time	CTGA	complete transposition of the great arteries
	clinical trial		
	clotting time		corrected transposition of the great arteries
	coagulation time		
	coated tablet	CTH	clot to hold
	compressed tablet	CTI	certification of terminal illness
	computed tomography		
	Coomb's test	CTICU	cardiothoracic intensive care unit
	corneal thickness		
	corneal transplant	CTL	cervical, thoracic, and lumbar
	corrective therapy		
	cytarabine and thioguanine		chronic tonsillitis
			cytotoxic T-lymphocytes
	cytoxic drug	CTM	Chlor-Trimeton®
C_t	concentration of drug in tissue		clinical trials materials
		CT/MPR	computed tomography with multiplanar reconstructions
CTA	catamenia (menses)		
	clear to auscultation		
C-TAB	cyanide tablet	CTN	calcitonin

C & T N, BLE	color and temperature normal, both lower extremities	CUPS	carcinoma of unknown primary site
cTNM	clinical-diagnostic staging of cancer	CUR	curettage cystourethrorectocele
CTP	comprehensive treatment plan	CUS	chronic undifferentiated schizophrenia
CTPN	central total parenteral nutrition		contact urticaria syndrome
CTR	carpal tunnel release carpal tunnel repair	CUSA	Cavitron ultrasonic suction aspirator
CTRS	Certified Therapeutic Recreation Specialist Conners Teachers Rating Scale	CUT	chronic undifferentiated type (schizophrenia)
		CV	cardiovascular cell volume
CT-RT	chemo-radiotherapy		cisplatin and etoposide
CTS	cardiothoracic surgeon carpal tunnel syndrome		coefficient of variation color vision
CTSP	called to see patient		common ventricle
CTW	central terminal of Wilson		consonant vowel
CTX	cerebrotendinous xanthomatosis		contrast venography *curriculum vitae*
	chemotherapy	C/V	cervical/vaginal
	cyclophosphamide (Cytoxan®)	CVA	cerebrovascular accident costovertebral angle
CTXN	contraction	CVAD	central venous access device
CTZ	chemoreceptor trigger zone	CVAH	congenital virilizing adrenal hyperplasia
	co-trimoxazole (sulfamethoxazole and trimethoprin)	CVAT	costovertebral angle tenderness
CU	cause undetermined	CVB	group B coxsackievirus
	cause unknown chronic undifferentiated color unit	CVC	central venous catheter chief visual complaint consonant vowel consonant
	convalescent unit Cuprophan (filter)	CVD	cardiovascular disease collagen vascular disease
Cu	copper		
CUA	clean urinalysis	CVEB	cisplatin, vinblastine, etoposide, and bleomycin
CUC	chronic ulcerative colitis Clinical Unit Clerk		
CUD	cause undetermined controlled unsterile delivery	CVF	cardiovascular failure central visual field cervicovaginal fluid
		CVG	coronary vein graft
CUFCM	Century Ultrafiltration Control Machine	CVHD	chronic valvular heart disease
CUG	cystourethrogram	CVI	carboplatin, etoposide, ifosfamide, and mesna uroprotection
CUP	carcinoma of unknown primary (site)		

	cerebrovascular insufficiency	CVSCU	cardiovascular special care unit
	common variable immunodeficiency (disease)	CVSU	cardiovascular specialty unit
	continuous venous infusion	CVTC	central venous tunneled catheter
CVICU	cardiovascular intensive care unit	CVU	clean voided urine
CVID	common variable immune deficiency	CVUG	cysto-void urethrogram
CVINT	cardiovascular intermediate	CVVH	continuous venovenous hemofiltration
CVL	central venous line	CW	careful watch
	clinical vascular laboratory		case worker
CVM	Center for Veterinary Medicine		chest wall
			clockwise
CVMT	cervical-vaginal, motion tenderness		compare with
CVN	central venous nutrient	C/W	consistent with
CVNSR	cardiovascular normal sinus rhythm		crutch walking
CVO	central vein occlusion	CWAF	Chemical Withdrawal Assessment Flowsheet
	conjugate diameter of pelvic inlet	CWAP	continuous wave arthroscopy pump
CvO₂	mixed venous oxygen content	CWD	cell wall defective
CVOR	cardiovascular operating room	CWE	cotton wool exudates
		CWL	Caldwell-Luc
CVP	central venous pressure	CWMS	color, warmth, movement, and sensation
	cyclophosphamide, vincristine, and prednisone	CWP	centimeters of water pressure
CVPP	lomustine, vinblastine, procarbazine, and prednisone		childbirth without pain
			coal worker's pneumoconiosis
CVR	cerebral vascular resistance		cold wet packs
		CWR	clockwise rotation
	cerebrovascular resuscitation	CWS	comfortable walking speed
CVRI	coronary vascular resistance index		cotton wool spots
CVS	cardiovascular surgery	CWT	compensated work training
	cardiovascular system	CWV	closed wound vacuum
	challenge virus standard	CX	cancel
	chorionic villi sampling		cervix
	clean voided specimen		chronic
	continuing vegetative state		culture
			cylinder axis
			cystectomy
		CXA	circumflex artery
		CxBx	cervical biopsy
		CxMT	cervical motion tenderness

CXR	chest x-ray		diminished
CXTX	cervical traction		diopter
CY	cyclophosphamide		distal
C&Y	Children with Youth (program)		distance
			divorced
CYA	cover your ass	$D_{0(2/7/95)}$	Day zero (the day treatment begins, February 7th, 1995)
CyA	cyclosporine		
CyADIC	cyclophosphamide, doxorubicin (Adriamycin), and dacarbazine	D_1	day one (first day of treatment)
		D-1 to D-12	dorsal vertebrae 1 to 12
Cyclo C	cyclocytidine HCl		dorsal nerves 1-12
CYL	cylinder	D_1	first diagonal branch (coronary artery)
CYP	cytochrome P-450		
CYRO	cryoprecipitate	D_2	second diagonal branch (coronary artery)
CYSTA	cystathionine		
CYSTO	cystogram		ergocalciferol
	cystoscopy	2/d	twice a day (this is a dangerous abbreviation)
CYT	cyclophosphamide		
CYVA DIC	cyclophosphamide, vincristine, Adriamycin®, and dacarbazine	2-D	two-dimensional
		3-D	three-dimensional
		D_3	cholecalciferol
		D-3+7	cytarabine and daunorubicin
CZE	capillary zone electrophoresis	4D	4 prism diopters
		5xD	five times a day (this is a dangerous abbreviation)
CZI	crystalline zinc insulin (regular insulin)		
		D50	50% dextrose injection
CZN	chlorzotocin	$D_{5/.45}$	dextrose 5% in 0.45% sodium chloride injection
CZP	clonazepam		
		DA	Debtors Anonymous
			degenerative arthritis
			delivery awareness
			Dental Assistant
	D		diagnostic arthroscopy
			direct admission
			direct agglutination
			diversional activity
			dopamine
D	daughter		drug addict
	day		drug aerosol
	dead	D/A	discharge and advise
	decay	DAA	dead after arrival
	depression		dissection aortic aneurysm
	dextrose	DA/A	drug/alcohol addiction
	dextro	DAB	days after birth
	diarrhea		diamino benzidine
	diastole	DAC	day activity center
	dilated		

71

	disabled adult child		drug abuse reporting program
	Division of Ambulatory Care	DAS	day of admission surgery
DACL	Depression Adjective Checklists		developmental apraxia of speech
DACT	dactinomycin		died at scene
DAD	diffuse alveolar damage	DASE	dobutamine-atropine stress echocardiography
	diode array detector	DAT	daunorubicin, cytarabine, (ara-C), and thioguanine
	dispense as directed		
	drug administration device		definitely abnormal tracing (electrocardiogram)
	father		dementia of the Alzheimer type
DAE	diving air embolism		
DAF	decay-accelerating factor		diet as tolerated
	delayed auditory feedback		diphtheria antitoxin
DAFE	Dial-A-Flow Extension®		direct agglutination test
DAFM	double aerosol face mask		direct antiglobulin test
DAG	diacylglyerol	DAU	daughter
	dianhydrogalactitol		drug abuse urine
DAH	diffuse alveolar hemorrhage	DAUNO	daunorubicin
		DAVA	vindesine sulfate
	disordered action of the heart	DAW	dispense as written
DAI	diffuse axonal injury	DAWN	Drug Abuse Warning Network
DAL	drug analysis laboratory	dB	decibel
DALM	dysplasia-associated lesion or mass	DB	date of birth
			deep breathe
DALY	disability-adjusted life year(s)		demonstration bath
			dermabrasion
DAM	diacetylmonoxime		diaphragmatic breathing
DAMA	discharged against medical advice		direct bilirubin
			double blind
DANA	drug induced antinuclear antibodies	DB & C	deep breathing and coughing
DAo	descending aorta	DBD	milolactol (dibromodulicitol)
DAP	dapsone		
	Draw-A-Person	DBE	deep breathing exercise
	diabetes-associated peptide	DBED	penicillin G benzathine
		dBEMCL	decibel effective masking contralateral
	diastolic augmentation pressure		
		D_5BES	dextrose in balanced electrolyte solution
	distending airway pressure		
		DBI®	phenformin HCl
DAPT	Draw-A-Person Test	DBIL	direct bilirubin
DAR	daily affective rhythm	DBL	double beta-lactam
DARE	data, action, response, and evaluation	DBMT	displacement bone marrow transplantation
DARP	drug abuse rehabilitation program		

DBP	D-binding protein
	diastolic blood pressure
	di-n-butyl phthalate
DBPCFC	double-blind, placebo-controlled food challenge
DBPT	dacarbazine (DTIC), carmustine (BCNU), cisplatin (Platinol), and tamoxifen
DBQ	debrisoquin
DBS	diminished breath sounds
DBW	dry body weight
DBZ	dibenzamine
DC	daunorubicin and cytarabine
	decrease
	dextrocardia
	diagonal conjugate
	direct Coombs (test)
	discharge
	Doctor of Chiropractic
D&C	dilation and curettage
	direct and consensual
d/c	discontinue
DC65®	Darvon Compound 65®
DCA	directional coronary atherectomy
	disk/condyle adhesion
	double cup arthroplasty
	sodium dichloroacetate
DCAG	double coronary artery graft
DC&B	dilation, currettage, and biopsy
DCBE	double contrast barium enema
DCC	day care center
DCCF	dural carotid-cavernous fistula
DCCT	Diabetes Control and Complications Trial (questionnaire)
DC'd	discontinued
DCE	delayed contrast-enhancement
	designated compensable event
DCF	data collection form
	2'-deoxycoformycin
	dichlorofluorescein
	pentostatin (deoxycoformycin)
DCFS	Department of Children and Family Services
DCH	delayed cutaneous hypersensitivity
DCIA	deep circumflex iliac artery (flap)
DCIS	ductal carcinoma *in situ*
DCLH®	diaspirin cross-linked hemoglobin
DCM	dilated cardiomyopathy
DCMXT	dichloromethotrexate
DCN	Darvocet N®
DCNU	chlorozotocin
DCO	diffusing capacity of carbon monoxide
DCP	dynamic compression plate
DCP®	calcium phosphate, dibasic
DCPM	daunorubicin, cytarabine, prednisolone, and mercaptopurine
DCPN	direction-changing positional nystagmus
DCR	dacryocystorhinostomy
	delayed cutaneous reaction
DCRF	data case report forms
DCS	decompression sickness
	dorsal column stimulator
DCSA	double contrast shoulder arthrography
DCT	daunorubicin, cytarabine, and thioguanine
	deep chest therapy
	direct (antiglobulin) Coombs test
DCTM	delay computer tomographic myelography
DCU	day care unit
DCUS	duplex color ultrasonography
DCW	direct care worker
DCYS	Department of Children and Youth Services

DD	delivery date	DDST	Denver Development
	dependent drainage		Screening Test
	Descemet's detachment	DDT	chlorophenothane
	detrusor dyssynergia	DDTP	drug dependence
	developmentally delayed		treatment program
	dialysis dementia	DDx	differential diagnosis
	died of the disease	DE	digitalis effect
	differential diagnosis	D_5E_{48}	5% Dextrose and
	discharge diagnosis		Electrolyte 48
	disk diameter	D_5E_{75}	5% Dextrose and
	Doctor of Divinity		Electrolyte 75
	down drain	2DE	two-dimensional
	dry dressing		echocardiography
	dual disorder	D&E	dilation and evacuation
	Duchenne's dystrophy	DEA#	Drug Enforcement
D/D	diarrhea/dehydration		Administration number
D→D	discharge to duty		(physician's Federal
D & D	debridement and dressing		narcotic number)
	diarrhea and dehydration	DEAE	diethylaminoethyl
	drilling and drainage	DEB	dystrophic epidermolysis
DDA	dideoxyadenosine		bullosa
DDAVP®	desmopressin acetate	DEC	deciduous (primary teeth)
DDC	zalcitabine (dideoxy-		decrease
	cytidine; Hivid)		diethylcarbamazine
DDD	defined daily doses	DECA	nandrolone decanoate
	degenerative disk disease	DECAFS	Department of Children
	dense deposit disease		and Family Services
	fully automatic pacing	DECEL	deceleration
DDDR	rate-adaptive DDD	decub	decubitus
	pacemaker device	DED	died in emergency
DDE	dichlorodiphenylethylene		department
DDGB	double-dose gallbladder	DEEDS	drugs, exercise, education,
	(test)		diet, and self-monitoring
DDHT	double dissociated	DEEG	deteriorating
	hypertropia		electroencephalogram
DDI	didanosine	DEET	diethyltoluamide
	(dideoxyinosine)	DEF	decayed, extracted, or
DDIs	drug-drug interactions		filled
DDNS	digestive disease and		defecation
	nutrition service		deficiency
DDP	cisplatin	DEFT	defendant
DDRA	dead despite resuscitation	DEG	diethylene glycol
	attempt	degen	degenerative
DDS	dialysis disequilibrium	DEL	delivery
	syndrome		delivered
	Doctor of Dental Surgery		deltoid
	double decidual sac (sign)	DEM	drug evaluation matrix
	4, 4-diaminodiphenyl-	DEP ST	depressed ST segment
	sulfone (dapsone)	SEG	

DER	disulfiram-ethanol reaction		distal femoral epiphysis
		DFG	direct forward gaze
DERM	dermatology	DFI	disease-free interval
DES	desflurane	DFM	decreased fetal movement
	diethylstilbestrol		deep finger massage
	diffuse esophageal spasm		deep friction massage
	disequilibrium syndrome	DFMC	daily fetal movement count
	dry eye syndrome		
DESAT	desaturation	DFMO	eflornithine (difluoro-methylorithine)
DESI	Drug Efficacy Study Implementation (Project)		
		DFMR	daily fetal movement record
DET	diethyltryptamine	DFO	deferoxamine
	dipyridamole echocardiography test	DFOM	deferoxamine
		DFP	diastolic filling period
DETOX	detoxification		isoflurophate (diisopropyl flurophosphate)
DEV	deviation		
	duck embryo vaccine	DFR	diabetic floor routine
DEVR	dominant exudative vitreoretinopathy	DFRC	deglycerolized frozen red cells
DEX	dexamethasone	DFS	disease-free survival
	dexter (right)		Division of Family Services
	dexverapamil		
DEXA	dual-energy x-ray absorptiometry		Doppler flow studies
		DFU	dead fetus in uterus
DF	day frequency (of voiding)	DFV	diarrhea, fever, and vomiting
	decayed and filled	DFW	Dexide face wash
	deferred	DG	diagnosis
	defibrotide		dorsal glides
	degree of freedom		downward gaze
	dengue fever	DGE	delayed gastric emptying
	dexfenfluramine	DGGE	denaturing gradient gel electrophoresis
	diabetic father		
	diastolic filling	DGI	disseminated gonococcal infection
	dorsiflexion		
	drug free	DGR	duodenogastric reflux
	dye free	DGM	ductal glandular mastectomy
DFA	delayed feedback audiometry		
		DH	delayed hypersensitivity
	diet for age		Dental Hygienist
	difficulty falling asleep		dermatitis herpetiformis
	direct fluorescent antibody		developmental history
			diaphragmatic hernia
	distal forearm	D+H	delusions and hallucinations
DFD	defined formula diets		
	degenerative facet disease	DHA	dihydroxyacetone
DFE	dilated fundus examination		docosahexaenoic acid

DHAC	dihydro-5-azacytidine	
DHAD	mitoxantrone HCl	
DHBV	duck hepatitis B virus	
DHCA	deep hypothermia circulatory arrest	
DHCC	dihydroxycholecalciferol	
DHD	dissociated horizontal deviation	
DHE 45®	dihydroergotamine mesylate	
DHEA	dehydroepiandrosterone	
DHEAS	dehydroepiandrosterone sulfate	
DHF	dengue hemorrhagic fever	
DHFR	dihydrofolate reductase	
DHHS	Department of Health and Human Services	
DHI	dynamic hyperinflation	
DHIC	detrusor hyperactivity with impaired contractility	
DHL	diffuse histocytic lymphoma	
DHP-1	dehydropeptidase-1	
DHPG	ganciclovir	
DHPR	erythrocyte dihydropteridine reductase	
DHR	delayed hypersensitivity reaction	
DHS	Department of Human Services	
	duration of hospital stay	
	dynamic hip screw	
DHST	delayed hypersensitivity test	
DHT	dihydrotachysterol	
	dihydrotestosterone	
	dissociated hypertropia	
	Dobhoff tube	
DHTF	Dobhoff tube feeding	
DI	(Beck) Depression Inventory	
	date of injury	
	Debrix Index	
	detrusor instability	
	diabetes insipidus	

	diagnostic imaging	
	dorsal interossei	
	drug interactions	
D&I	debridement and irrigation	
	dry and intact	
DIA	drug-induced agranulocytosis	
diag.	diagnosis	
DIAP-PERS	(causes of transient incontinence) delirium/confusion, infection, (urinary), atrophic urethritis/vaginitis, pharmaceuticals, psychological, excessive excretion (e.g., CHF, hyperglycemia) restricted mobility, and stool impaction	
DIAS	diastolic	
DIAS BP	diastolic blood pressure	
Diath SW	diathermy short wave	
DIAZ	diazepam	
DIB	disability insurance benefits	
DIBC	drug-induced blood cytopenias	
DIC	dacarbazine	
	differential interference contrast	
	disseminated intravascular coagulation	
	drug information center	
DICC	dynamic infusion cavernosometry and cavernosography	
DICLOX	dicloxacillin	
DICP	demyelinated inflammatory chronic polyneuropathy	
DICT	dose-intensive chemotherapy	
DID	delayed ischemia deficit	
	drug-induced disease	
di,di	dichorionic, diamniotic	
DIE	died in emergency department	
DIED	died in emergency	

	department	DIR	directions
DIF	differentiation-inducing factor	DIRD	drug-induced renal disease
DIFF	differential blood count	DIS	Diagnostic Interview Schedule (questionnaire)
DIG	digoxin (this is a dangerous abbreviation)		digital imaging spectrophotometer
DIH	died in hospital		dislocation
DIJOA	dominantly inherited juvenile optic atrophy	disch.	discharge
DIL	daughter-in-law	DISCUS	Dyskinesia Indentification System Condensed User Scale
	dilute		
	drug-induced lupus	DISH	diffuse idiopathic skeletal hyperostosis
DILC	dose-intensity limiting criterium	DISI	dorsal intercalated segmental (segment) instability
DILD	diffuse infiltrative lung disease		
	drug-induced liver disease	DISIDA	diisopropyl imino diacetic acid
DILE	drug induced lupus erythematosus	D_5ISOM	5% Dextrose and Isolyte M
DIM	diminish	D_5ISOP	5% Dextrose and Isolyte P
D_5IMB	Ionosol MB with 5% dextrose injection		
		DISR	drug-induced skin reactions
DIMD	drug induced movement disorders	DIST	distal
			distilled
DIMOAD	diabetes insipidus, diabetes mellitus, optic atrophy, and deafness	DIT	diiodotyrosine
			drug-induced thrombocytopenia
DIMS	disorders of initiating and maintaining sleep	DIU	death in utero
DIND	delayed ischemic neurologic deficit	DIV	double inlet ventricle
		DIVA	digital intravenous angiography
DIOS	distal ileal obstruction syndrome	Div ex	divergence excess
	distal intestinal obstruction syndrome	DJD	degenerative joint disease
		DK	dark
DIP	desquamative interstitial pneumonia		diabetic ketoacidosis
			diseased kidney
	diplopia	DKA	diabetic ketoacidosis
	distal interphalangeal		didn't keep appointment
	drip infusion pyelogram	DKB	deep knee bends
	drug-induced parkinsonism	DKC	double knee to chest
		dl	deciliter (100 mL)
DIPC	dynamic infusion pharmacocavemosometry	DL	danger list
			deciliter
DIPJ	distal interphalangeal joint		diagnostic laparoscopy
			direct laryngoscopy

	drug level	DMAS	Drug Management and
D_L	maximal diffusing		Authorization Section
	capacity	DMAT	disaster medical
DLB	direct laryngoscopy and		assistance team
	bronchoscopy	DMBA	dimethylbenzanthracene
DLC	double lumen catheter	DMC	dactinomycin,
DLCO sb	diffusion capacity of		methotrexate, and
	carbon monoxide,		cyclophosphamide
	single breath		diabetes management
DLD	date of last drink		center
DLE	discoid lupus	DMD	disciform macular
	erythematosus		degeneration
	disseminated lupus		Doctor of Dental
	erythematosis		Medicine
DLF	digitalis-like factor		Duchenne's muscular
DLIF	digoxin-like		dystrophy
	immunoreactive factors	DMD w/	disciform macular
DLIS	digoxin-like	SRNM	degeneration with
	immunoreactive		subretinal neovascular
	substance		membrane
DLMP	date of last menstrual	DME	durable medical
	period		equipment
DLNG	dl-norgestrel	DMF	decayed, missing, or filled
DLNMP	date of last normal		Drug Master File
	menstrual period	DMFS	decayed, missing, or filled
DLP	dislocation of patella		surfaces
DLPD	diffuse lymphocytic	DMI	desipramine
	poorly differentiated		diaphragmatic myocardial
D5LR	dextrose 5% in lactated		infarction
	Ringer's injection	DM Isch	diaphragmatic myocardial
DLS	daily living skills		ischemia
	digitalis-like substances	DMKA	diabetes mellitus
DLSC	double lumen subclavian		ketoacidosis
	catheter	DMO	dimethadone
DLT	dose-limiting toxicity	DMOOC	diabetes mellitus out of
	double-lung transplant		control
DLU	diffused lung uptake	DMP	dimethyl phthalate
DLV	delavirdine (Rescriptor)	DMPA	depot-medroxypro-
DM	dehydrated and		gesterone acetate
	malnourished	D-MRI	dynamic magnetic
	dermatomyositis		resonance imaging
	dextromethorphan	DMS	dimethylsulfide
	diabetes mellitus	DMSA	succimer
	diabetic mother		(dimercaptosuccinic
	diastolic murmur		acid)
DMAD	disease-modifying	DMSO	dimethyl sulfoxide
	antirheumatic drug	DMT	dimethyltryptamine
DMARD	disease modifying	DMV	Doctor of Veterinary
	antirheumatic drug		Medicine

DMVP	disk, macula, vessel, periphery		saline (0.9% sodium chloride) injection
DMX	diathermy, massage, and exercise	DNT	did not test
		DO	diet order
DN	diabetic nephropathy		distocclusal
	dicrotic notch		Doctor of Osteopathy
	down		doctor's order
	dysplastic nevus	D/O	disorder
D & N	distance and near (vision)	✓DO	check doctor's order
D5NS	dextrose 5% in 0.9% sodium chloride injection	DO₂	oxygen delivery
		DOA	date of admission
			dead on arrival
D₅ 1/2NS	dextrose 5% in 0.45% sodium chloride injection		driver of automobile
			duration of action
		DOA-DRA	dead on arrival despite resuscitative attempts
DNA	deoxyribonucleic acid		
	did not answer	DOB	dangle out of bed
	did not attend		date of birth
	does not apply		dobutamine
DNCB	dinitrochlorobenzene		doctor's order book
DNC	did not come	DOC	date of conception
DND	died a natural death		diabetes out of control
DNEPTE	did not exist prior to enlistment		died of other causes
			diet of choice
DNFC	does not follow commands		drug of choice
		DOCA	desoxycorticosterone acetate
DNI	do not intubate		
DNIC	diffuse noxious inhibitory control	DOCP	desoxycorticosterone pivalate
		DOD	date of death
DNIF	duties not including flying		dead of disease
DNKA	did not keep appointment		Department of Defense
DNN	did not nurse	DODD	demand oxygen delivery device
DNP	did not pay		
	dinitrophenylhydrazine	DOE	dyspnea on exertion
	do not publish	DOES	disorders of excessive somnolence
DNR	daunorubicin		
	did not respond	DOH	Department of Health
	do not report	DOI	date of implant (pacemaker)
	do not resuscitate		
	dorsal nerve root		date of injury
DNS	deviated nasal septum	DO₂I	oxygen delivery index
	doctor did not see patient	DOJ	Department of Justice
	do not show	DOL	days of life
	dysplastic nevus syndrome	DOL #2	second day of life
		DOLV	double outlet left ventricle
D₅ 1/4 NS	dextrose 5% in 1/4 normal saline (0.225% sodium chloride) injection	DOM	Doctor of Oriental Medicine
			domiciliary
D₅NS	5% dextrose in normal		

	domiciliary care	DPDL	diffuse poorly differentiated lymphocytic lymphoma
DON	Director of Nursing		
DOOC	diabetes out of control		
DOP	dopamine	2,3-DPG	2,3-diphosphoglyceric acid
DOPS	diffuse obstructive pulmonary syndrome		
	dihydroxyphenylserine	DPH	Department of Public Health
	Director of Pharmacy Service(s)		diphenhydramine
DOR	date of release		Doctor of Public Health
DORV	double-outlet right ventricle		phenytoin (diphenylhydantoin)
DORx	date of treatment	DPI	dietary protein intake
DOS	date of surgery		dry powder inhaler
	doctor's order sheet	DPIL	dextrose (percentage), protein (grams per kilogram) Intralipid® (grams per kilogram)
DOSA	day of surgery admission		
DOSS	docusate sodium (dioctyl sodium sulfosuccinate)		
		DPL	diagnostic peritoneal lavage
DOT	date of transcription		
	date of transfer	D5PLM	dextrose 5% and Plasmalyte M® injection
	died on table		
	directly observed therapy		
	Doppler ophthalmic test	DPM	distintegrations per minute (dpm)
DOTS	directly observed treatment, short course		
			Doctor of Podiatric Medicine
DOV	distribution of ventilation		
DOX	doxepin		drops per minute
	doxorubicin	DPN	diabetic peripheral neuropathy
doz	dozen		
DP	dental prosthesis	DPP	dorsalis pedal pulse
	diastolic pressure	DPPC	colfosceril palmitate (dipalmitoylphosphati-dylcholine)
	disability pension		
	discharge planning		
	dorsalis pedis (pulse)	DPT	Demerol®, Phenergan®, and Thorazine® (this is a dangerous abbreviation)
DPA	Department of Public Assistance		
	dipropylacetic acid		
	dual photon absorptiometry		diphtheria, pertussis, and tetanus (immunization)
	durable power of attorney		Driver Performance Test
DPAP	diastolic pulmonary artery pressure	DPTPM	diphtheria, pertussis, tetanus, poliomyelitis, and measles
DPB	days postburn		
DPBS	Dulbecco's phosphate-buffered saline	DPU	delayed pressure urticaria
		DPUD	duodenal peptic ulcer disease
DPC	delayed primary closure		
	discharge planning coordinator	DPVSs	dilated perivascular spaces
	distal palmar crease	DPXA	dual-photon x-ray

80

	absorptiometry	D&S	diagnostic and surgical
D/Q	deep quiet		dilation and suction
D&Q	deep and quiet	D5S	dextrose 5% in 0.9%
Dr	doctor		sodium chloride
DR	delivery room		(saline) injection
	diabetic retinopathy	D$_5$-1/2S	5% dextrose in 0.45%
	diagnostic radiology		sodium chloride
	dining room		(saline) injection
	diurnal rhythm	DSA	digital subtraction
DRA	drug-related admissions		angiography
DRAPE	drug-related adverse		(angiocardiography)
	patient event	DSAP	disseminated superficial
DRE	digital rectal examination		actinic porokeratosis
DRESS	depth resolved surface	DSB	drug-seeking behavior
	coil spectroscopy	DSC	Down's syndrome child
DREZ	dorsal root entry zone	DSD	discharge summary
DRG	diagnosis-related groups		dictated
DRGE	drainage		dry sterile dressing
DRI	Discharge Readiness	DSDB	direct self-destructive
	Index		behavior
	dopamine reuptake	DSF	doxorubicin, streptozocin,
	inhibitor		and fluorouracil
DRM	drug-related morbidity	DSG	desogestrel
DRN	drug-related neutropenia		dressing
DRP	drug-related problem	DSG	deoxyspergualin
DRPLA	dentatorubral-	DSHR	delayed skin
	pallidolluysian atrophy		hypersensitivity
DRR	drug regimen review		reaction
DRS	Disability Rating Scale	DSHS	Department of Social and
	Duane's retraction		Health Services
	syndrome	DSI	deep shock insulin
DRSG	dressing		Depression Status
DRSP	drug-resistant		Inventory
	Streptococcus	DSIAR	double-stapled ileoanal
	pneumoniae		reservoir
DRT	drug-related	DSM	disease state management
	thrombocytopenia		drink skim milk
DRUB	drug screen-blood	DSM III	Diagnostic & Statistical
DRUJ	distal or radial ulnar joint		Manual, 3rd Edition
DS	deep sleep	DSM-IV	Diagnostic and Statistical
	Dextrostix®		Manual of Mental
	discharge summary		Disorders, 4th Edition
	disoriented	DSO	distal-lateral subungual
	double strength		onychomycosis
	Down's syndrome	DSP	digital signal processor
	drug screen	D-SPINE	dorsal spine
D/S	5% dextrose and 0.9%	DSRF	drainage subretinal fluid
	sodium chloride	DSS	dengue shock syndrome
	(saline) injection		Disability Status Scale

	discharge summary sheet	D TIME	dream time
	disease-specific survival	DTM	deep tissue massage
	distal splenorenal shunt		dermatophyte test medium
	docusate sodium	DTO	deodorized tincture of
DSST	Digit-Symbol Substitution		opium (warning: this is
	Test		*NOT* paregoric)
DST	daylight saving time	DTOGV	dextral-transposition of
	dexamethasone		great vessels
	suppression test	DTP	distal tingling on
	digit substitution test		percussion (+Tinel's
	donor-specific (blood)		sign)
	transfusion	DTPA	pentetic acid
DSU	day stay unit		(diethylenetriaminepen-
	day surgery unit		taacetic acid)
DSUH	direct suggestion under	DTR	deep tendon reflexes
	hypnosis		Dietetic Technician
DSV	digital subtraction		Registered
	ventriculography	DTs	delirium tremens
DSWI	deep surgical wound	DTS	donor specific transfusion
	infection	DTT	diphtheria tetanus toxoid
DT	delirium tremens		dithiothreitol
	dietary thermogenesis	DTUS	diathermy, traction, and
	dietetic technician		ultrasound
	diphtheria and tetanus	DVG	double vein graft
	toxoids, pediatric	DTV	due to void
	strength	DTwP	diphtheria and tetanus
	discharge tomorrow		toxoids with whole-cell
d/t	due to		pertussis vaccine
d4T	stavudine (Zerit®)	DTX	detoxification
D/T	due to	DU	decubitus ulcer
D & T	diagnosis and treatment		developmental unit
	dictated and typed		diabetic urine
DTaP	diphtheria and tetanus		diagnosis undetermined
	toxoids with acellular		duodenal ulcer
	pertussis vaccine		duroxide uptake
DTBC	tubocurarine	DUB	Dubowitz (score)
	(D-tubocurarine)		dysfunctional uterine
DTBE	Division of Tuberculosis		bleeding
	Elimination	DUD	dihydrouracil
DTC	day treatment center		dehydrogenase
	diticarb (diethyldithio-	DUE	drug use evaluation
	carbamate)	D&UE	dilation and uterine
	tubocurarine		evacuation
	(D-tubocurarine)	DUF	Doppler ultrasonic
DTD #30	dispense 30 such doses		flowmeter
DTF	deep transverse friction	DUI	driving under the
DTH	delayed-type		influence
	hypersensitivity	DUID	driving under the
DTIC	dacarbazine		influence of drugs

82

DUII	driving under the influence of intoxicants	DVR	Division of Vocational Rehabilitation
DUIL	driving under the influence of liquor		double valve replacement
		DVSA	digital venous subtraction angiography
DUN	dialysate urea nitrogen		
DUNHL	diffuse undifferentiated non-Hodgkins lymphoma	DVT	deep vein thrombosis
		DVTS	deep venous thromboscintigram
DUO	Duotube®	DVVC	direct visualization of vocal cords
DUR	drug utilization review		
	duration	DW	daily weight
DUS	distal urethral stenosis		deionized water
	Doppler ultrasound stethoscope		detention warrant
			dextrose in water
DUSN	diffuse unilateral subacute neuroretinitis		diffusion-weighted (imaging)
			distilled water
DV	distance vision		doing well
	double vision	D/W	dextrose in water
D&V	diarrhea and vomiting		discussed with
	disks and vessels	D₅W	5% dextrose (in water) injection
DVA	Department of Veterans Affairs		
		D10W	10% dextrose (in water) injection
	distance visual acuity		
	vindesine	D20W	20% dextrose (in water) injection
DVC	direct visualization of vocal cords		
		D50W	50% dextrose (in water) injection
D V® Cream	dienestrol vaginal cream		
		D70W	70% dextrose (in water) injection
DVD	dissociated vertical deviation		
		5 DW	5% dextrose (in water) injection
	double vessel disease		
DVI	atrioventricular sequential pacing	DWDL	diffuse well differentiated lymphocytic lymphoma
	digital vascular imaging	DWI	driving while intoxicated
DVIU	direct vision internal urethrotomy		driving while impaired
		DWRT	delayed work recall test
DVM	Doctor of Veterinary Medicine	Dx	diagnosis
			disease
DVMP	disks, vessels, and macula periphery	DXA	dual energy x-ray absorptiometry
DVP	cyclophosphamide, vincristine, and prednisone	DxLS	diagnosis responsible for length of stay
		DXM	dexamethasone
DVP-Asp	daunorubicin, vincristine, prednisone, and asparaginase	DXR	delayed xenograft rejection
		DXT	deep x-ray therapy
DVPA	daunorubicin, vincristine, prednisone, and asparaginase	DXRT	deep x-ray therapy
		DXS	Dextrostix®

DY	dysprosium			excitatory amino acid
DYF	drag your feet (author's note: see you in court)	EAB		elective abortion Ethical Advisory Board
DYFS	Division of Youth and Family Services	EAC		erythema annulare centrifugum
DZ	diazepam			external auditory canal
	disease	EACA		aminocaproic acid
	dizygotic			(epsilon-aminocaproic
	dozen			acid)
DZP	diazepam	EADs		early after-depolarizations
DZT	dizygotic twins	EAE		experimental autoimmune encephalomyelitis
		EAHF		eczema, allergy, and hay fever

E

		EAL		electronic artificial larynx
		EAM		external auditory meatus
		EAP		Employment (employee) Assistance Programs
E	edema			erythrocyte acid phosphatase
	effective			etoposide, doxorubicin
	eloper			(Adriamycin), and
	enema			cisplatin (Platinol)
	engorged	EARLIES		early decelerations
	eosinophil	EAS		external anal sphincter
	esophoria for distance	EAST		external rotation, abduction stress test
	evaluation	EAT		Eating Attitudes Test
	expired			ectopic atrial tachycardia
	eye	EAU		experimental autoimmune uveitis
E'	elbow			
	esophoria for near	EB		epidermolysis bullosa
E₁	estrone			Epstein-Barr
E2	estradiol	EBA		epidermolysis bullosa acquisita
E3	estriol			
4E	4 plus edema	EBB		equal breath bilaterally
E20	Enfamil 20®	EBBS		equal bilateral breath sounds
E → A	say E,E,E, comes out as A,A,A upon auscultation of lung showing consolidation	EBC		esophageal balloon catheter
		EBCT		electron-beam computed tomography
EA	early amniocentesis			
	elbow aspiration	EBE		equal bilateral expansion
	enteral alimentation	EBEA		Epstein-Barr (virus) early antigen
	esophageal atresia			
E&A	evaluate and advise	EBF		erythroblastosis fetalis
EAA	electrothermal atomic absorption	EBL		estimated blood loss
		EBL-1		European bat lyssavirus 1
	essential amino acids	EBM		expressed breast milk

EBNA	Epstein-Barr (virus) nuclear antigen		photophoresis
		ECD	endocardial cushion defect
EBP	epidural blood patch		
EBR	external beam radiotherapy		equivalent current dipole
		ECDB	encourage to cough and deep breathe
EBRs	evidence-based recommendations		
		ECE	extracapsular extension
EBRT	external beam radiation therapy	ECEMG	evoked compound electromyography
EBS	epidermolysis bullosa	ECF	epirubicin, cisplatin, and fluorouracil
EBSB	equal breath sounds bilaterally		
			extended care facility
EBV	Epstein-Barr virus		extracellular fluid
EBVCA	Epstein-Barr viral capsid antigen	ECF-A	eosinophil chemotactic factors of anaphylaxis
EBVEA	Epstein-Barr virus, early antigen	ECG	electrocardiogram
		ECHINO	echinocyte
EBVNA	Epstein-Barr virus, nuclear antigen	ECHO	echocardiogram
			enterocytopathogenic human orphan (virus)
EC	ejection click		
	endocervical		etoposide, cyclophosphamide, doxorubicin (hydroxydaunomycin), and vincristine (Oncovin)
	enteric coated		
	Escherichia coli		
	extracellular		
	eye care		
	eyes closed		
ECA	enteric coated aspirin (tablets)	ECHO/ RV	echocardiography/ radionuclide ventriculography
	Epidemiological Catchment Area	ECI	extracorporeal irradiation
		ECIB	extracorporeal irradiation of blood
	ethacrynic acid		
	external carotid artery	ECIC	extracranial to intracranial (anastamosis)
ECASA	enteric coated aspirin (tablets)		
			external carotid and internal carotid
ECBD	exploration of common bile duct		
		EC/IC	extracranial/intracranial
ECC	edema, clubbing, and cyanosis	ECL	electrochemiluminescence
			enterochromaffin-like
	embryonal cell cancer		extend of cerebral lesion
	emergency cardiac care		extracapillary lesions
	endocervical curettage	ECM	erythema chronicum migrans
	estimated creatinine clearance		
			extracellular mass
	external cardiac compression		extracellular matrix
		ECM/ BCM	extracellular mass, body cell mass ratio
	extracorporeal circulation		
ECCE	extracapsular cataract extraction	ECMO	extracorporeal membrane oxygenation
ECCP	extracorporeal		

	(oxygenator)		of x-rays
ECN	extended care nursery	EDB	ethylene dibromide
ECochG	electrocochleography		extensor digitorum brevis
ECOG	Eastern Cooperative Oncology Group	EDC	effective dynamic compliance
ECoG	electrocochleography electrocorticogram		electrodesiccation and curettage
ECP	extracorporeal photochemotherapy		end diastolic counts
ECPD	external counterpressure device		estimated date of conception
ECR	emergency chemical restraint		estimated date of confinement
	extensor carpi radialis		extensor digitorium communis
ECRB	extensor carpi radialis brevis	EDCF	endothelium-derived constricting factor
ECRL	extensor carpi radialis longus	EDCP	eccentric dynamic compression plates
ECS	electrocerebral silence	EDD	esophageal detector device
ECT	electroconvulsive therapy		expected date of delivery
	emission computed tomography	EDENT	edentulous
	enhanced computed tomography	EDF	elongation, derotation, and flexion
ECU	electrocautery unit	EDH	epidural hematoma
	emotional care units	EDHF	endothelium-derived hyperpolarizing factor
	extensor carpi ulnaris		
ECV	external cephalic version	EDI	Eating Disorders Inventory
ECVE	extracellular volume expansion	EDITAR	extended-duration topical arthropod repellent
ECW	extracellular water	EDL	extensor digitorum longus
ED	education	ED/LD	emotionally disturbed and learning disabled
	elbow disarticulation		
	emergency department	EDLS	endogenous digitalis-like substance
	emotional disorder		
	epidural	EDM	early diastolic murmur
	erectile dysfunction		esophageal Doppler monitor
	ethynodiol diacetate		
	extensive disease	EDNO	endothelium-related nitric oxide
ED$_{50}$	median effective dose		
EDAM	edatrexate	EDP	emergency department physician
EDAP	Emergency Department Approved for Pediatrics		end diastolic pressure
EDAS	encephalodural arterio-synangiosis	EDQ	extensor digiti quinti (tendon)
EDAT	Emergency Department Alert Team	EDQV	extensor digiti quinti five
		EDR	edrophonium
EDAX	energy-dispersive analysis	EDRF	endothelium derived

	relaxing factor (nitric oxide)		extended-field (radiotherapy)
EDS	Ehlers-Danlos syndrome	EFA	essential fatty acid
	excessive daytime somnolence	EFAD	essential fatty acid deficiency
EDTA	edetic acid (ethylenedi-aminetetraacetic acid)	EFBW	estimate fetal body weight
EDU	eating disorder unit	EFD	episode free day
EDV	end-diastolic volume	EFE	endocardial fibroelastosis
	epidermal dysplastic verruciformis	EFF	effacement
EDW	estimated dry weight	EFR	effective filtration rate
EDX	edatrexate	EFS	event-free survival
EE	end to end	EFHBM	eosinophilic fibrohistiocytic lesion of bone marrow
	equine encephalitis		
	ethinyl estradiol		
	external ear	EFM	electronic fetal monitor(ing)
E & E	eyes and ears		external fetal monitoring
EEA	electroencephalic audiometry	EFMM	external fetal maternal monitor
	elemental enteral alimentation	EFMT	electric field mediated transfer
	end-to-end anastomosis	EFN	effusion
	energy expended with activity	EFW	estimated fetal weight
EEC	ectrodactyly-ectodermal dysplasia, cleft	EF/WM	ejection fraction/wall motion
Syn-		e.g.	for example
drome	syndrome	EGA	esophageal gastric (tube) airway
EEE	Eastern equine encephalomyelitis		estimated gestational age
	edema, erythema, and exudate	EGBUS	external genitalia, Bartholin, urethral, and Skene's glands
	external eye examination		
EEG	electroencephalogram	EGC	early gastric carcinoma
EEN	estimated energy needs	EGFR	epidermal growth factor receptor
EENT	eyes, ears, nose, and throat	EGD	esophagogastroduodenoscopy
EEP	end expiratory pressure	EGDT	esophagogastric devascularization and transection
EER	extended endocardial resection		
EES®	erythromycin ethylsuccinate	EGF	epidermal growth factor
		EGF-R	epidermal growth factor receptor
EET	early exercise testing		
EEV	encircling endocardial ventriculotomy	EGG	electrogastrography
		EGJ	esophagogastric junction
EF	eccentric fixation	EGL	eosinophilic granuloma of the lung
	ejection fraction		
	endurance factor	EGS	ethylene glycol succinate
	erythroblastosis fetalis	EGSs	external guide sequences

EGTA	esophageal gastric tube airway	EIDC	extreme intervertebral disk collapse
	ethyleneglycoltetracetic acid	EIEC	enteroinvasive *Escherichia coli*
EH	educationally handicapped	EIL	elective induction of labor
	enlarged heart	EIOA	excessive intake of alcohol
	essential hypertension		
	extramedullary hematopoiesis	EIP	elective interruption of pregnancy
EHB	elevate head of bed		end-inspiratory pressure
	extensor hallucis brevis		extensor indicis proprius
EHBA	extrahepatic biliary atresia	EIR	entomological inoculation rate
EHBF	extrahepatic blood flow	EIS	endoscopic injection scleropathy
EHC	enterohepatic circulation		
EHDA	etidronate sodium	EITB	enzyme-linked immunoelectrotransfer blot
EHDP	etidronate disodium		
EHE	epithelioid hemangioen-dothelioma	EIV	external iliac vein
EHEC	enterohemorrhagic *Escherichia coli*	EJ	ejection
			elbow jerk
EHF	epidemic hemorrhagic fever		external jugular
		EJB	ectopic junctional beat
	extremely high frequency	EJV	external jugular vein
EHH	esophageal hiatal hernia	EN	erythrokinase
EHL	electrohydraulic lithotripsy	EK	erythrokinase
			Ektachem 400 (analysis for potassium, carbon dioxide, chloride, glucose, and blood urea nitrogen)
	extensor hallucis longus		
EHN	ethotoin		
EHO	extrahepatic obstruction		
EHPH	extrahepatic portal hypertension		
		EKC	epidemic keratoconjunctivitis
EHS	employee health service	EKG	electrocardiogram
EHT	electrohydrothermosation	EKO	echoencephalogram
E/I	expiratory to inspiratory (ratio)	EKY	electrokymogram
		E-L	external lids
E & I	endocrine and infertility	ELAD	extracorporeal liver-assist device
EIA	enzyme immunoassay		
	exercise induced asthma	ELAM	endothelial leukocyte adhesion molecule
EIAB	extracranial-intracranial arterial bypass		
		ELB	early light breakfast
EIB	exercise induced bronchospasm		elbow
		ELBW	extremely low birth weight (less then 1000 g)
EIC	extensive intraduct component		
EICA	extra-intracranial artery (bypass)	ELC	earlobe creases
		ELCA	excimer laser coronary angioplasty
EID	electroimmunodiffusion		
	electronic infusion device		

ELEC	elective	EMB	endometrial biopsy
ELF	elective low forceps		endomyocardial biopsy
	epithelial lining fluid		ethambutol
	etoposide, leucovorin, and		Explanation of Medicare
	fluorouracil		Benefits
ELH	endolymphatic hydrops	EMC	encephalomyocarditis
ELI	endomyocardial		endometrial currettage
	lymphocytic infiltrates		essential mixed
ELIG	eligible		cryoglobulinemia
ELISA	enzyme-linked	EMD	electromechanical
	immunosorbent assay		dissociation
Elix	elixir	EMDR	eye movement
ELLIP	ellipotocytosis		desensitization and
ELND	elective lymph node		reprocessing
	dissection	EME	extreme medical
ELO	enteroviral leukemic		emergency
	oncogene	EMEA	European Medicines
ELOP	estimated length of		Evaluations Agency
	program	EMF	elective mid forceps
ELOS	estimated length of stay		electromagnetic field(s)
ELP	electrophoresis		electromagnetic flow
ELPS	excessive lateral pressure		endomyocardial fibrosis
	syndrome		erythrocyte maturation
ELS	Eaton-Lambert syndrome		factor
ELSI	ethical, legal, and social		evaporated milk formula
	implications	EMG	electromyograph
ELSS	emergency life support		emergency
	system		essential monoclonal
ELT	euglobulin lysis time		gammopathy
ELVIS™	Enzyme Linked Virus	EMI	elderly and mentally
	Inducible System		infirm
EM	early memory	EMIC	emergency maternity and
	ejection murmur		infant care
	electron microscope	E-MICR	electron microscopy
	emergency medicine	EMIT	enzyme multiplied
	emmetropia		immunoassay technique
	erythema migrans		(test)
	erythema multiforme	EMLA®	eutectic mixture of local
	estramustine		anesthetics (lidocaine
	extensive metabolizers		and prilocaine in an
	external monitor		emulsion base)
E&M	Evaluation and	EMLB	erythromycin lactobionate
	Management (coding	EMMV	extended mandatory
	system)		minute ventilation
EMA	early morning awakening	EMP	electromolecular
	endomysial antibody		propulsion
EMA-CO	etoposide, methotrexate,		estramustine phosphate
	dactinomycin, and	EMR	educable mentally
	leucovorin		retarded

	electrical muscle stimulation	ENF	Enfamil®
	electronic medical record	ENF c Fe	Enfamil® with iron
	emergency mechanical restraint	ENG	electronystagmogram engorged
	empty, measure, and record	ENL	erythema nodosum leprosum
	eye movement recording	ENMG	electroneuromyography
EMS	early morning specimen	ENS	exogenous natural surfactant
	early morning stiffness		
	electrical muscle stimulation	ENP	extractable nucleoprotein
	emergency medical services	ENT	ears, nose, throat
	eosinophilia myalgia syndrome	ENVD	elevated new vessels on the disk
EMSU	early morning specimen of urine	ENVE	elevated new vessels elsewhere
EMT	emergency medical technician	ENVT	environment
EMTA	Emergency Medical Technician, Advanced	EO	elbow orthosis embolic occlusion eosinophilia
EMTC	emergency medical trauma center		ethylene oxide eyes open
EMT-D	emergency medical technician-defibrillation	EOA	erosive osteoarthritis esophageal obturator airway
EMTP	Emergency Medical Technician, Paramedic		examine, opinion, and advice
EMU	early morning urine electromagnetic unit		external oblique aponeurosis
EMV	eye, motor, verbal (grading for Glasgow coma scale)	EOAE	evoked otoacoustic emissions
EMVC	early mitral valve closure	EOB	edge of bed end of bed
EMW	electromagnetic waves	EOC	enema of choice
EN	enema		epithelial ovarian cancer
	enteral nutrition	EOD	every other day (this is a dangerous abbreviation)
	erythema nodosum		
E/N	eggnog		extent of disease
E 50% N	extension 50% of normal	EOE	extraosseous Ewing's sarcoma
ENA	extractable nuclear antigen	EOFAD	early-onset form of familial Alzheimer's disease
ENB	esthesioneuroblastoma		
ENC	encourage	EOG	electro-oculogram
ENDO	endodontia		Ethrane®, oxygen, and gas (nitrous oxide)
	endodontics		
	endoscopy	EOL	end of file
	endotracheal	EOM	error of measurement
ENOG	electroneurography		external otitis media extraocular movement

	extraocular muscles		epinephrine
EOMI	extraocular muscles intact		epirubicin
EOO	external oculomotor ophthalmoplegia		epitheloid cells
			exercise pressure index
EOR	emergency operating room		exocrine pancreatic insufficiency
	end of range	EPIC	etoposide, ifosfamide, and cisplatin (Platinol)
EORA	elderly onset rheumatoid arthritis	EPID	epidural
EOS	end of study	EPIG	epigastric
	eosinophil	EPIS	episiotomy
EP	ectopic pregnancy	epith.	epithelial
	electrophysiologic	EPL	extensor pollicis longus (tendon)
	elopement precaution		
	endogenous pyrogen	EPM	electronic pacemaker
	Episcopal	EPN	estimated protein needs
	esophageal pressure	EPO	epoetin alfa (erythropoietin)
	etoposide and cisplatin (Platinol)		evening primrose oil
	evoked potentials		exclusive provider organization
E&P	estrogen and progesterone	EPP	erythropoietic protoporphyria
EPA	eicosapentaenoic acid		
	Environmental Protection Agency	EPR	electrophrenic respiration
EPAB	extracorporeal pneumoperititoneal access bubble		emergency physical restraint
			epirubicin
E-Panel	electrolyte panel (potassium, sodium, carbon dioxide, and chloride)		estimated protein requirement
		EPS	electrophysiologic study
			expressed prostatic secretions
EPAP	expiratory positive airway pressure		extrapulmonary shunt
EPB	extensor pollicis brevis		extrapyramidal syndrome (symptom)
EPC	erosive prephloric changes	EPSCCA	extrapulmonary small cell carcinoma
	external pneumatic compression	EPSDT	early periodic screening, diagnosis, and treatment
EPD	electrode placement device		
	equilibrium peritoneal dialysis	EPSE	extrapyramidal side effects
EPEC	enteropathogen *Escherichia coli*	EPSP	excitatory postsynaptic potential
EPEG	etoposide	EPSS	E point septal separation
EPF	Enfamil Premature Formula®	EPT®	early pregnancy test
		EPTE	existed prior to enlistment
EPG	electronic pupillography	EPTS	existed prior to service
EPI	echoplanar imaging	ER	emergency room

	estrogen receptors
	extended release
	external resistance
	extended external rotation
E & R	equal and reactive
	examination and report
ER+	estrogen receptor-positive
ERA	estrogen receptor assay
	evoked response audiometry
%ERAD	eradication rates
ERBD	endoscopic retrograde biliary drainage
ERC	endoscopic retrograde cholangiography
ERCP	endoscopic retrograde cholangiopancreatography
ERCT	emergency room computerized tomography
ERD	early retirement with disability
ERE	external rotation in extension
ERF	external rotation in flexion
ERFC	erythrocyte rosette forming cells
ERG	electroretinogram
ERL	effective refractory length
ERMS	exacerbating-remitting multiple sclerosis
ERNA	equilibrium radionuclide angiocardiography
ERP	effective refractory period
	emergency room physician
	endocardial resection procedure
	endoscopic retrograde pancreatography
	event-related potentials
	estrogen receptor protein
ERPF	effective renal plasma flow
ER/PR	estrogen receptor/ progesterone receptor
ERS	endoscopic retrograde sphincterotomy

	evacuation of retained secundines (afterbirth)
ERT	estrogen replacement therapy
ERTD	emergency room triage documentation
ERUS	endorectal ultrasound
ERV	expiratory reserve volume
ES	electrical stimulation
	emergency service
	endoscopic sphincterotomy
	end-to-side
	ex-smoker
	extra strength
ESA	end-to-side anastomosis
	ethmoid sinus adenocarcinoma
ESADDI	estimated safe and adequate daily dietary intake
ESAP	evoked sensory (nerve) action potential
ESAT	extrasystolic atrial tachycardia
ESC	end systolic counts
ESD	Emergency Services Department
	esophagus, stomach, and duodenum
ESF	external skeletal fixation
ESFT	Ewing's sarcoma family of tumors
ESI	epidural steroid injection
ESI-MS	electrospray ionization- mass spectrometry
ESL	English as a second language
ESLD	end-stage liver disease
	end-stage lung disease
ESM	ejection systolic murmur
	endolymphatic stromal myosis
	ethosuximide
ESN	educationally subnormal
ESN(M)	educationally subnormal- moderate
ESN(S)	educationally subnormal- severe

ESO	esophagus	
	esotropia	
ESP	endometritis, salpingitis, and peritonitis	
	end systolic pressure	
	especially	
	extrasensory perception	
ESR	erythrocyte sedimentation rate	
ESRD	end-stage renal disease	
ESRF	end-stage renal failure	
ESS	emotional, spiritual, and social	
	endoscopic sinus surgery	
	essential	
EST	Eastern Standard Time	
	endoscopic spincterotomy	
	electroshock therapy	
	electrostimulation therapy	
	estimated	
	exercise stress test	
E-stim	electrical stimulation	
ESU	electrosurgical unit	
ESWL	extracorporeal shockwave lithotripsy	
ET	ejection time	
	embryo transfer	
	endotoxin	
	endothelin	
	endotracheal	
	endotracheal tube	
	enterostomal therapy (therapist)	
	esotropia	
	essential thrombocythemia	
	essential tremor	
	eustachian tube	
	Ewing's tumor	
	exchange transfusion	
	exercise treadmill	
et	and	
ET′	esotropia at near	
E(T)	intermittent esotropia at infinity	
E(T′)	intermittent esotropia at near	
ET @ 20′	esotropia at 6 meters (infinity)	
ETA	endotracheal airway	

		ethionamide
et al		and others
ETC		and so forth
		Emergency and Trauma Center
		estimated time of conception
$ETCO_2$		end tidal carbon dioxide
ETD		eustachian tube dysfunction
ETDLA		esophageal-tracheal double lumen airway
ETE		end-to-end
ETEC		enterotoxigenic *Escherichia coli*
ETF		eustachian tubal function
ETH		elixir terpin hydrate
		ethanol
		Ethrane®
ETHc̄C		elixir terpin hydrate with codeine
ETI		ejective time index
		endotracheal intubation
ETKTM		every test known to man
ETO		estimated time of ovulation
		ethylene oxide
		etoposide
		eustachian tube obstruction
ETOH		alcohol
		alcoholic
ETOP		elective termination of pregnancy
ETP		elective termination of pregnancy
ETS		elevated toilet seat
		endoscopic transthoracic sympathectomy
		endotracheal suction
		end-to-side
		environmental tobacco smoke
		erythromycin topical solution
ETT		endotracheal tube
		esophageal transit time
		exercise tolerance test

	exercise treadmill test	EVS	endoscopic variceal
	extrathyroidal thyroxine		sclerosis
ETT-Tl	exercise treadmill test with thallium	ew	elsewhere
ETU	emergency and trauma unit	EWB	estrogen withdrawal bleeding
	emergency treatment unit	EWCL	extended wear contact lens
ETX	edatrexate	EWHO	elbow-wrist-hand orthosis
EU	Ehrlich units		
	equivalent units	EWL	estimated weight loss
	esophageal ulcer		
	etiology unknown	EWSCLs	extended-wear soft contact lenses
	European Union		
	excretory urography	EWT	erupted wisdom teeth
EUA	examine under anesthesia		
EUCD	emotionally unstable character disorder	ex	examined
			example
EUD	external urinary device		excision
EUG	extrauterine gestation		exercise
EUL	extra uterine life	exam.	examination
EUM	external urethral meatus	EXEF	exercise ejection fraction
EUP	extrauterine pregnancy		
EUS	endoscopic ultrasonography	EXGBUS	external genitalia, Bartholin (gland), urethral (gland), and Skene (gland)
	external urethral sphincter		
EV	epidermodysplasia verruciformis		
	esophageal varices	EXH VT	exhaled tidal volume
	etoposide and vincristine	EXL	elixir
eV	electron volt (unit of radiation energy)	EXOPH	exophthalmos
EVA	ethylene vinyl acetate	EXP	experienced
	etoposide, vinblastine, and doxorubicin (Adriamycin)		expired
			exploration
			expose
		expect	expectorant
EVAC	evacuation	exp. lap.	exploratory laparotomy
EVAc	ethylene-vinyl acetate copolymer	EXT	extension
			external
eval	evaluate		extract
EXC	excision		extraction
EVD	external ventricular (ventriculostomy) drain		extremities
			extremity
		Ext mon	external monitor
EVE	evening	extrav	extravasation
EXEC 22	Executive 22 chemistry profile (see SMA-23)	ext. rot.	external rotation
		EXTUB	extubation
EVER	eversion	EX U	excretory urogram
EVG	endovascular grafting	EZ	Edmonston-Zagreb (vaccine)
EVL	endoscopic variceal		

EZ-HT	Edmonston-Zagreb high-titer (vaccine)

	forearm
	functional activities
FAA	febrile antigen agglutination
	folic acid antagonist
FAAP	family assessment adjustment pass
FAA SOL	formalin, acetic, and alcohol solution
FAAN	Fellow of the American Academy of Nursing
FAAP	Fellow of the American Academy of Pediatrics
FAB	digoxin immune Fab (Digibind®)
	French-American-British Cooperative group
	functional arm brace
FABER	flexion, abduction, and external rotation
FABF	femoral artery blood flow
FAC	fluorouracil doxorubicin (Adriamycin), and cyclophosphamide
	fractional area concentration
FACA	Fellow of the American College of Anaesthetists
FACAG	Fellow of the American College of Angiology
FACAL	Fellow of the American College of Allergists
FACAN	Fellow of the American College of Anesthesiologists
FACAS	Fellow of the American College of Abdominal Surgeons
FACC	Fellow of the American College of Cardiology
FACCP	Fellow of the American College of Chest Physicians
FACCPC	Fellow of the American College of Clinical Pharmacology & Chemotherapy
FACD	Fellow of the American College of Dentists

F

F	facial
	Fahrenheit
	fair
	false
	fasting
	father
	feces
	female
	finger
	firm
	flow
	fluoride
	French
	fundi
	fundus
F/	full upper denture
/F	full lower denture
(F)	final
°F	degrees Fahrenheit
F=	firm and equal
F_1	offspring from the first generation
F_2	offspring from the second generation
F_3	Fluothane
14 F	14-hour fast required
F II	factor II (two)
F VIII	factor VIII (eight)
F IX	factor IX (nine)
FA	fatty acid
	femoral artery
	fetus active
	first aid
	fluorescein angiogram
	fluorescent antibody
	folic acid

95

FACEM	Fellow of the American College of Emergency Medicine		flavin adenine dinucleotide
FACEP	Fellow of the American College of Emergency Physicians	FAE	fetal alcohol effect
		FAGA	full-term appropriate for gestational age
FACGE	Fellow of the American College of Gastroenterology	FAH	fumarylacetoacetase hydrolase
FACH	forceps to after-coming head	FAI	Functional Assessment Inventory
FACLM	Fellow of the American College of Legal Medicine	FAK	focal adhesion kinase
		FAL	femoral arterial line
		FALL	fallopian
FACN	Fellow of the American College of Nutrition	FALS	familial amyotrophic lateral sclerosis
FACNP	Fellow of the American College of Neuropsychopharmacology	FAM	family
			fluorouracil, doxorubicin (Adriamycin®), and mitomycin
FACOG	Fellow of the American College of Obstetricians & Gynecologists	FAMA	fluorescent antibody to membrane antigen
		FAME	fluorouracil, doxorubicin (Adriamycin), and semustin (methyl CCNU)
FACOS	Fellow of the American College of Orthopedic Surgeons		
FACP	Fellow of the American College of Physicians	FAM-S	fluorouracil, doxorubicin (Adriamycin), mitomycin, and streptozotocin
FACPRM	Fellow of the American College of Preventive Medicine	FAMTX	fluorouracil, doxorubicin (Adriamycin), and methotrexate
FACR	Fellow of the American College of Radiologists	FANA	fluorescent antinuclear antibody
FACS	Fellow of the American College of Surgeons	FANG	fluorescent angiography
	fluorescent-activated cell sorter	FANSS&M	fundus anterior, normal size and shape and mobile
FACSM	Fellow of the American College of Sports Medicine	FAP	familial adenomatous polyposis
			familial amyloid polyneuropathy
FACT-G	Functional Assessment Cancer Therapy		femoral artery pressure
FAD	familial Alzheimer's disease		fibrillating action potential
	Family Assessment Device	FAQ	frequently asked question(s)
	fetal abdominal diameter	F-ara-A	fludarabine phosphate
	fetal activity determination	FAS	fetal alcohol syndrome
		FASC	fasciculations

FASHP	Fellow of the American Society of Health-Systems Pharmacists
FAST	fetal acoustic stimulation testing
	fluorescent allergosorbent technique
FAT	Fetal Activity Test
	fluorescent antibody test
	food awareness training
FAV	facio-auricular vertebral
FAZ	foveal avascular zone
FB	fasting blood (sugar)
	finger breadth
	flexible bronchoscope
	foreign body
F/B	followed by
	forward/backward
	forward bending
FBC	full (complete) blood count
FBCOD	foreign body, cornea, right eye
FBCOS	foreign body, cornea, left eye
FBD	fibrocystic breast disease
	functional bowel disease
FBF	forearm blood flow
FBG	fasting blood glucose
	foreign-body-type granulomata
FBH	hydroxybutyric dehydrogenase
FBI	flossing, brushing, and irrigation
	full bony impaction
FBL	fecal blood loss
FBM	felbamate
	fetal breathing motion
	foreign body, metallic
FBRCM	fingerbreadth below right costal margin
FBS	failed back syndrome
	fasting blood sugar
	fetal bovine serum
	foreign body sensation (eye)
FBU	fingers below umbilicus
FBW	fasting blood work

FC	family conference
	febrile convulsion
	female child
	fever, chills
	financial class
	finger clubbing
	finger counting
	flexion contractor
	flucytosine
	foam cuffed (tracheal or endotracheal tube)
	Foley catheter
	follows commands
	foster care
	functional capacity
	functional class
5FC	flucytosine (this is a dangerous abbreviation as it can look like 5FU)
F + C	flare and cells
F & C	foam and condom
F. cath.	Foley catheter
FCBD	fibrocystic breast disease
FCC	familial colonic cancer
	family centered care
	femoral cerebral catheter
	follicular center cells
	fracture compound comminuted
FCCA	Final Comprehensive Consensus Assessment
FCCC	fracture complete, compound, and comminuted
FCCL	follicular center cell lymphoma
FCCU	family centered care unit
FCD	feces collection device
	fibrocystic disease
FCDB	fibrocystic disease of the breast
FCE	fluorouracil, cisplatin, and etoposide
	functional capacity evaluation
FCFD	fluorescence capillary-fill device
FCH	familial combined hyperlipidemia

	fibrosing cholestatic hepatitis
FCHL	familial combined hyperlipemia
FCL	fibular collateral ligament
F-CL	fluorouracil and calcium leucovorin
FCMC	family centered maternity care
FCMD	Fukiyama's congenital muscular dystrophy
FCMN	family centered maternity nursing
F/C/N/V	fever, cough, nausea, and vomiting
FCOU	finger count, both eyes
FCP	formocresol pulpotomu
FCR	flexor carpi radialis
	fractional catabolic rate
FCRB	flexor carpi radialis brevis
FCRT	fetal cardiac reactivity test
FCS	fever, chills, and sweating
FCSNVD	fever, chills, sweating, nausea, vomiting, and diarrhea
FCU	flexor carpi ulnaris (tendon)
FCV	feline calicivirus
FD	familial dysautonomia
	fetal demise
	fetal distress
	focal distance
	forceps delivery
	free drain
	full denture
	fully dilated
F & D	fixed and dilated
FDA	Food and Drug Administration
	fronto-dextra anterior
FDB	flexor digitorum brevis
FDBL	fecal daily blood loss
FDE	fixed-drug eruption
FDF	flexor digitorum profundus (tendon)
FDG	feeding
	fluorine-18-labeled deoxyglucose (fluoro-fluorodeoxyglucose)

FDG-PET	positron emission tomography with ^{18}fluorodeoxyglucose
FDGS	feedings
FDIU	fetal death in utero
FDL	flexor digitorum longus
FDLMP	first day of last menstrual period
FDM	fetus of diabetic mother
	flexor digiti minimi
FDP	fibrin-degradation products
	flexor digitorum profundus
FDQB	flexor digiti quinti brevis
FDR	first-dose reaction
FDS	flexor digitorum superficialis
	for duration of stay
FDT	fronto-dextra transversa (right frontotransverse)
Fe	female
	iron
FEB	febrile
FEC	fluorouracil, etoposide, and cisplatin
	forced expiratory capacity
FECG	fetal electrocardiogram
FeCh	ferrochelatase
FECP	free erythrocyte coproporphyrin
FECT	fibroelastic connective tissue
FED	fish eye disease
FEES	fiberoptic endoscopic evaluation of swallowing
FEF	forced expiratory flow rate
$FEF_{25\%-75\%}$	forced expiratory flow during the middle half of the forced vital capacity
FEF_{x-y}	forced expiratory flow between two designated volume points in the forced vital capacity
FEL	familial erythrophagocytic lymphohistiocytosis

FeLV	feline leukemia virus	F&F	fixes and follows
FEM	femoral	F→F	finger to finger
FEM-FEM	femoral femoral (bypass)	FF1/U	fundus firm 1 cm above umbilicus
FEM-POP	femoral popliteal (bypass)		
FEM-TIB	femoral tibial (bypass)	FF2/U	fundus firm 2 cm above umbilicus
FERGs	focal electroretinograms		
FEN	fluid, electrolytes, and nutrition	FF@u	fundus firm at umbilicus
		FFA	free fatty acid
FENa	fractional extraction of sodium		fundus fluorescein angiogram
FEN-PHEN	fenfluramine and phentermine	FFAT	Free Floating Anxiety Test
FEOM	full extraocular movements	FFB	flexible fiberoptic bronchoscopy
FEP	free erythrocyte porphyrins	FFD	fat-free diet
			focal-film distance
	free erythrocyte protoporphyrin	FFDM	freedom from distant metastases
FER	flexion, extension, and rotation	FFE	free-flow electrophoresis
		FFI	fast food intake
FES	fat embolism syndrome		fatal familial insomnia
	functional electrical stimulation	FFM	fat-free mass
			five finger movement
FeSO₄	ferrous sulfate		freedom from metastases
FESS	functional endonasal sinus surgery	FFP	fresh frozen plasma
		FFROM	full, free range of motion
	functional endoscopic sinus surgery	FFS	failure-free survival
			fee-for-service
FET	fixed erythrocyte turnover		Fight For Sight
FETI	fluorescence (fluorescent) energy transfer immunoassay		flexible fiberoptic sigmoidoscopy
		FFT	fast-Fourier transforms
FEUO	for external use only		flicker fusion threshold
FEV₁	forced expiratory volume in one second	FFTP	first full-term pregnancy
		FFU/1	fundus firm 1 cm below umbilicus
FEV₁%VC	forced expiratory volume in one second as percent of forced vital capacity	FFU/2	fundus firm 2 cm below umbilicus
		FG	fibrin glue
		FGC	full gold crown
FF	fat free	FGF	fibroblast growth factor
	fecal frequency	FGP	fundic gland polyps
	filtration fraction	FGS	fibrogastroscopy
	finger to finger		focal glomerulosclerosis
	flat feet	FH	family history
	force fluids		familial hypercholester-olemia
	foster father		
	forward flexion		favorable histology
	fundus firm		fetal head
	further flexion		

	fetal heart	FIN	flexible intramedullary nail
	fundal height		
FH+	family history positive	FIND	follow-up intervention for normal development
FH−	family history negative		
FHA	filamentous hemagglutinin	FiO₂	fraction of inspired oxygen
FHC	familial hypertrophic cardiomyopathy		
	family health center	FIP	flatus in progress
FHD	family history of diabetes	FIRI	fasting insulin resistance index
FHF	fulminant hepatic failure		
FHH	familial hypocalciuric hypercalcemia	FISH	fluorescent (fluorescence) *in situ* hybridization
	fetal heart heard	FISP	fast imaging with steady state precision
FHI	frontal horn index		
	Fuch's heterochromic iridocyclitis	FITC	fluorescein isothiocyanate
FHL	flexor hallucis longus	FIV	feline immunodeficiency virus
FHN	family history negative		
FHNH	fetal heart not heard	FIVC	forced inspiratory vital capacity
FHO	family history of obesity		
FHP	family history positive	FIX	factor IX (nine)
FHR	fetal heart rate	FJB	facet joint block
FHRB	fetal heart rate baseline	FJN	familial juvenile nephrophthisis
FHRV	fetal heart rate variability	FJP	familial juvenile polyposis
FHS	fetal heart sounds	FJROM	full joint range of motion
	fetal hydantoin syndrome	FJS	finger joint size
FHT	fetal heart tone	FK506	tacrolimus
FHVP	free hepatic vein pressure	FKBP	FK-506 binding protein (tacrolimus)
FHx	family history		
FIAC	fiacitabine	FKD	Kinetic Family Drawing
FIAU	fialuridine	FKE	full knee extension
FIB	fibrillation	FL	fatty liver
	fibula		femur length
FICA	Federal Insurance Contributions Act (Social Security)		fetal length
			fluid
			fluorescein
FiCO₂	fraction of inspired carbon dioxide		flutamide and leuprolide acetate
			full liquids
FID	father in delivery	fL	femtoliter (10⁻¹⁵ liter)
	free induction decay	F/L	father-in-law
FIF	forced inspiratory flow	FLA	free-living amebic (ameba)
FIGLU	formiminoglutamic acid		low-friction arthroplasty
FIGO	International Federation of Gynecology and Obstetrics	FLAIR	fluid attenuated inversion recovery
FIL	father-in-law	FLAP	5-lipoxygenase activating protein
FIM	functional independence measure	FLASH	fast low-angle shot
		FLB	funny looking beat

FLBS	funny looking baby syndrome (see note under FLK)	
FLD	fatty liver disease	
	fluid	
	flutamide and leuprolide acetate depot	
	full lower denture	
FL Dtr	full lower denture	
FLe	fluorouracil and levamisole	
flexsig	flexible sigmoidoscopy	
FLF	funny looking facies (see note under FLK)	
FLGA	full-term, large for gestational age	
FLIC	Functional Living Index–Cancer	
FLIE	Functional Living Index—Emesis	
FLK	funny looking kid (should never be used: unusual facial features, is a better expression)	
FLM	fetal lung maturity	
fl. oz.	fluid ounce	
FL REST	fluid restriction	
FLS	flashing lights and/or scotoma	
FLT	fluorothymidine	
FLU	fluconazole	
FLU A	influenza A virus	
FLUO	Fluothane	
fluoro	fluoroscopy	
FLUT	flutamide	
FLV	Friend leukemia virus	
FLW	fasting laboratory work	
FLZ	flurazepam	
FM	face mask	
	fat mass	
	fetal movements	
	fine motor	
	floor manager	
	fluorescent microscopy	
	foster mother	
F & M	firm and midline (uterus)	
FMC	fetal movement count	
FMD	family medical doctor	
	fibromuscular dysplasia	

	foot and mouth disease	
FME	full mouth extraction	
FMF	familial Mediterranean fever	
	fetal movement felt	
	forced midexpiratory flow	
FMG	fine mesh gauze	
	foreign medical graduate	
FMH	family medical history	
	fibromuscular hyperplasia	
FmHx	family history	
FML®	fluorometholone	
FMN	first malignant neoplasm	
	flavin mononucleotide	
FMOL	femtomole	
FMP	fasting metabolic panel	
	first menstrual period	
FMPA	full mouth periapicals	
FMR	fetal movement record	
	functional magnetic resonance (imaging)	
FMRD	full mouth restorative dentistry	
fMRI	functional magnetic resonance imaging	
FMS	fluorouracil, mitomycin, and streptozocin	
	full mouth series	
FMT	functional muscle test	
FMU	first morning urine	
FMV	fluorouracil, semustine (methyl-CCNU), and vincristine	
FMX	full mouth x-ray	
FN	facial nerve	
	false negative	
	febrile neutropenia	
	finger-to-nose	
	flight nurse	
F/N	fluids and nutrition	
F to N	finger to nose	
FNA	fine-needle aspiration	
FNa	filtered sodium	
FNAB	fine-needle aspiration biopsy	
FNAC	fine-needle aspiratory cytology	
FNCJ	fine needle catheter jejunostomy	

FNF	femoral-neck fracture		future order screen
	finger nose finger	FOT	form of thought
FNH	focal nodular hyperplasia		frontal outflow tract
FNP	Family Nurse Practitioner	FOV	field of view
FNR	false negative rate	FOVI	field of vision intact
FNS	food and nutrition services	FOW	fenestration of oval window
	functional neuromuscular stimulation	FP	fall precautions
			false positive
F/NS	fever and night sweats		family planning
FNT	finger to nose test		family practice
FNTC	fine needle transhepatic cholangiography		family practitioner
			fibrous proliferation
FO	foot orthosis		flat plate
	foramen ovale		food poisoning
	foreign object		frozen plasma
	fronto-occipital	F/P	fluid/plasma (ratio)
FOB	father of baby	F-P	femoral popliteal
	fecal occult blood	fpA	fibrinopeptide A
	feet out of bed	FPAL	full term, premature, abortion, living
	fiberoptic bronchoscope		
	foot of bed	FPB	femoral-popliteal bypass
FOBT	fecal occult blood test		flexor pollicis brevis
FOC	father of child	FPC	familial polyposis coli
	fluid of choice		family practice center
	fronto-occipital circumference	FPD	feto-pelvic disproportion
			fixed partial denture
FOD	fixing right eye	FPDL	flashlamp-pumped pulsed dye laser
	free of disease		
FOEB	feet over edge of bed	FPE	first-pass effect
FOG	Fluothane, oxygen and gas (nitrous oxide)	FPG	fasting plasma glucose
		FPHx	family psychiatric history
	full-on gain	FPIA	fluorescence-polarization immunoassay
FOH	family ocular history		
FOI	flight of ideas	FPL	flexor pollicis longus (tendon)
FOIA	Freedom of Information Act		
		FPM	full passive movements
FOID	fear of impending doom	FPNA	first-pass nuclear angiocardiography
FOM	floor of mouth		
FOMi	fluorouracil, Oncovin, (vincristine), and mitomycin	FPOR	follicle puncture for oocyte retrieval
		FPU	family participation unit
FOOB	fell out of bed	FPZ	fluphenazine
FOOSH	fell on outstretched hand	FPZ-D	fluphenazine decanoate
FOPS	fiberoptic proctosigmoid-oscopy	FQ	fluoroquinolones
		FR	fair
FORMIL	foreign military		father
FOS	fiberoptic sigmoidoscopy		Father (priest)
	fixing left eye		flow rate

	fluid restriction
	fluid retention
	fractional reabsorption
	frequent relapses
	Friends
	full range
F & R	force and rhythm (pulse)
FRA	fluorescent rabies antibody
FRAC	fracture
FRACTS	fractional urines
FRAG	fragment
FRAP	Family risk assessment program
FRC	frozen red cells
	functional residual capacity
FRE	flow-related enhancement
FRF	filtration replacement fluid
FRJM	full range of joint movement
FROA	full range of affect
FROM	full range of motion
FRP	follicle regulatory protein
	functional refractory period
FS	fetoscope
	fibromyalgia syndrome
	fingerstick
	flexible sigmoidoscopy
	foreskin
	fractional shortenings
	frozen section
	full strength
	functional status
F & S	full and soft
FSALO	Fletcher suite after loading ovoids
FSALT	Fletcher suite after loading tandem
FSB	fetal scalp blood
	full spine board
FSBG	fingerstick blood glucose
FSBM	full strength breast milk
FSBS	fingerstick blood sugar
FSC	flexible sigmoidoscopy
	fracture, simple, and comminuted

	fracture, simple and complete
FSCC	fracture, simple, complete, and comminuted
FSD	focal-skin distance
	fracture, simple and depressed
FSE	fast spin-echo
	fetal scalp electrode
FSF	fibrin stabilizing factor
FSG	fasting serum glucose
	focal and segmental glomerulosclerosis
FSGA	full-term, small for gestational age
FSGN	focal segmental glomerulonephritis
FSGS	focal segmental glomerulosclerosis
FSH	facioscapulohumeral
	follicle stimulating hormone
FSHMD	facioscapulohumeral muscular dystrophy
FSIQ	Full-Scale Intelligence Quotient (part of Wechsler test)
FSL	fasting serum level
FSM	functional status measures
F-SM/C	fungus, smear and culture
FSME	Frühsommer-meningoencephalitis
FSOP	French Society of Pediatric Oncology
FSP	fibrin split products
FSS	fetal scalp sampling
	French steel sound (dilated to #24FSS)
	frequency-selective saturation
	full scale score
FSW	feet of sea water (pressure)
	field service worker
FT	family therapy
	feeding tube
	filling time
	finger tip
	flexor tendon

103

	fluidotherapy		failed to respond
	follow through		for the record
	foot (ft)	FTRAM	free transverse rectus
	free testosterone		abdominis
	full term		myocutaneous (flap)
F_3T	trifluridine	FTSD	full-term spontaneous
FT_3	free triiodothyronine		delivery
FT_4	free thyroxine	FTSG	full-thickness skin graft
FT_4I	free thyroxine index	FTT	failure to thrive
FTA	fluorescent titer antibody		fetal tissue transplant
	fluorescent treponemal	Ftube	feeding tube
	antibody	FTUPLD	full-term uncomplicated
FTB	fingertip blood		pregnancy, labor, and
FTBD	full-term born dead		delivery
FTC	frames to come	FTV	functional trial visit
	full to confrontation	FTW	failure to wean
FTD	failure to descend	FU	fraction unbound
	full-term delivery		fluorouracil
FTEs	full-time equivalents	F & U	flanks and upper
FTF	finger-to-finger		quadrants
	free thyroxine fraction	F/U	follow-up
FTFTN	finger-to-finger-to-nose		fundus at umbilicus
FTG	full thickness graft	F↑U	fingers above umbilicus
FTI	free thyroxine index	F↓U	fingers below umbilicus
F TIP	finger tip	5-FU	fluorouracil
FTIUP	full-term intrauterine	FUB	function uterine bleeding
	pregnancy	FUCO	fractional uptake of
FTKA	failed to keep		carbon monoxide
	appointment	FUD	full upper denture
FTLB	full-term living birth	FUDR®	floxuridine
FTLFC	full-term living female	FU Dtr	full upper denture
	child	FUFA	fluorouracil and
FTLMC	full-term living male child		leucovorin (folinic
FTM	fluid thioglycollate		acid)
	medium	FU/FL	full upper denture, full
FTN	finger-to-nose		lower denture
	full-term nursery	FULG	fulguration
FTNB	full-term newborn	5FU/LV	fluorouracil and
FTND	Fagerstrom Test for		leucovorin
	Nicotine Dependence	FUN	follow-up note
	full-term normal delivery	FUNG-C	fungus culture
FTNSD	full-term, normal,	FUNG-S	fungus smear
	spontaneous delivery	FUO	fever of undetermined
FTO	full-time occlusion (eye		origin
	patch)	FUOV	follow-up office visit
FTP	failure to progress	FU/LP	full upper denture, partial
	full-term pregnancy		lower denture
FTR	father	FUP	follow-up
	failed to report	FUS	fusion

FUV	follow-up visit			gravida
FV	femoral vein			guaiac
FVC	false vocal cord(s)			guanine
	forced vital capacity		G +	gram-positive
FVFR	filled voiding flow rate			guaiac positive
FVH	focal vascular headache		G –	gram-negative
F VIII	factor VIII (eight)			guaiac negative
FVL	femoral vein ligation		↑g	increasing
	flow volume loop		↓g	decreasing
FVR	feline viral rhinotracheitis		G1–4	grade 1–4
	forearm vascular		G-11	hexachlorophene
	resistance		GA	Gamblers Anonymous
FW	fetal weight			gastric analysis
F/W	followed with			general anesthesia
F waves	fibrillatory waves			general appearance
	flutter waves			gestational age
FWB	full weight bearing			ginger ale
FWD	fairly well developed			granuloma annulare
FWS	fetal warfarin syndrome			glucose/acetone
FWW	front wheel walker		Ga	gallium
Fx	fractional urine		⁶⁷Ga	gallium citrate Ga 67
	fracture		GABA	gamma-aminobutyric acid
Fx-BB	fracture both bones		GABHS	group A beta hemolytic
Fx-dis	fracture-dislocation			streptococci
F XI	Factor XI (eleven)		GAD	generalized anxiety
FXN	function			disorder
FXR	fracture			glutamic acid
FYC	facultative yeast carrier			decarboxylase
FYI	for your information		GAF	geographic adjustment
FZ	flutamide and goserelin			factors
	acetate (Zoladex®)		GAG	glycosaminoglycan
			Gal	gallon
FZRC	frozen red (blood) cells		G'ale	ginger ale
			GALI-PUT	galactose-1-phosphate uridye transferase enzyme
			GAR	gonnococcal antibody reaction
	G		GAS	general adaption syndrome
				ginseng-abuse syndrome
				Glasgow Assessment Schedule
				Global Assessment Scale
G	gallop			group A streptococci
	gastrostomy		Gas Anal F&T	gastric analysis, free and total
	gauge			
	gingiva		Ga scan	gallium scan
	good		Gastroc	gastrocnemius
	grade			
	gram (g)			

GAT	geriatric assessment team	GCE	general conditioning exercise
	group adjustment therapy	GCDFP	gross cystic disease fluid protein
GATB	General Aptitude Test Battery		
GAU	geriatric assessment unit	GCI	General Cognitive Index
Gaw	airway conductance	GCIIS	glucose control insulin infusion system
GB	gallbladder		
	Guillain-Barré (syndrome)	GCM	good central maintained
G & B	good and bad	GCMD	generalized cardiovascular metabolic disease
GBA	gingivobuccoaxial		
	ganglionic-blocking agent	GC-MS	gas chromatography-mass spectroscopy
GBBS	group B beta hemolytic streptococcus	GCP	good clinical practices
		GCR	gastrocolonic response
GBE	*Ginkgo biloba* extract	GCS	Glasgow Coma Scale
GBG	gonadal-steroid binding globulin	G-CSF	filgrastrim (granulocyte colony-stimulating factor)
GBH	gamma benzene hexachloride (lindane)		
		GCST	Gibson-Cooke sweat test
GBIA	Guthrie bacterial inhibition assay	GCT	general care and treatment
			germ cell tumor
GBM	glioblastoma multiforme		giant cell tumor
	glomerular basement membrane		granulosa cell tumor
		GCU	gonococcal urethritis
GBMI	guilty but mentally ill	GCV	great cardiac vein
GBP	gated blood pool (imaging)	GCVF	great cardiac vein flow
		GD	gestational diabetes
	gastric bypass		good
GBPS	gated blood pool scan		Graves' disease
GBR	good blood return	Gd	gadolinium
GBS	gallbladder series	G & D	growth and development
	gastric bypass surgery	GDA	gastroduodenal artery
	group B streptococci	GDB	Guide Dogs for the Blind
	Guillain-Barré syndrome		
GBW	generalized body weakness	Gd-BOPTA	gadolinium benzyloxypropionic tetra acetate
GBX	gall bladder extraction (cholecystectomy)		
		Gd-DTPA	gadopentetate
GC	gas chromatography	Gd-DTPA-BMA	gadodiamide
	geriatric chair (Gerichair®)		
		GD FA	grandfather
	gingival curettage	GDH	glutamic dehydrogenase
	gonococci (gonorrhea)	Gd-HPD03A	gadoteridol
	good condition		
	graham crackers	g/dl	grams per deciliter
G−C	gram-negative cocci	GDM	gestational diabetes mellitus
G+C	gram-positive cocci		
GCA	giant cell arteritis	GDNF	glial-derived neurotrophic factor
GCBP	gated cardiac blood pool		

GDP	gel diffusion precipitin	GFM	good fetal movement
GD MO	grandmother	GFR	glomerular filtration rate
GDS	Global Deterioration Scale		grunting, flaring, and retractions
GE	gainfully employed	GFS	glaucoma filtering surgery
	gastric emptying	GG	gamma globulin
	gastroenteritis		guaifenesin (glyceryl guaiacolate)
	gastroesophageal	G=G	grips equal and good
GEA	gastroepiploic artery	GGE	Gastrografin enema
GEC	galactose elimination capacity		generalized glandular enlargement
GED	General Educational Development (Test)	GGS	glands, goiter, and stiffness
GEE	Global Evaluation of Efficacy	GGT	gamma-glutamyl transferase
	glycine ethyl ester	GGTP	gamma-glutamyl transpeptidase
	graft-enteric erosion	GH	general health
GEF	graft-enteric fistula		gingival hyperplasia
GEM	gemcitabine (Gemzar)		glenohumeral
GEMU	geriatric evaluation and management unit		good health
GEN	genital		growth hormone
GEN/ ENDO	general anesthesia with endotracheal intubation	GHB	gamma hydroxybutyrate
GENT	gentamicin	GHb	glycosylated hemoglobin
GENTA/P	gentamicin-peak	GHD	growth hormone deficiency
GENTA/T	gentamicin-trough	GHDA	growth hormone deficiency (syndrome) in adults
GEP	gastroenteropancreatic		
GEQ	generic equiavalent	GHJ	glenohumeral joint
GER	gastroesophageal reflux	G-H jt	glenohumeral joint
GERD	gastroesophageal reflux disease	GHP(S)	gated heart pool (scan)
		GHQ	General Health Questionnaire
GES	gastric emptying scan		
GET	gastric emptying time	GHRF	growth hormone releasing factor
	graded exercise test		
GET 1/2	gastric emptying half-time	GI	gastrointestinal
GETA	general endotracheal anesthesia		granuloma inguinale
		GIB	gastric ileal bypass
GEU	geriatric evaluation unit		gastrointestinal bleeding
GF	gastric fistula	GIC	general immunocompetence
	gluten free		
	grandfather	GID	gastrointestinal distress
GFAP	glial fibrillary acid protein		gender identity disorder
GF-BAO	gastric fluid, basal acid output	GIDA	Gastrointestinal Diagnostic Area
GFCL	Goldmann fundus contact lens		
GFD	gluten-free diet		
GFJ	grapefruit juice		

GIFD #3	colonoscope	GLU 5	five hour glucose tolerance test
GIFT	gamete intrafallopian (tube) transfer	GLUC	glucose
GIH	gastrointestinal hemorrhage	GLYCOS Hb	glycosylated hemoglobin
GIK	glucose-insulin-potassium	GM	general medicine
GIL	gastrointestinal (tract) lymphoma		geometric mean
			gram (g)
GING	gingiva		grand mal
	gingivectomy		grandmother
G1K	greater than one thousand	GM +	gram-positive
GIP	gastric inhibitory peptide	GM −	gram-negative
	giant cell interstitial pneumonia	gm %	grams per 100 milliliters
		GMC	general medical clinic
GIS	gas in stomach	GMCD	grand mal convulsive disorder
	gastrointestinal series		
GIT	gastrointestinal tract	GM-CSF	sargramostim (granulo-cyte-macrophage colony-stimulating factor)
GITS	gastrointestinal therapeutic system		
	gut-derived infectious toxic shock		
		GME	gaseous microemboli
GITSG	Gastrointestinal Tumor Study Group	GMF	general medical floor
		GMH	germinal matrix hemorrhage
GITT	glucose insulin tolerance test		
		GMP	general medical panel
GIWU	gastrointestinal work-up		Good Manufacturing Practices
giv	given		
GJ	gastrojejunostomy		guanosine monophosphate
GJT	gastrojejunostomy tube	GMS	general medical services
G1K	greater than one thousand		general medicine and surgery
GL	gastric lavage		
	glaucoma		Gomori methenamine silver
	greatest length		
GLA	gamolenic acid	GM&S	general medicine and surgery
	gingivolinguoaxial		
	glucose-lowering agents	GMTs	geometric mean antibody titers
GLC	gas-liquid chromatog-raphy		
		GN	glomerulonephritis
GLIO	glioblastoma		graduate nurse
GLN	glomerulonephritis		gram-negative
GLOC	gravity induced loss of consciousness	GNB	ganglioneuroblastoma
			gram-negative bacilli
GLP	Gambro Liendia Plate		gram-negative bacteremia
	Good Laboratory Practice (Principles of)	GNBM	gram-negative bacillary meningitis
	group-living program	GNC	gram-negative cocci
GLP-1	glucagon-like peptide-1	GND	gram-negative diplococci
GLR	gravity lumbar reduction	GNID	gram-negative intracellular diplococci
GLU	glucose		

GNP	Geriatric Nurse Practitioner		living children (p = para)
GNR	gram-negative rods	GPA	global program on AIDS
GnRH	gonadotropin-releasing hormone		pregnant, birth, and miscarriage
GNS	gram-negative sepsis	GPB	gram-positive bacilli
GnSAF	gonadotropin surge attenuating factor	GPC	giant papillary conjunctivitis
GNT	Graduate Nurse Technician		glycerophosphorylcholine G-protein coupled
GO	Graves' ophthalmopathy Greek Orthodox	GPCR	gram-positive cocci G protein-coupled receptors
GOBI	growth monitoring, oral rehydration, breast feeding, and immunization	GPC/TP	glycerylphosphorylcholine to total phosphate
GOCS	Global Obsessive-Compulsive Scale	G6PD	glucose-6-phosphate dehydrogenase
GOD	glucose oxidase	GPI	general paralysis of the insane
GOG	Gynecologic Oncology Group		glucose-6-phosphate isomerase
GOK	God only knows	G-PLT	giant platelets
GOMER	get out of my emergency room	GPMAL	gravida, para, multiple births, abortions, and
GON	gonococcal ophthalmia neonatorum		live births
		GPN	graduate practical nurse
	greater occipital neuritis	GPO	group purchasing organization
GOO	gastric outlet obstruction		
GOR	gastro-oesophageal reflux	GPS	Goodpasture's syndrome
	general operating room	GPT	glutamic pyruvic transaminase
GOS	Glasgow Outcome Scale		
GOT	glucose oxidase test	GR	gastric resection
	glutamic-oxaloacetic transaminase (aspartate aminotransferase)	gr	grain (approximately 60 mg) (this is a dangerous abbreviation)
	goals of treatment	G−R	gram-negative rods
GP	gabapentin	G+R	gram-positive rods
	general practitioner	GRAS	generally recognized as safe
	globus pallidus		
	glucose polymers	GRASS	gradient recalled acquisition in a steady state
	glycoprotein		
	gram-positive		
	grandparent	Grav.	gravid (pregnant)
	gutta percha	GRD	gastroesophageal reflux disease
G/P	gravida/para		
G4P3104	four pregnancies (gravid), 3 went to term, one premature, no abortion (or miscarriage), and 4	GRD DTR	granddaughter
		GRD SON	grandson
		GRE	graded resistive exercise gradient-recalled echo

	gradient refocused echo	GST	glutathione S-transferase
GR-FR	grandfather		gold sodium thiomalate
GR-MO	grandmother	GSTM	gold sodium thiomalate
GRN	granules	GSUI	genuine stress urinary
	green		incontinence
GRP	group	GSW	gunshot wound
$Gr_1P_0AB_1$	one pregnancy, no births, and one abortion	GSWA	gunshot wound to abdomen
GRT	gastric residence time	GT	gait
	glandular replacement therapy		gait training
	Graduate Respiratory Therapist		gastrotomy tube
GRTT	Graduate Respiratory Therapist Technician		glucose tolerance
GS	gallstone		great toe
	generalized seizure		group therapy
	general surgery	GTA	glutaraldehyde
	gluteal sets	GTB	gastrointestinal tract bleeding
	Gram stain	GTC	generalized tonic-clonic (seizure)
	grip strength	GTCS	generalized tonic-clonic seizure
G/S	5% dextrose (glucose) and 0.9% sodium chloride (saline) injection	GTD	gestational trophoblastic disease
		GTE	general therapeutic exercise
GSAP	greatest single allergen present	GTF	gastrostomy tube feedings
GSCV	geriatric skilled care unit		glucose tolerence factor
GSD	glucogen storage disease	GTH	gonadotropic hormone
GSD-1	glycogen storage disease, type 1	GTN	gestational trophoblastic neoplasms
GSE	genital self-examination		glomerulo-tubulo-nephritis
	gluten sensitive enteropathy		glyceryl trinitrate (name for nitroglycerin in the United Kingdom)
	grip strong and equal	GTP	glutamyl transpeptidase
GSH	glutathione		guanosine triphosphate
GSI	genuine stress incontinence	GTR	granulocyte turnover rate
GSMD	gestational sack and maternal date		gross total resection
GSP	general survey panel		guided tissue regeneration
GSPN	greater superficial petrosal neurectomy	GTS	Gilles de la Tourette syndrome
GSR	galvanic skin resistance (response)	GTT	drop
	gastrosalivary reflex		glucose tolerance test
GSS	Gerstmann-Straüssler-Scheinker (syndrome)	GTT agar	gelatin-tellurite-taurocholate agar
		GTT3H	glucose tolerance test 3 hours (oral)
		GTTS	drops
		G-tube	gastrostomy tube

GU genitourinary
gonococcal urethritis
GUAR guarantor
GUD genital ulcer disease
GUI genitourinary infection
GUS genitourinary sphincter
genitourinary system
GUSTO Global Utilization of Streptokinase and TPA for Occluded Arteries
GV gentian violet
GVF Goldmann visual fields
good visual fields
GVG vigabatrin (gamma-vinyl GABA)
GVHD graft-versus-host disease
GVN gentamicin, vancomycin, and nystatin
GVS gastric vertical stapling
G/W dextrose (glucose) in water
G&W glycerin and water (enema)
GWA gunshot wound of the abdomen
GWD Guinea worm disease
GWS Gulf war syndrome
GWT gunshot wound of the throat
GWX guide wire exchange
GXP graded exercise program
GXT graded exercise test
Gy gray (radiation unit)
GYN gynecology
GZTS Guilford-Zimmerman Temperament Survey

H

H *Haemophilis*
heart
head
height
Helicobacter
heroin
Hispanic
hour
husband
hydrogen
hyperopia
hypermetropia
hyperphoria
hypodermic
objective angle
H′ hip
Ⓗ hypodermic injection
H^2 hiatal hernia
H_2 hydrogen
3H high, hot, and a helluva lot
HA headache
hearing aid
heart attack
hemadsorption
hemolytic anemia
hospital admission
hyaluronan
hyaluronic acid
hyperalimentation
hypermetropic astigmatism
hypothalmic amenorrhea
H/A head-to-abdomen (ratio)
HA-1A® nebacumab
HAA hepatitis-associated antigen
HAAB hepatitis A antibody
HABF hepatic artery blood flow
HAc acetic acid
HACE hepatic artery chemoembolization
high-altitude cerebral edema
HACS hyperactive child syndrome
HAD human adjuvant disease
HADS Hospital Anxiety and Depression Scale
HAE hearing aid evaluation
hepatic artery embolization

	hereditary angioedema		hyperacute rejection
HAF	hyperalimentation fluid	HARH	high altitude retinal
HAGG	hyperimmune antivariola		hemorrhage
	gamma globulin	HARS	Hamilton Anxiety Rating
HAH	high-altitude headache		Scale
HAI	hemagglutination	HAS	Hamilton Anxiety
	inhibition assay		(Rating) Scale
	hepatic arterial infusion		home assessment service
HAIC	hepatic arterial infusional		hyperalimentation solution
	chemotherapy	HASCVD	hypertensive
HAK	hyperalimentation kit		arteriosclerotic
HAL	hyperalimentation		cardiovascular disease
HALO	halothane	HASHD	hypertensive
HALRI	hospital-acquired lower		arteriosclerotic heart
	respiratory infections		disease
HAM	HTLV-1-associated	HAT	head, arms, and trunk
	myelopathy		heterophile antibody titer
	human albumin		hospital arrival time
	microspheres	HAV	hallux abducto valgus
HAMA	human anti-murine		hepatitis A virus
	(anti-mouse) antibody	HAZWO-	Hazardous Waste
HAM-A	Hamilton Anxiety (scale)	PER	Operations and
HAM D	Hamilton Depression		Emergency Response
	(scale)	HB	heart-beating (donor)
HAMS	hamstrings		heart block
HAN	heroin associated		heel to buttock
	nephropathy		hemoglobin (Hb)
HANE	hereditary angioneurotic		hepatitis B
	edema		high calorie
HAO	hearing aid orientation		hold breakfast
HAP	hearing aid problem		housebound
	heredopathia atactica	1^0HB	first degree heart block
	polyneuritiformis	HB1°	first degree heart block
	hospital-acquired	HB2°	second degree heart
	pneumonia		block
HAPC	hospital-acquired	HB3°	third degree heart block
	penetration contact	HBAB	hepatitis B antibody
HAPD	home-automated	Hb A$_{lc}$	glycosylated hemoglobin
	peritoneal dialysis	HBAC	hyperdynamic
HAPE	high altitude pulmonary		beta-adrenergic
	edema		circulatory
HAPS	hepatic arterial perfusion	HbAS	sickle cell trait
	scintigraphy	HBBW	hold breakfast for blood
HAPTO	haptoglobin		work
HAQ	Headache Assessment	HBcAb	hepatitis B core antibody
	Questionnaire		(antigen)
	Health Assessment	HBc AB	hepatitis B core antibody
	Questionnaire	HBc Ag	hepatitis B core antigen
HAR	high altitude retinopathy	HB core	hepatitis B core antigen

HbCV	*Haemophilus* b conjugate vaccine	HBVP	high biological value protein
HBD	has been drinking hydroxybutyrate dehydrogenase	HBW	high birth weight
		H/BW	heart-to-body weight (ratio)
HBDH	hydroxybutyrate dehydrogenase	HC	hairy cell
HBF	fetal hemoglobin hepatic blood flow		handicapped head circumference heart catheterization
HBGA	had it before, got it again		heel cords Hickman catheter
HBGM	home blood glucose monitoring		home care hot compress
HBH	Health Belief Model		housecall
HBHC	hospital based home care		Huntington's chorea
HBI	Harvey-Bradshaw Index hemibody irradiation		hydrocephalus hydrocortisone
HBID	hereditary benign intraepithelial dyskeratosis	4-HC	4-hydroperoxycyclo-phosphamide
		H & C	hot and cold
HBIG	hepatitis B immune globulin	HCA	health care aide heterocyclic antidepres-sant
Hb Kansas	mutant hemoglobin with a low affinity for oxygen	H-CAP	altretamine (hexamethyl-melamine),
HBLV	B-lymphotropic virus human		cyclophosphamide, doxorubicin
HBM	human bone marrow		(Adriamycin), and
HBO	hyperbaric oxygen		cisplatin (Platinol)
HbO₂	hyperbaric oxygen hemoglobin, oxygenated	HCC	hepatocellular carcinoma
HBOC	hemoglobin-based oxygen carrier	HCD	herniate cervical disk
HBOT	hyperbaric oxygen treatment		hydrocolloid dressing
HBP	high blood pressure	HCFA	Health Care Financing Administration
HBPM	home blood pressure monitoring	HCFC	hydrochlorofluorocarbon
HBS	Health Behavior Scale	HCG	human chorionic gonadotropin
HbS	sickle cell hemoglobin	HCH	hexachlorocyclohexane
HBsAg	hepatitis B surface antigen	HCI	home care instructions
HbSC	sickle cell hemoglobin C	HCL	hairy cell leukemia
HBSS	Hank's balanced salt solution	HCl	hydrochloric acid hydrochloride
HbSS	sickle cell anemia	HCLF	high carbohydrate, low fiber (diet)
HBT	hydrogen breath test	HCLs	hard contact lenses
HBV	hepatitis B vaccine hepatitis B virus honey-bee venom	HCLV	hairy cell leukemia variant
		HCM	health care maintenance

	heterogeneous cation-exchange membrane		Heller-Dor (procedure)
			heloma durum
	hypercalcemia of malignancy		hemodialysis
			herniated disk
	hypertropic cardiomyopathy		high dose
			hip disarticulation
HCMV	human cytomegalovirus		Hodgkin's disease
HCO₃	bicarbonate		hospital day
HCP	handicapped		hospital discharge
	healthcare provider		house dust
	hearing conservation programs		Huntington's disease
		HD-AC	high-dose cytarabine
	hereditary coporphyria	HD-ara-C	high-dose cytarabine (ara-C)
	hexachlorophene		
HCPCS	Health Care Common Procedure Coding System	HDBQ	Hilton Drinking Behavior Questionnaire
		HDC	high-dose chemotherapy
HCQ	hydroxychloroquine	HDCC	high-dose combination chemotherapy
HCR	health care review		
HCS	human chorionic somatomammotropin	HD-CPA	high-dose cyclophosphamide
17-HCS	17-hydroxycorticosteroids	HDCPT	high-dose cyclophosphamide therapy
HCT	head computerized (axial) tomography	HDC-SCR	high-dose chemotherapy with stem-cell rescue
	hematocrit		
	histamine challenge test	HDCT	high-dose chemotherapy
	human chorionic thyrotropin	HDCV	rabies virus vaccine, human diploid (human diploid cell vaccine)
	hydrochlorothiazide (this is a dangerous abbreviation)		
		HDH	high-density humidity
		HDI	high-definition imagine
	hydrocortisone	HDL	high-density lipoprotein
HCTU	home cervical traction unit	HDLW	hearing distance for watch to be heard in left ear
HCTZ	hydrochlorothiazide (this is a dangerous abbreviation)	HDM	home-delivered meals
			house dust mite
HCV	hepatitis C virus	HDMEC	human dermal microvascular endothelial cells
HCVD	hypertensive cardiovascular disease		
		HD-MTX	high-dose methotrexate
HCWs	health-care workers	HD-MTX-CF	high-dose methotrexate and leucovorin (citrovorum factor)
HCY	homocysteine		
HCYS	homocysteine		
HD	haloperidol decanoate	HD-MTX/LV	high-dose methotrexate and leucovorin
	Hansen's disease		
	hearing distance	HDN	hemolytic disease of the newborn
	heart disease		heparin dosing nomogram

	high-density nebulizer	HELLP Syndrome	hemolysis, elevated liver enzymes, and low platelet count
HDNS	Hodgkin's disease, nodular sclerosis		
HDP	high-density polyethylene	HEMA	hydroxyethylmethacrylate
	hydroxymethyline diphosphonate	HEMI	hemiplegia
		HEMOSID	hemosiderin
HDPAA	heparin-dependent platelet-associated antibody	HEMPAS	hereditary erythrocytic multinuclearity with positive acidified serum test
HDPC	hand piece		
HDR	heparin dose response	HEMS	helicopter emergency medical services
	husband to delivery room		
HDRA	histoculture drug response assay	HEN	hemorrhages, exudates, and nicking
HDRB	high-dose rate brachytherapy	HEP	hemoglobin electrophoresis
HDRS	Hamilton Depression Rating Scale		heparin
			hepatic
HDRW	hearing distance for watch to be heard in right ear		hepatoerythropoietic porphyria
HDS	Hamilton Depression (Rating) Scale		hepatoma
			histamine equivalent prick
	herniated disk syndrome		home exercise program
HDSCR	health deviation self-care requisite	HEPA	hamster egg penetration assay
HDU	hemodialysis unit		high-efficiency particulate air (filter)
HDV	hepatitis D virus		
HDW	hearing distance (with) watch	hep cap	heparin cap
		HERP	human exposure (dose)/rodent potency (dose)
HDYF	how do you feel		
HE	hard exudate		
	hepatic encephalopathy	HES	hetastarch (hydroxyethyl starch)
H&E	hematoxylin and eosin		
	hemorrhage and exudate		hypereosinophilic syndrome
	heredity and environment		
HEA	health	HEs	hypertensive emergencies
HEAR	hospital emergency ambulance radio	HETF	home enteral tube feeding
		HEV	hepatitis E virus
HEAT	human erythrocyte agglutination test		hepato-encephalomyelitis virus
HEB	hydrophilic emollient base		high endothelial venule
HEC	Health Education Center	Hex	altretamine (hexamethylmelamine)
HeCOG	Hellenic Cooperative Oncology Group		
		Hexa-CAF	altretamine (hexamethylmelamine), cyclophosphamide, methotrexate (amethopterin), and fluorouracil
HEENT	head, eyes, ears, nose, and throat		
HEK	human embryonic kidney		
HEL	human embryonic lung		
HeLa	Helen Lake (tumor cells)		

HF	Hageman factor	HGES	handgrasp equal and strong
	hard feces	HGF	hepatocyte growth factor
	hay fever	HGG	human gamma globulin
	head of fetus	HGH	human growth hormone
	heart failure	HGI	Human Genome Initiative
	high frequency	HGM	home glucose monitoring
	Hispanic female	HGN	hypogastric nerve
	hot flashes	HGO	hepatic glucose output
	house formula		hip guidance orthosis
HFA	health facility administrator	HGPRT	hypoxanthine-guanine phosphoribosyl-transferase
	hydrofluoroalkane-134a		
HFAS	hereditary flat adenoma syndrome	HGSIL	high-grade squamous intraepithelial lesion
HFB	high frequency band	HGV	hepatitis G virus
HFC	hydrofluorocarbon	HH	hard of hearing
HFD	high fiber diet		head hood
	high forceps delivery		hiatal hernia
HFHL	high-frequence hearing loss		home health
			homonymous hemiopia
HFI	hereditary fructose intolerance		household
			hypogonadotropic hypogonadism
HFJV	high frequency jet ventilation		hypoeninemic hypoaldosteronism
H flu	*Haemophilus influenzae*	H/H	hemoglobin/hematocrit
HFO	high-frequency oscillation	H&H	hematocrit and hemoglobin
HFOV	high-frequency oscillatory ventilation	HHA	health hazard appraisal
HFPPV	high-frequency positive pressure ventilation		hereditary hemolytic anemia
			home health agency
HFRS	hemorrhagic fever with renal syndrome		home health aid
		HHC	home health care
HFSH	human follicle-stimulating hormone	HHD	home hemodialysis
			hypertensive heart disease
HFST	hearing-for-speech test	HHFM	high-humidity face mask
HFUPR	hourly fetal urine production rate	HHM	high-humidity mask
			humoral hypercalcemia of malignancy
HFV	high-frequency ventilation		
HFX RT	hyperfractionated radiation therapy	HHN	hand held nebulizer
		HHNC	hyperosmolar hyperglycemic nonketotic coma
HG	handgrasp		
	handgrip		
	hemoglobin	HHNK	hyperglycemic hyperosmolar nonketotic (coma)
Hg	mercury		
Hgb	hemoglobin		
Hgb F	fetal hemoglobin	HHS	Health and Human
Hgb S	sickle cell hemoglobin		
HGE	human granulocytic ehrlichiosis		

		HILP	hyperthermic isolated limb perfusion
	Service (US Department of)	HIM	health information management
HHT	hereditary hemorrhagic telangiectasis	HINI	hypoxic-ischemic neuronal injury
HHTC	high-humidity trach collar	HIP	health insurance plan
HHTM	high-humidity trach mask	HIPC	hormone-independent prostate cancer
HHTS	high-humidity tracheostomy shield	hi-pro	high protein
HHV-6	human herpesvirus 6	HIR	head injury routine
HI	head injury	HIS	Hanover Intensive Score
	health insurance		Health Intention Scale
	hearing impaired		high intermittent suction
	hemagglutination inhibition		histidine
	human insulin		Home Incapacity Scale
	hospital insurance		hospital information system
HIA	hemagglutination inhibition antibody	HISMS	How I See Myself Scale
HIAA	hydroxyindoleacetic acid	HISTO	histoplasmosis
5-HIAA	5-hydroxyindoleacetic acid		histoplasmin skin test
HIB	*Haemophilus influenzae* type b (vaccine)	HIT	heparin induced thrombocytopenia
HIB-C	*Haemophilus-influenzae* B vaccine conjugate		histamine inhalation test
hi-cal	high caloric		home infusion therapy
HID	headache, insomnia, and depression	HITTS	heparin-induced thrombotic thrombocytopenia syndrome
	herniated intervertebral disk		
HIDA	hepato-iminodiacetic acid (lidofenin)	HIU	head injury unit
HIDS	hyperimmunoglobulinemia D syndrome	HIV	human immunodeficiency virus
HIE	hyperimmunoglobuline-mia E	HIV-1	human immunodeficiency virus type 1
	hypoxic-ischemic encephalopathy	HIV-2	human immunodeficiency virus type 2
HIF	*Haemophilus influenzae*	HIVAT	home intravenous antibiotic therapy
	higher integrative functions	HIVD	herniated intervertebral disk
HIHA	high impulsiveness, high anxiety	hi-vit	high vitamin
HIIC	heated intraoperative intraperitoneal chemotherapy	HIVMP	high-dose intravenous methylprednisolone
		HJB	Howell-Jolly bodies
HIL	hypoxic-ischemic lesion	HJR	hepato-jugular reflux
HILA	high impulsiveness, low anxiety	HK	hand-to-knee
			heel-to-knee
			hexokinase

HKAFO	hip-knee-ankle-foot orthosis			Hispanic male
				Holter monitor
HKAO	hip-knee-ankle orthosis			human milk
HKO	hip-knee orthosis			human semisynthetic insulin
HKS	heel-knee-shin (test)			humidity mask
HKT	heterotopic kidney transplant		HMA	hemorrhages and microaneurysms
HL	hairline		HMB	homatropine methylbromide
	half-life		HMBA	hexamethylene bisacetamide
	hallux limitus			
	haloperidol		HMD	hyaline membrane disease
	harelip		HME	heat and moisture exchanger
	hearing level			
	hearing loss			heat, massage, and exercise
	heavy lifting			
	hemilaryngectomy			home medical equipment
	heparin lock		HMDP	hydroxymethyline diphosphonate
	hepatic lipase			
	Hickman line		HMETSC	heavy metal screen
H&L	heart and lung		HMG	human menopausal gonadotropin
HLA	human leukocyte antigen			
	human lymphocyte antigen		HMG CoA	hepatic hydroxymethyl glutaryl coenzyme A
HLA nega-tive	heart, lungs, and abdomen negative		HMI	healed myocardial infarction
HLB	head, limbs, and body			history of medical illness
HLD	haloperidol decanoate		HMIS	hospital medical information system
	herniated lumbar disk			
HLDP	hypoglossia-limb deficiency phenotype		HMK	homemaking
			HM & LP	hand motion and light perception
HLGR	high-level gentamicin resistance			
			HMM	altretamine (hexamethyl-melamine)
HLH	hemophagocytic lymphohistiocytosis			
			HMO	Health Maintenance Organization
	human luteinizing hormone			
			HMP	health maintenance plan
HLHS	hypoplastic left heart syndrome			hexose monophosphate
				hot moist packs
HLK	heart, liver, and kidneys		HMPAO	hexylmethylpropylene amineoxine
HLP	hyperlipoproteinemia			
HLT	heart-lung transplantation (transplant)		HMR	histocytic medullary reticulosis
			¹H-MRS	proton magnetic resonance spectroscopy
HLV	herpes-like virus			
	hypoplastic left ventricle		HMS	hyperactive malarial splenomegaly
HM	hand motion			
	head movement			hypodermic morphine
	heart murmur			
	heavily muscled			
	heloma molle			

118

	sulfate (this is a dangerous abbreviation)		heterotropic ossification
			hip orthosis
HMS®	medrysone		house officer
HMSN I	hereditary motor and sensory neuropathy type I	H/O	history of
		H₂O	water
HMSR	high medical-social risk	H₂O₂	hydrogen peroxide
HMSS	hyperactive malarial splenomegaly syndrome	HOA	hip osteoarthritis
		HOB	head of bed
HMWK	high molecular weight kininogen	HOB UPSOB	head of bed up for shortness of breath
HMX	heat massage exercise	HOC	Health Officer Certificate
HN	head and neck	HOCM	high-osmolality contrast media
	head nurse		
	high nitrogen		hypertrophic obstructive cardiomyopathy
	home nursing		
H&N	head and neck	HOG	halothane, oxygen, and gas (nitrous oxide)
HN₂	mechlorethamine HCl		
HNC	head and neck cancer	HOH	hard of hearing
	human neutrophil collagenase	HOI	hospital onset of infection
		HOM	high-osmolar contrast media
	hyperosmolar nonketotic coma		
		HONK	hyperosmolar nonketotic (coma)
HNCa	head and neck cancer		
HNE	human neutrophil elastase	HOPI	history of present illness
HNI	hospitalization not indicated	HORF	high-output renal failure
		HORS	Hemiballism/Hemichorea Outcome Rating Score
HNKDC	hyperosomolar nonketotic diabetic coma		
		HOSP	hospital
HNKDS	hyperosmolar nonketotic diabetic state		hospitalization
		HP	hard palate
HNLN	hospitalization no longer necessary		Harvard pump
			Helicobacter pylori
HNN	hybrid neural network		hemipelvectomy
HNP	herniated nucleus pulposus		hemiplegia
			high-protein (supplement)
HNPCC	heredity nonpolyposis colorectal cancer		hot packs
			house physician
HNRNA	heterogeneous nuclear ribonucleic acid		hydrogen peroxide
			hydrophilic petrolatum
HNS	head and neck surgery	H&P	history and physical
	head, neck, and shaft	HPA	hypothalamic-pituitary-adrenal (axis)
HNSCC	squamous cell carcinoma of the head and neck		
		HPAT	home parenteral antibiotic therapy
HNSN	home, no services needed		
HNV	has not voided	HPB	Health Protection Branch (the Canadian equivalent of the U.S. Food and Drug Administration)
HNWG	has not worn glasses		
HO	hand orthosis		
	Hemotology-Oncology		

HPC	history of present condition (complaint)	hPTH	human parathyroid hormone I$_{34}$ (teriparatide)
HPCE	high performance capillary electrophoresis	HPTM	home prothrombin time monitoring
HPD	high protein diet	HPV	human papilloma virus
	home peritoneal dialysis		human parvovirus
HP&D	hemoprofile and differential	*H pylori*	*Helicobacter pylori*
		HPZ	high pressure zone
HPE	hemorrhage, papilledema, exudate	HQC	hydroquinone cream
		HQL	health-related quality of life
	history and physical examination	HR	hallus rigidus
HPET	*Helicobacter pylori* eradication therapy		Harrington rod
			hazard ratio
HPF	high-power field		heart rate
HPFH	hereditary persistence of fetal hemoglobin		hemorrhagic retinopathy
			hospital record
HPG	human pituitary gonadotropin		hour
		Hr 0	zero hour (when treatment starts)
HPI	history of present illness		
HPL	human placenta lactogen	Hr -2	minus two hours (two hours prior to treatment)
	hyperplexia		
HPLC	high-pressure (performance) liquid chromatography		
		H & R	hysterectomy and radiation
HPM	hemiplegic migraine	HRA	high right atrium
HPN	home parenteral nutrition		histamine releasing activity
HPNS	high pressure nervous syndrome		
		H2RA	H2-receptor antagonist
HPO	hydrophilic ointment	HRC	Human Rights Committee
	hypertrophic pulmonary osteoarthropathy	HRCT	high-resolution computed tomography
HPOA	hypertrophic pulmonary osteoarthropathy	HRD	human retroviral disease
		HRE	high-resolution electrocardiography
2HPP	2-hour postprandial (blood sugar)		
		HRF	Harris return flow
2HPPBS	2-hour postprandial blood sugar		health-related facility
			histamine releasing factor
HPPM	hyperplastic persistent pupillary membrane	HRIF	histamine inhibitory releasing factor
HPS	hantavirus pulmonary syndrome	HRL	head rotated left
		HRLA	human reovirus-like agent
	hypertrophic pyloric stenosis	HRLM	high-resolution light microscopy
HPT	heparin protamine titration	hRLX-2	synthetic human relaxin
	histamine provocation test	HRMPC	hormone-refractory metastatic prostate cancer
	hyperparathyroidism		

HRNB	Halstead-Reitan Neuropsychological Battery		hypersomnia-sleep apnea
		HSB	husband
HRP	high-risk pregnancy	HSBG	heel stick blood gas
	horseradish peroxidase	HSC	hematopoietic stem cell
HRP-2	histidine-rich protein-2	HSCL	Hopkins Symptom Check List
HRPC	hormone-refractory prostate cancer	HSD	hypoactive sexual desire (disorder)
HRQL	health-related quality of life	HSE	herpes simplex encephalitis
HRQOL	health-related quality of life	HSES	hemorrhagic shock and encephalopathy
HRR	head rotated right	HSG	herpes simplex genitalis
HRRC	Human Research Review Committee		hysterosalpingogram
HRS	Haw River syndrome	H-SIL	high-grade squamous intraepithelial lesions
	hepatorenal syndrome	HSK	herpes simplex keratitis
HRSD	Hamilton Rating Scale for Depression	HSL	herpes simplex labialis
			hormone sensitive lipase
HRST	heat, reddening, swelling, or tenderness	HSM	hepatosplenomegaly
			holosystolic murmur
HRT	heart rate	HSN	Hansen-Street nail
	heparin response test		heart sounds normal
	high-risk transfer	HSP	heat shock protein
	hormone replacement therapy		Henoch-Schönlein purpura
HS	bedtime		hysterosalpingography
	half strength	HSPE	high-strength pancreatic enzymes
	hamstrings		
	hamstring sets	HSQ	Health Status Questionnaire
	Hartman's solution (lactated Ringer's)	HSR	heated serum reagin
	heart size	HSSE	high soap suds enema
	heart sounds	HS-tk	herpes simplex thymidine kinase
	heavy smoker		
	heel spur	HSV	herpes simplex virus
	heel stick		highly selective vagotomy
	hereditary spherocytosis	HSV1	herpes simplex virus type 1
	herpes simplex		
	high school	HSV2	herpes simplex virus type 2
	hippocampal sclerosis		
	Hurlers syndrome	HSVE	herpes simplex virus encephalitis
H→S	heel to shin		
H&S	hearing and speech	HT	hammertoe
	hemorrhage and shock		hearing test
	hysterectomy and sterilization		heart
			heart transplant
HSA	Health Systems Agency		height
	human serum albumin		high temperature

	hormonotherapy		hypertensive urgencies
	hyperthermia		hydroxyurea
	Hubbard tank	Hu	Hounsfield units
	hypermetropia	HUCB	human umbilical cord blood
	hyperopia		
	hypertension	HUH	Humana Hospital
	hyperthyroid	HUIFM	human leukocyte interferon meloy
H/T	heel and toe (walking)		
H&T	hospitalization and treatment	HUK	human urinary kallikrein
H(T)	intermittent hypertropia	HUM	heat, ultrasound, and massage
5-HT	serotonin (5-hydroxytryptamine)	HUM 70/30	human insulin, regular 30 units/mL with human insulin isophane suspension 70 units/mL (Humulin® 70/30 insulin)
ht. aer.	heated aerosol		
HTAT	human tetanus antitoxin		
HTB	hot tub bath		
HTC	heated tracheostomy collar	HUM L	human insulin zinc suspension (Humulin® L Insulin)
	hypertensive crisis		
HTF	house tube feeding	HUM N	human insulin isophane suspension (Humulin® N Insulin)
HTGL	hepatic triglyceride lipase		
HTK	heel to knee		
HTL	hearing threshold level	HUM R	human insulin, regular (Humulin® R Insulin)
	human T-cell leukemia		
	human thymic leukemia	HUR	hydroxyurea
HTLV III	human T-cell lymphotrophic virus type III	HUS	head ultrasound
			hemolytic uremic syndrome
HTM	*Haemophilus* test medium		husband
	high threshold mechanoceptors	husb	husband
HTN	hypertension	HUT	hyperplasia of usual type
HTO	high tibia osteotomy		
HTP	House-Tree-Person-test	HUVEC	human umbilical vein endothelial cells
5-HTP	serotonin (5-hydroxytryptophan)		
HTS	head traumatic syndrome	HV	hallux valgus
	heel-to-shin		Hantavirus
	Hematest® stools		has voided
HTSCA	human tumor stem cell assay		Hemovac®
			hepatic vein
H-TSH	human thyroid-stimulating hormone		herpesvirus
			home visit
HTT	hand thrust test	H&V	hemigastrecotomy and vagotomy
HTV	herpes-type virus		
HTVD	hypertensive vascular disease	HVA	homovanillic acid
		HVD	hypertensive vascular disease
HTX	hemothorax		
HU	head unit	HVDO	hypovitaminosis D osteopathy

HVE	high voltage electrophoresis	HZO	herpes zoster ophthalmicus
HVES	high voltage electrical stimulation	HZV	herpes zoster virus
HVF	Humphrey visual field		
HVGS	high volt galvanic stimulation		
HVL	half value layer hippocampal volume loss		**I**
HVOO	hepatic venous outflow obstruction		
HVPC	high voltage pulsed current		
HVPG	hepatic venous pressure gradient	I	impression incisal
HYPT	hyperventilation provocation test		independent initial
HVS	hyperventilation syndrome		inspiration intact (bag of waters)
HW	heparin well homework		intermediate iris
	housewife		one
HWB	hot water bottle	I_2	iodine
HWFE	housewife	I^{131}	radioactive iodine
HWG	has worn glasses	I-3+7	idarubicin and cytarabine
HWH	halfway house	IA	incidental appendectomy
HWP	hot wet pack		incurred accidentally
HWPG	has worn prescription glasses		intra-amniotic intra-arterial
Hx	history hospitalization	I & A	irrigation and aspiration
HXM	altretamine (hexamethylmelamine)	IAA	ileoanal anastomosis insulin autoantibodies
Hx & Px	history and physical (examination)		interrupted aortic arch
Hy	hypermetropia	IAB	incomplete abortion induced abortion
HYDRO	hydronephrosis hydrotherapy	IABC	intra-aortic balloon counterpulsation
HYG	hygiene	IABP	intra-aortic balloon
Hyper Al	hyperalimentation		counterpulsation
Hyper K	hyperkalemia		intra-aortic balloon pump
HYPER T & A	hypertrophic tonsils and adenoids	IAC	internal auditory canal intra-arterial
HYPO	hypodermic injection injection		chemotherapy isolated adrenal cell
Hypo K	hypokalemia	IAC-CPR	interposed abdominal
hypopit	hypopituitarism		compressions—cardio-
Hyst	hysterectomy		pulmonary resuscitation
Hz	Hertz	IACG	intermittent angle-closure
HZ	herpes zoster		glaucoma

IACP	intra-aortic counterpulsation	IBC	invasive bladder cancer
			iron binding capacity
IAD	intractable atopic dermatitis	IBD	infectious bursal disease
			inflammatory bowel disease
IADHS	inappropriate antidiuretic hormone syndrome	IBDQ	Inflammatory Bowel Disease Questionnaire
IADL	Instrumental Activities of Daily Living	IBG	iliac bone graft
IA DSA	intra-arterial digital subtraction arteriography	IBI	intermittent bladder irrigation
		ibid	at the same place
IAGT	indirect antiglobulin test	IBILI	indirect bilirubin
IAHA	immune adherence hemagglutination	IBM	inclusion body myositis
		IBMI	initial body mass index
IAHD	idiopathic acquired hemolytic disease	IBMTR	International Bone Marrow Transplant Registry
IAI	intra-abdominal infection intra-amniotic infection	IBNR	incurred but not reported
IAM	internal auditory meatus	IBOW	intact bag of waters
IAN	intern's admission note	IBPS	Insall-Burstein posterior stabilizer
IAO	immediately after onset	IBR	immediate breast reconstruction
IAP	independent adjudicating panel		infectious bovine rhinotracheitis
	intermittent acute porphyria	IBRS	Inpatient Behavior Rating Scale
IARC	International Agency for Research on Cancer	IBS	irritable bowel syndrome
IART	intra-atrial reentrant tachycardia	IBT	ink blot test (Rorschach test)
IAS	intermittent androgen suppression	IBTR	intra-breast tumor recurrence
	internal anal sphincter idiopathic ankylosing spondylitis	IBU	ibuprofen
IASD	interatrial septal defect	IBW	ideal body weight
IAT	immunoaugmentive therapy	IC	between meals
			immune complex
	indirect antiglobulin test		immunocompromised
IAV	intermittent assist ventilation		incipient cataract (grade 1+ to 4+)
IB	ileal bypass		incomplete
	insulin receptor binding test		indirect calorimetry
			indirect Coombs (test)
	isolation bed		individual counseling
IBAM	idiopathic bile acid malabsorption		inspiratory capacity
			intensive care
IBBB	intra-blood-brain barrier		intercostal
IBBBB	incomplete bilateral bundle branch block		intercourse
			intermediate care

124

	intermittent catheterization		Classification of Diseases, 9th Revision, Clinical Modification
	interstitial changes		
	interstitial cystitis	ICDO	International Classification of Diseases for Oncology
	intracerebral		
	intracranial		
	intraincisional	ICE	ice, compression, and elevation
	irritable colon		
I/C	imipenem-cilastatin (Primaxin®)		ifosfamide, carboplatin, and etoposide
ICA	ileocolic anastomosis		individual career exploration
	intermediate care area		
	internal carotid artery		interleukin-1 alpha converting enzyme
	intracranial aneurysm		
	islet-cell antibody		interleukin-1 beta converting enzyme
ICAM	intracellular adhesion molecule	+ ice	add ice
ICAM-1	intercellular adhesion molecule-1	ICES	ice, compression, elevation, and support
ICAO	internal carotid artery occlusion	ICF	intermediate care facility
			intracellular fluid
ICAS	intermediate coronary artery syndrome	ICG	indocyanine green
		ICGA	indocyanine green angiography
ICAT	infant cardiac arrest tray		
ICB	intracranial bleeding	ICH	immunocompromised host
ICBG	iliac crest bone graft		intracerebral hemorrhage
ICBT	intercostobronchial trunk		intracranial hemorrhage
ICC	immunocytochemistry	ICIT	intensified conventional insulin therapy
	Indian childhood cirrhosis		
	intraclass correlation coefficient	ICL	intracorneal lens
		ICLE	intracapsular lens extraction
	islet cell carcinoma		
ICCE	intracapsular cataract extraction	ICM	intercostal muscle
			intracostal margin
ICCU	intensive coronary care unit	ICN	infection control nurse
			intensive care nursery
	intermediate coronary care unit	ICN2	neonatal intensive care unit level II
ICD	implantable cardioverter defibrillator	ICP	intracranial pressure
		ICPP	intubated continuous positive pressure
	indigocarmine dye		
	instantaneous cardiac death	ICR	intercostal retractions
			intrastromal corneal ring
	isocitrate dehydrogenase	ICRF-159	razoxane
	irritant contact dermatitis	ICS	inhaled corticosteroid(s)
ICDB	incomplete database		ileocecal sphincter
ICDC	implantable cardioverter defibrillator catheter		intercostal space
		ICSH	interstitial cell-stimulating hormone
ICD 9 CM	International		

ICSI	intracytoplasmic sperm injection	IDCF	immunodiffusion complement fixation
ICSR	intercostal space retractions	IDD	iodine-deficiency disorders
ICT	icterus		insulin-dependent diabetes
	indirect Coombs' test	IDDM	insulin-dependent diabetes mellitus
	inflammation of connective tissue	IDDS	implantable drug delivery system
	intensive conventional therapy	IDE	Investigational Device Exemption
	intermittent cervical traction	IDFC	immature dead female child
	intracranial tumor	IDH	isocitric dehydrogenase
	intracutaneous test	IDI	Interpersonal Dependency Inventory
	islet cell transplant		
ICTX	intermittent cervical traction		intrathecal drug infusion
ICU	intensive care unit	IDK	internal derangement of knee
	intermediate care unit	IDL	intermediate-density lipoprotein
ICV	intracerebroventricular		
ICVH	ischemic cerebrovascular headache	IDM	infant of a diabetic mother
ICW	in connection with	IDMC	immature dead male child
	intercellular water	IDP	initiate discharge planning
ID	identification		inosine diphosphate
	identify	IDPN	intradialytic parenteral nutrition
	idiotype		
	ifosfamide, mesna uroprotection, and doxorubicin	IDR	idarubicin
			idiosyncratic drug reaction
	immunodiffusion		intradermal reaction
	induction delivery	IDS	infectious disease service
	infectious disease (physician or department)		integrated delivery system
		IDT	intradermal test
	initial diagnosis	IDTP	immunodiffusion tube precipitin
	initial dose		
	intradermal	IDU	idoxuridine
id	the same		infectious disease unit
I & D	incision and drainage		injecting drug user
IDA	idarubicin	IDV	indinavir (Crixivan)
	iron deficiency anemia		intermittent demand ventilation
IDAM	infant of drug abusing mother	IDVC	indwelling venous catheter
IDB	incomplete database	IE	immunoelectrophoresis
IDC	idiopathic dilated cardiomyopathy		induced emesis
			infective endocarditis
	invasive ductal cancer		inner ear

	international unit (European abbreviation)	IFNB	interferon beta-1 b (Betaseron®)
I & E	ingress and egress (tubes)	IFO	ifosfamide
i.e.	that is	IFOS	ifosfamide
I&E	internal and external	IFP	inflammatory fibroid polyps
IEC	independent ethics committee	IFSE	internal fetal scalp electrode
	inpatient exercise center	IgA	immunoglobulin A
IEF	isoelectric focusing	IGCS	inpatient geriatric consultation services
IEL	intestinal-intraepithelial lymphocyte	IgD	immunoglobulin D
IEM	immune electron microscopy	IGDE	idiopathic gait disorders of the elderly
	inborn errors of metabolism	IGDM	infant of gestational diabetic mother
iEMG	integrated electromyography	IgE	immunoglobulin E
IEP	immunoelectrophoresis	IGF-I	insulin-like growth factor I
	Individualized Education Plan	IgG	immunoglobulin G
IEPA	immunoelectrophoresis analysis	IGIM	immune globulin intramuscular
I:E ratio	inspiratory to expiratory time ratio	IGIV	immune globulin intravenous
IET	infantile estropia	IgM	immunoglobulin M
IF	idiopathic flushing	IGP	interstitial glycoprotein
	ifosfamide	IGR	intrauterine growth retardation
	immunofluorescence	IGT	impaired glucose tolerance
	injury factor		
	interferon	IGTN	ingrown toenail
	interfrontal	IH	indirect hemagglutination
	intermaxillary fixation		infectious hepatitis
	internal fixation		inguinal hernia
	intrinsic factor	IHA	immune hemolytic anemia
	involved field (radiotherapy)		indirect hemagglutination
IFA	indirect fluorescent antibody immunofluorescent assay		infusion hepatic arteriography
		IHC	idiopathic hypercalciuria
IFAT	immunofluorescence antibody test (technique)		immobilization hypercalcemia
			immunohistochemistry
IFE	immunofixation electrophoresis		inner hair cell (in cochlea)
	in-flight emergency	IHD	intraheptic duct (ule)
IFM	internal fetal monitoring		ischemic heart disease
IFN	interferon	IHDN	integrated health delivery network
		IHH	idiopathic hypogona-

	dotrophic hypogo-		interleukin (1, 2, and 3)
	nadism		intralesional
IHO	idiopathic hypertrophic		Intralipid®
	osteoarthropathy	ILA	insulin-like activity
IHP	idiopathic hypoparathy-	ILBBB	incomplete left bundle
	roidism		branch block
IHPH	intrahepatic portal	ILBW	infant, low birth weight
	hypertension	ILC	invasive lobular cancer
IHR	inguinal hernia repair	ILD	intermediate density
	intrinsic heart rate		lipoproteins
IHS	Indian Health Service		interstitial lung disease
	Iodiopathic Headache		ischemic leg disease
	Score	ILE	infantile lobar emphysema
IHs	iris hamartomas	ILF	indicated low forceps
IHSA	iodinated human serum	ILFC	immature living female
	albumin		child
IHSS	idiopathic hypertrophic	ILM	internal limiting
	subaortic stenosis		membrane
IHT	insulin hypoglycemia test	ILMC	immature living male
IHW	inner heel wedge		child
II	internal iliac (artery)	ILMI	inferolateral myocardial
IIA	internal iliac artery		infarct
IICP	increased intracranial	ILP	interstitial laser
	pressure		photocoagulation
IICU	infant intensive care unit	ILQTS	idiopathic long QT
IIH	idiopathic infantile		(interval) syndrome
	hypercalcemia	ILVEN	inflammatory linear
IIH	iodine-induced		verrucal epidermal
	hyperthyroidism		nevus
IIHT	iodide-induced	IM	ice massage
	hyperthyroidism		infectious mononucleosis
IIP	idiopathic interstitial		intermetatarsal
	pneumonitis		internal medicine
IIPF	idiopathic interstitial		intramedullary
	pulmonary fibrosis		intramuscular
IJ	ileojejunal	IMA	inferior mesenteric
	internal jugular		artery
I&J	insight and judgment		internal mammary artery
IJC	internal jugular catheter	IMAC	ifosfamide, mesna
IJD	inflammatory joint disease		uroprotection,
IJO	idiopathic juvenile		doxorubicin
	osteoporosis		(Adriamycin), and
IJP	internal jugular pressure		cisplatin
IJR	idiojunctional rhythm	IMAE	internal maxillary artery
IJT	idiojunctional tachycardia		embolization
IJV	internal jugular vein	IMAG	internal mammary artery
IK	immobilized knee		graft
	interstitial keratitis	IMARD	immunomodulating
IL	immature lungs		antirheumatic drugs

IMB	intermenstrual bleeding		immunosuppressants
IMC	intermittent catheterization	IMT	inspiratory muscle training
	intramedullary catheter		intima to media (wall) thickness
IMCU	intermediate care unit		
IME	independent medical examination	IMU	intermediate medicine unit
IMF	idiopathic myelofibrosis	IMV	inferior mesenteric vein
	ifosfamide, mesna uroprotection, methotrexate, and fluorouracil		intermittent mandatory ventilation
			intermittent mechanical ventilation
	immobilization	IMVP-16	ifosfamide, mesna uroprotection, methotrexate, and etoposide
	mandibular fracture		
	inframammary fold		
	intermaxillary fixation		
IMG	internal medicine group	IN	insulin
IMGU	insulin-mediated glucose uptake		intranasal
IMH	idiopathic myocardial hypertrophy	In	inches
			indium
IMH test	indirect microhemagglutination test	INAD	in no apparent distress
		INC	incisal
IMI	imipramine		incision
	impending myocardial infarction		incomplete
			incontinent
	inferior myocardial infarction		increase
			inside-the-needle catheter
	intramuscular injection	Inc Spir	incentive spirometer
^{131}I-MIBG	iodine^{131}-metaiodobenzylguanidine (iobenguane ^{131}I)	IND	induced
			Investigational New Drug (application)
IMIG	intramuscular immunoglobulin	INDA	Investigational New Drug Application
IMLC	incomplete mitral leaflet closure	INDM	infant of nondiabetic mother
IMM	immunizations	INDO	indomethacin
IMN	internal mammary (lymph) node	^{111}In-DTPA	indium pentetate
IMP	impacted	INE	infantile necrotizing encephalomyelopathy
	important		
	impression	INEX	inexperienced
	improved	INF	infant
	inosine monophoshate		infarction
IMPX	impaction		infected
IMR	infant mortality rate		infection
IMRA	immunoradiometric assay		inferior
IMS	incurred in military service		information
			infused

	infusion		intraoperative
	intravenous nutritional		cholangiogram
	fluid	IOCG	intraoperative
INFC	infected		cholangiogram
	infection	IOD	interorbital distance
ING	inguinal	IODM	infant of diabetic
✔ ing	checking		mother
INH	isoniazid	IOF	intraocular fluid
INI	intranuclear inclusion	IOFB	intraocular foreign body
inj	injection	IOFNA	intraoperative fine needle
	injury		aspiration
INK	injury not known	IOH	idiopathic orthostatic
INN	International		hypotension
	Nonproprietary Name	IOI	intraosseous infusion
INO	internuclear ophthal-	IOL	intraocular lens
	moplegia	IOLI	intraocular lens
INOP	internodal ophthal-		implantation
	moplegia	ION	ischemic optic neuropathy
inpt	inpatient	IONIS	indirect optic nerve injury
INQ	inferior nasal quadrant		syndrome
INR	international normalized	IONTO	iontophoresis
	ratio (for anticoagulant	IOP	intraocular pressure
	monitoring)	IOR	ideas of reference
INS	idiopathic nephrotic		inferior oblique recession
	syndrome	IO-RB	intraocular retinoblastoma
	insurance	IORT	intraoperative radiation
INST	instrumental delivery		therapy
INT	intermittent needle	IOS	intraoperative sonography
	therapy	IOT	intraocular tension
	internal	IOUS	intraocular ultrasound
Int mon	internal monitor	IOV	initial office visit
INTERP	interpretation	IP	ice pack
Int Med	internal medicine		incubation period
intol	intolerance		individualized plan
int-rot	internal rotation		in plaster
int trx	intermittent traction		interphalangeal
intub	intubation		interstitial pneumonia
inver	inversion		intestinal permeability
INVOS	in vivo optical		intraperitoneal
	spectroscopy	I/P	iris/pupil
IO	inferior oblique	IP3	inositol triphosphate
	initial opening	IPA	independent practice
	intestinal obstruction		association
	intraocular pressure		interpleural analgesia
	intra-Ommaya		invasive pulmonary
	intraoperative		aspergillosis
I&O	intake and output		isopropyl alcohol
IOA	intact on admission	IPAA	ileo-pouch anal
IOC	intern on call		anastamosis

IPAP	inspiratory positive airway pressure	IPN	infantile periarteritis nodosa
IPB	infrapopliteal bypass		intern's progress note
IPC	indirect pulp cavity		interstitial pneumonia
	intermittent pneumatic compression (boots)	IPOF	immediate postoperative fitting
	intraperitoneal chemotherapy	IPOP	immediate postoperative prosthesis
IPCD	idiopathic paroxysmal cerebral dysrhythmia	IPP	inflatable penile prosthesis
	infantile polycystic disease		intrapleual pressure
IPCK	infantile polycystic kidney (disease)		isolated pelvic perfusion
IPD	idiopathic Parkinson's disease	IPPA	inspection, palpation, percussion, and auscultation
	immediate pigment darkening	IPPB	intermittent positive pressure breathing
	inflammatory pelvic disease	IPPF	immediate postoperative prosthetic fitting
	intermittent peritoneal dialysis	IPPI	interruption of pregnancy for psychiatric indication
	interpupillary distance	IPPV	intermittent positive pressure ventilation
IPF	idiopathic pulmonary fibrosis	IPS	infundibular pulmonic stenosis
	interstitial pulmonary fibrosis		initial prognostic score
IPFD	intrapartum fetal distress		intermittent photic stimulation
IPG	impedance plethysmography	IPSF	immediate postsurgical fitting
	individually polymerized grass	IPSID	immunoproliferative small intestinal disease
IPH	idiopathic pulmonary hemosiderosis	IPSP	inhibitory postsynaptic potential
	interphalangeal	I PSY	intermediate psychiatry
	intraparenchymal hemorrhage	IPT	intermittent pelvic traction
IPHP	intraperitoneal hyperthermic chemotherapy	iPTH	parathyroid hormone by radioimmunoassay
IPI	International Prognostic Index	IPTX	intermittent pelvic traction
IPJ	interphalangeal joint	IPV	inactivated poliovirus vaccine
IPK	intractable plantar keratosis	IPVC	interpolated premature ventricular contraction
IPM	intrauterine pressure monitor	IPW	interphalangeal width
		IQ	intelligence quotient
IPMI	inferoposterior myocardial infarct	IQR	interquartile range
		IR	immediate-release (tablets)

	inferior rectus	IROS	ipsilateral routing of
	infrared		signals
	insulin resistance	IRR	infrared radiation
	internal reduction		intrarenal reflux
	internal resistance		irregular rate and rhythm
	internal rotation	IRRC	Institutional Research
I&R	insertion and removal		Review Committee
IRA-EEA	ileorectal anastomoses	irreg	irregular
	with end-to-end	IRR	irreversible hydrocolloid
	anastomosis	HYDRO	
IRAP	interleukin-1 receptor	IRS	Information and Referral
	antagonist protein		Society
IRB	Institutional Review	IRSB	intravenous regional
	Board		sympathetic block
IRBBB	incomplete right bundle	IRT	immunoreactive trypsin
	branch block	IRV	inspiratory reserve
IRBC	immature red blood cell		volume
	irradiated red blood cells		inverse ratio ventilation
IRBP	interphotoreceptor	IS	incentive spirometer
	retinoid-binding protein		induced sputum
IRC	indirect radionuclide		*in situ*
	cystography		intercostal space
	Institutional Review		inventory of systems
	Committee (Board)		ipecac syrup
IRCU	intensive respiratory care	I-S	Ionescu-Shiley (prosthetic
	unit		heart valve)
IRD	immune renal disease(s)	I/S	instruct/supervise
IRDM	insulin-resistant diabetes	ISA	ileosigmoid anastomosis
	mellitus		Incest Survivors
IRDS	idiopathic respiratory		Anonymous
	distress syndrome		intrinsic sympathomimetic
	infant respiratory distress		activity
	syndrome	ISADH	inappropriate secretion of
IRE	internal rotation in		antidiuretic hormone
	extension	ISB	incentive spirometry
IRED	infrared emission		breathing
	detection	ISBP	interscalen brachial plexus
IRF	internal rotation in	ISC	indwelling subclavian
	flexion		catheter
IRH	intraretinal hemorrhage		infant servo-control
IRI	immunoreactive insulin		infant skin control
IRIV	immunopotentiating		intermittent straight
	reconstituted influenza		catheterization
	virosomes		isolette servo-control
IRMA	immunoradiometric assay	I/SCN	urinary iodine/thiocyanate
	intraretinal microvascular		ratio
	abnormalities	ISCOM	immunostimulating
IRMS	isotope-ratio mass		complex
	spectrometry	ISCs	irreversible sickle cells

ISD	inhibited sexual desire	ISU	intermediate surgical unit
	initial sleep disturbance	ISW	interstitial water
	isosorbide dinitrate	IS10W	10% invert sugar injection (in water)
	intrinsic (urethral) sphincter deficiency	ISWI	incisional surgical wound infection
ISDN	isosorbide dinitrate	IT	incentive therapy
ISE	ion-sensitive electrode		individual therapy
ISEL	*in situ* end labeling		inferior-temporal
ISF	interstitial fluid		Inhalation Therapist
ISG	immune serum globulin (immune globulin)		inhalation therapy
			intensive therapy
ISH	isolated systolic hypertension		intermittent traction
			intertrochanteric
ISHT	isolated systolic hypertension		intertuberous
			intrathecal (dangerous)
ISI	International Sensitivity Index		intratracheal (dangerous, could be interupted as intrathecal)
ISK	isokinetic	ITA	individual treatment assessment
ISMA	infantile spinal muscular atrophy		inferior temporal artery
ISMN	isosorbide mononitrate	ITAG	internal thoracic artery graft
ISMO®	isosorbide mononitrate		
ISO	isodose	ITB	iliotibial band
	isolette	ITC	Incontinence Treatment Center
	isoproterenol		
ISOE	isoetharine	ITCP	idiopathic thrombocytopenic purpura
ISOK	isokinetic		
ISOM	isometric	ITCU	intensive thoracic cardiovascular unit
ISOs	isoenzymes		
ISP	interspace	ITE	insufficient therapeutic effect
ISQ	as before; continue on (*in status quo*)		in-the-ear (hearing aid)
		ITFF	intertrochanteric femoral fracture
ISR	integrated secretory response		
		ITGV	intrathoracic gas volume
ISS	idiopathic short stature	ITMTX	intrathecal methotrexate
	Injury Severity Score	ITOP	intentional termination of pregnancy
	Individual Self-Rating Scale		
		ITP	idiopathic thrombocytopenic purpura
	irritable stomach syndrome		
			interim treatment plan
	Integrated Summary of Safety	ITPA	Illinois Test of Psycholinguistic Ability
IS10S	10% invert sugar in 0.9% sodium chloride (saline) injection	ITQ	inferior temporal quadrant
		ITR	isotretinoin
IST	injection sclerotherapy	ITRA	itraconazole
	insulin sensitivity test		
	insulin shock therapy		

ITSCU	infant-toddler special care unit	IVA	Intervir-A
ITT	identical twins (raised) together	IVAD	implantable venous access device
	insulin tolerance test		implantable vascular access device
	intention-to-treat (analysis)	IVBAT	intravascular bronchoalveolar tumor
ITU	infant-toddler unit	IVC	inferior vena cava
ITVAD	indwelling transcutaneous vascular access device		inspiratory vital capacity
			intravenous chemotherapy
ITX	immunotoxin(s)		intravenous cholangio-gram
IU	international unit (this is a dangerous abbreviation as it is read as intravenous)		intraventricular catheter
		IVCD	intraventricular conduction defect (delay)
IUC	intrauterine catheter		
IUCD	intrauterine contraceptive device	IVCP	inferior vena cava pressure
IUD	intrauterine death	IVCV	inferior venacavography
	intrauterine device	IVD	intervertebral disk
IUDR	idoxuridine		intravenous drip
IUFB	intrauterine foreign body	IVDA	intravenous drug abuse
IUFD	intrauterine fetal death	IVDSA	intravenous digital subtraction angiography
	intrauterine fetal distress		
IUFT	intrauterine fetal transfusion	IVDU	intravenous drug user
		IVET	*in vivo* expression technology
IUGR	intrauterine growth retardation		
		IVF	intervertebral foramina
IUI	intrauterine insemination		*in vitro* fertilization
IUP	intrauterine pregnancy		intravenous fluid(s)
IUPC	intrauterine pressure catheter	IVFA	intravenous fluorescein angiography
IUPD	intrauterine pregnancy delivered	IVFE	intravenous fat emulsion
		IVF-ET	*in vitro* fertilization-embryo transfer
IUP,TBCS	intrauterine pregnancy, term birth, cesarean section		
		IVFT	intravenous fetal transfusion
IUP,TBLC	intrauterine pregnancy, term birth, living child	IVGG	intravenous gamma globulin
IUR	intrauterine retardation	IVGTT	intravenous glucose tolerance test
IUT	intrauterine transfusion		
IUTD	immunizations up to date	IVH	intravenous hyperalimen-tation
IV	four		
	interview		intraventricular hemorrhage
	intravenous (i.v.)		
	intravertebral	IVIG	intravenous immunoglob-ulin
	invasive		
	symbol for class 4 controlled substances	IVJC	intervertebral joint complex

IVL	intravenous lock	IWMI	inferior wall myocardial infarct
IVLBW	infant of very low birth weight	IWML	idiopathic white matter lesion
IVO	intraoral vertical osteotomy	IWT	ice-water test
IVOX	intravascular oxygenator (oxygenation)		impacted wisdom teeth
IVP	intravenous push (this is a dangerous meaning as it is read as intravenous pyelogram)		
	intravenous pyelogram		
IVPB	intravenous piggyback		
IVPF	isovolume pressure flow		
IVPU	intravenous push		
IVR	idioventricular rhythm		
	intravenous retrograde		

J

	intravenous rider (this is a dangerous abbreviation as it has been read as IVP-IV push)	J	Jaeger measure of near vision with 20/20 about equal to J1
	isovolumic relaxation (time)		jejunostomy
IVRAP	intravenous retrograde access port		Jewish
			joint
IVRG	intravenous retrograde		joule
IV-RNV	intravenous radionuclide venography		juice
IVRO	intraoral vertical ramus osteotomy	Jack	jacknife position
		JAMA	*Journal of the American Medical Association*
IVS	intraventricular septum	JAMG	juvenile autoimmune myasthenia gravis
	irritable voiding syndrome		
IVSD	intraventricular septal defect	JAR	junior assistant resident
IVSE	interventricular septal excursion	JARAN	junior assistant resident admission note
IVSO	intraoral vertical segmental osteotomy	JBE	Japanese B encephalitis
		JC	junior clinicians (medical students)
IVSS	intravenous Soluset®		
IVT	intravenous transfusion	JCAHO	Joint Commission on Accreditation of Healthcare Organizations
IVTTT	intravenous tolbutamide tolerance test		
IVU	intravenous urography (urogram)		
		JCOG	Japanese Clinical Oncology Group
IVUC	intravenous ultrasound catheter	JD	jaundice
IVUS	intravascular ultrasound	JDG	jugulodigastric
IWI	inferior wall infarction	JDM	juvenile diabetes mellitus
IWL	insensible water loss		

JDMS	juvenile dermatomyositis	JRAN	junior resident admission note
JE	Japanese encephalitis		
JEB	junctional escape beat	Jr BF	junior baby food
JEJ	jejunum	JRC	joint replacement center
JER	junctional escape rhythm	JT	jejunostomy tube
JET	junctional ectopic tachycardia		joint
			junctional tachycardia
JF	joint fluid	JTF	jejunostomy tube feeding
JFS	Jewish Family Service	JTP	joint projection
JGCT	juvenile granulosa cell tumor	JTPS	juvenile tropical pancreatitis syndrome
JHR	Jarisch-Herxheimer reaction	J-Tube	jejunostomy tube
		JUV	juvenile
JI	jejunoileal	JV	jugular vein
JIB	jejunoileal bypass	JVC	jugular venous catheter
JIS	juvenile idiopathic scoliosis	JVD	jugular venous distention
		JVP	jugular venous pressure
JJ	jaw jerk		jugular venous pulsation
JLP	juvenile laryngeal papillomatosis		jugular venous pulse
		JVPT	jugular venous pulse tracing
JM-9	iproplatin		
JMS	junior medical student	JW	Jehovah's Witness
JNCL	juvenile-onset neuronal ceroid lipofuscinosis	Jx	joint
		JXG	juvenile xanthogranuloma
JND	just noticeable difference		
JNT	joint		
JNVD	jugular neck vein distention		
JODM	juvenile onset diabetes mellitus		
JOMAC	judgment, orientation, memory, abstraction, and calculation		
JOMACI	judgment, orientation, memory, abstraction, and calculation intact	**K**	
		K	cornea
			kelvin
JP	Jackson-Pratt (drain)		ketamine (Super K)
	Jobst pump		Kosher
	joint protection		potassium
JPB	junctional premature beats		thousand
			vitamin K
JP BS	Jackson-Pratt to bulb suction	K'	knee
		K+	potassium
JPC	junctional premature contraction	K_1	phytonadione
		K_3	menadione
JPS	joint position sense	K_4	menadiol sodium diphosphate
JR	junctional rhythm		
JRA	juvenile rheumatoid arthritis	17K	17-ketosteroids
		KA	keratoacanthoma

	ketoacidosis	KEVD	Krupin eye valve
Ka	first order absorption constant in hr.$^{-1}$		with disk
		KF	kidney function
KAB	knowledge, attitude, and behavior	KFA	kinetic fibrinogen assay
		KFAB	kidney-fixing antibodies
K-ABC	Kaufman Assessment Battery for Children	KFAO	knee-foot-ankle orthosis
		KFD	Kyasanur Forrest disease
KABINS	knowledge, attitude, behavior, and improvement in nutritional status	KFR	Kayser-Fleischer ring
		KFS	Klippel-Feil syndrome
		kg	kilogram
		K-G	Kimray-Greenfield (filter)
KAFO	knee-ankle-foot orthosis	KGF	keratinocyte growth factor
KAO	knee-ankle orthosis		
KAS	Katz Adjustment Scale	KGC	Keflin®, gentamicin, and carbenicillin
KASH	knowledge, abilities, skills, and habits		
		KHF	Korean hemorrhagic fever
kat	katal	K24H	potassium, urine 24 hour
K-A units	King-Armstrong units		
KB	ketone bodies	KI	karyopyknotic index
KC	keratoconjunctivitis		knee immobilizer
	keratoconus		potassium iodide
	knees to chest	KID	keratitis, ichthyosis, and deafness (syndrome)
	Korean conflict		
kcal	kilocalorie		kidney
KCCT	kaolin cephalin clotting time	kilo	kilogram
			thousand
kCi	kilocurie	KISS	saturated solution of potassium iodide
KCl	potassium chloride		
KCS	keratoconjunctivitis sicca	KIT	Kahn Intelligence Test
		KIU	kallikrein inhibitor units
KCZ	ketoconazole	KJ	kilojoule
KD	Kawasaki's disease		knee jerk
	Keto Diastix®	KK	knee kick
	kidney donors	KL-BET	Kleihauer-Betke
	knee disarticulation	KPE	Kemper phako-emulsification
Kd	kilodalton		
KDA	known drug allergies	Kleb	*Klebsiella*
KDC®	brand name of infant warmer	KLH	keyhole limpet hemocyanin
		K-Lor®	potassium chloride tablets
KDU	Kidney Dialysis Unit	KLS	kidneys, liver, and spleen
KE	first order elimination rate constant in hr.$^{-1}$	KM	kanamycin
		KMnO$_4$	potassium permanganate
KED	Kendrick extrication device	KMV	killed measles vaccine
		KN	knee
^{k}el	elimination rate constant	KNO	keep needle open
KET	ketoconazole	KO	keep open
	ketones		knee orthosis
17 Keto	17 ketosteroids		knocked out
keV	kilo-electron volts		

KOH	potassium hydroxide	K-wire	Kirschner wire
KOR	keep open rate		
KP	hot pack		
	keratoprecipitate		
	kinetic perimetry		
KPE	Kelman phacoemulsification		
KPM	kilopounds per minute		
KPS	Karnofsky performance status (scores)		
Kr	krypton		
K-rod	Küntscher rod	L	fifty
KS	Kawasaki syndrome		left
	Kaposi's sarcoma		lente insulin
	Klinefelter's syndrome		levorotatory
17-KS	17-ketosteroids		lingual
KSA	knowledge, skills, and abilities		liter
			liver
KSHV	Kaposi's sarcoma-associated herpesvirus		lumbar
			lung
KS/OI	Kaposi's sarcoma and opportunistic infections	l	levorotatory
		L'	lumbar
KSR	potassium chloride sustained release (tablets)	Ⓛ	left
		$L_1...L_5$	lumbar nerve 1 through 5 lumbar vertebra 1 through 5
KSW	knife stab wound		
KT	kidney transplant	LA	language age
	kinesiotherapy		latex agglutination
	known to		Latin American
KTC	knee to chest		left arm
KTP	potassium-titanyl-phosphate (laser)		left atrial
			left atrium
KTU	kidney transplant unit		linguoaxial
	known to us		local anesthesia
KUB	kidney(s), ureter(s), and bladder		long acting
			lupus anticoagulant
	kidney ultrasound biopsy	L + A	light and accommodation
			living and active
KUS	kidney(s), ureter(s), and spleen	LAA	left atrium and its appendage
KV	kilovolt	LAAM	levomethadyl acetate (L-alpha acetylmeth-adol)
KVO	keep vein open		
KVP	kilovolt peak		
KW	Keith-Wagener (ophthalmoscopic finding, graded I-IV)	LAB	laboratory
			left abdomen
		LABBB	left anterior bundle branch block
	Kimmelstiel-Wilson		
KWB	Keith, Wagener, Barker	LABC	locally advanced breast cancer
KWIC	keywork in context		

L

LAC	laceration	L-AMB	liposomal amphotericin B
	left atrial catheter	LANC	long arm navicular cast
	long arm cast	LAN	lymphadenopathy
LACT-ART	lactate arterial	LAO	left anterior oblique
		LAP	laparoscopy
LAD	left anterior descending		laparotomy
	left axis deviation		left atrial pressure
	leukocyte adhesion deficiency		leucine amino peptidase
			leukocyte alkaline phosphatase
LADA	left anterior descending (coronary) artery	LAP-APPY	laparoscopic appendectomy
LADCA	left anterior descending coronary artery	LAP CHOLE	laparoscopic cholecystectomy
LADD	left anterior descending diagonal	LAPMS	long arm posterior molded splint
LAD-MIN	left axis deviation minimal	LAPW	left atrial posterior wall
LAE	left atrial enlargement	LAQ	long arc quad
	long above elbow	LAR	left arm, reclining
LAEC	locally advanced esophageal cancer	LARM	left arm
		LAS	laxative abuse syndrome
LAF	laminar air flow		left arm, sitting
	Latin-American female		leucine acetylsalicylate
	low animal fat		long arm splint
	lymphocyte-activating factor		lymphadenopathy syndrome
			lymphangioscintigraphy
LAFB	left anterior fascicular block		lysine acetylsalicylate
LAFR	laminar airflow room	LASA	Linear Analogue Self-Assessment (scales)
LAG	lymphangiogram		
LAH	left anterior hemiblock		lipid-associated sialic acid
	left atrial hypertrophy	LASER	light amplification by stimulated emission of radiation
LAHB	left anterior hemiblock		
LAIT	latex agglutination inhibition test		
		LASIK	laser in situ keratomileusis
LAK	lymphokine-activated killer	L-ASP	asparaginase
LAL	left axillary line	LAST	left anterior small thoracotomy
	limulus amebocyte lysate		
		LAT	lateral
LALLS	low-angle laser light scattering		latex agglutination test
			left anterior thigh
LAM	laminectomy	LATCH	literature attached to chart
	laminogram	lat.men.	lateral meniscectomy
	Latin-American male	LATS	long-acting thyroid stimulator
lam✔	laminectomy check		
LAMB	mucocutaneous lentigines, atrial myxoma, and blue nevus (syndrome)	LAUP	laser-assisted uvula-palatoplasty

LAV	lymphadenopathy associated virus	LBO	large bowel obstruction
LAVA	laser-assisted vasal anastomosis	LBP	low back pain
			low blood pressure
LAVH	laparoscopically assisted vaginal hysterectomy	LBQC	large base quad cane
		LBS	low back syndrome
			pounds
LAW	left atrial wall	LBT	low back tenderness
LAWER	life-terminating acts without the explicit request		low back trouble
		LBV	left brachial vein
			low biological value
LAX	laxative	LBW	lean body weight
LB	large bowel		low birth weight
	lateral bend	LBWI	low birth weight infant
	left breast	LC	Laënnec's cirrhosis
	left buttock		laparoscopic cholecystectomy
	live births		
	low back		left circumflex
	lung biopsy		leisure counseling
	lymphoid body		level of consciousness
	pound		living children
L&B	left and below		low calorie
LB3	colonoscope		lung cancer
LBA	laser balloon angioplasty	3LC	triple lumen catheter
LBB	left breast biopsy	LCA	Leber's congenital amaurosis
	long back board		
LBBB	left bundle branch block		left circumflex artery
LBBx	left breast biopsy		left coronary artery
LBCD	left border of cardiac dullness		light contact assist
		LCAD	long-chain acyl-coenzyme A dehydrogenase
L/B/Cr	electrolytes, blood urea nitrogen, and serum creatinine		
		LCAL	large-cell anaplastic lymphoma
LBD	large bile duct	LCAT	lecithin cholesterol acyltransferase
	left border dullness		
	Lewy body dementia	LCB	left costal border
	low back disability	LCCA	left common carotid artery
LBE	long below elbow		
LBG	Landry-Guillain-Barré (syndrome)		leukocytoclastic angiitis
		LCCS	low cervical cesarean section
LBH	length, breadth, and height	LCD	coal tar solution (*liquor carbonis detergens*)
LBM	last bowel movement		
	lean body mass		localized collagen dystrophy
	loose bowel movement		low calcium diet
LBMI	last body mass index	LCDC	Laboratory Centre for Disease Control (Canada)
LBNA	lysis bladder neck adhesions		
LBNP	lower body negative pressure		

LCDCP	low-contact dynamic compression plate		low cervical transverse lymphocytotoxicity
LCDE	laparoscopic common duct exploration	LCTCS	low cervical transverse cesarean section
LCE	laparoscopic cholecystectomy	LCTD	low-calcium test diet
		LCV	leucovorin
	left carotid endarterectomy		leukocytoclastic vasculitis
LCF	left circumflex		low cervical vertical
LCFA	long-chain fatty acid	LCX	left circumflex coronary artery
LCFM	left circumflex marginal	LD	lactic dehydrogenase (formerly LDH)
LCGU	local cerebral glucose utilization		last dose
LCH	Langerhans' cell histiocytosis		latissimus dorsi
			learning disability
	local city hospital		learning disorder
LCIS	lobular cancer *in situ*		left deltoid
LCL	lateral collateral ligament		Legionnaire's disease
LCLC	large cell lung carcinoma		lethal dose
LCM	left costal margin		levodopa
	lower costal margin		Licensed Dietician
	lymphocytic choriomeningitis		liver disease
			living donor
LCMI	left ventricular mass index		loading dose
			long dwell
LCN	lidocaine		low density
LCO	low cardiac output		low dosage
LCP	long, closed, posterior (cervix)		Lyme disease
		L&D	labor and deliver
LCPD	Legg-Calvé-Perthes disease		liver and spleen
		L/D	labor and delivery
LCPUFAs	long-chain polyunsaturated fatty acids		light to dark (ratio)
		LD-1	lactic dehydrogenase 1
		LD-5	lactic dehydrogenase 5
LCR	late cortical response	LD_{50}	median lethal dose
	late cutaneous reaction	LDA	low density areas
	ligase chain reaction	LDB	Legionnaires disease bacterium
LCS	low constant suction		
	low continuous suction	LDCOC	low-dose combination oral contraceptive
LCSG	left cardiac sympathetic ganglionectomy	LDD	laser disk decompression
	lost child support group		Lee and Desu's D (test)
LCSS	Lung Cancer Symptom Score		light-dark discrimination
		LDDS	local dentist
LCSW	Licensed Clinical Social Worker	LDEA	left deviation of electrical axis
	low continuous wall suction	LDF	laser Doppler flowmetry
		LDH	lactic dehydrogenase
LCT	long chain triglyceride	LDIH	left direct inguinal hernia

LDL	low-density lipoprotein	LEP	leptospirosis
LDLC	low-density lipoprotein cholesterol		lower esophageal pressure
l-dopa	levodopa	LEP 2	leptospirosis 2
LD-PCR	limiting dilution polymerase chain reaction	LE prep	lupus erythematosus preparation
LDR	labor, delivery, and recovery	L-ERX	leukoerythroblastic reaction
	length-to-diameter ratio	LES	local excitatory state
LDR/P	labor, delivery, recovery, and postpartum		lower esophageal sphincter
LDT	left dorsotransverse		lupus erythematosus systemic
LD-T	lactic dehydrogenase total	LESG	Late Effects Study Group
LDUB	long double upright brace	LESI	lumbar epidural steroid injection
LDV	laser Doppler velocimetry	LESP	lower esophageal sphincter pressure
LE	left ear	LET	left esotropia
	left eye		leukocyte esterase test
	lens extraction		linear energy transfer
	live embryo	LEU	leucine
	lower extremities	LEV	levamisole
	lupus erythematosus		levator muscle
LEA	lower extremity amputation	LEVA	levamisole
	lumbar epidural anesthesia	LF	laparoscopic fundoplications
LEAD	lower extremity arterial disease		Lassa fever
			left foot
LEAP	Lower Extremity Amputation Prevention (program)		living female
			low fat
			low forceps
LEC	lens epithelial cell		low frequency
LED	liposomal encapsulated doxorubicin	LFA	left femoral artery
			left forearm
	lowest effective dose		left fronto-anterior
	lupus erythematosus disseminatus		leukocyte function-associated antigen
LEEP	loop electrosurgical excision procedure		low friction arthroplasty
			lymphocyte function-associated antigen
LEF	lower extremity fracture	LFA-1	leukocyte function-associated antigen-1
LEH	liposome-encapsulated hemoglobin		
LEHPZ	lower esophageal high pressure zone	LFB	low frequency band
		LFC	living female child
LEJ	ligation of the esophagogastric junction		low fat and cholesterol
		LFCS	low flap cesarean section
		LFD	lactose-free diet
LEM	lateral eye movements		low fat diet
	light electron microscope		low fiber diet

142

	low forceps delivery	LHH	left homonymous
	lunate fossa depression		hemianopsia
LFGNR	lactose fermenting	LHI	Labor Health Institute
	gram-negative rod	LHL	left hemisphere lesions
LFL	left frontolateral		left hepatic lobe
LFP	left frontoposterior	LHON	Leber's hereditary optic
LFS	leukemia-free survival		neuropathy
	Li-Fraumeni syndrome	LHP	left hemiparesis
	liver function series	LHR	leukocyte histamine
LFT	latex flocculation test		release
	left fronto-transverse	LHRH	luteinizing hormone-
	liver function tests		releasing hormone
	low flap transverse		(hypothalamic)
LFU	limit flocculation	LHRT	leukocyte histamine
	unit		release test
LG	large	LHS	left hand side
	laryngectomy		long-handled sponge
	left gluteal	LHSH	long-handled shoe horn
	linguogingival	LHT	left hypertropia
	lymphography	LI	lactose intolerance
LGA	large for gestational age		lamellar ichthyosis
	left gastric artery		large intestine
LGI	lower gastrointestinal		laser iridotomy
	(series)		learning impaired
LGIOS	low-grade intraosseous-		linguoincisal
	type osteosarcoma	Li	lithium
LGL	low-grade lymphoma(s)	LIA	laser interference acuity
	Lown-Ganong-Levine		left iliac artery
	(syndrome)	LIB	left in bottle
LGLS	Lown-Ganong-Levine	LIC	left iliac crest
	syndrome		left internal carotid
LGM	left gluteus medius		leisure interest class
	(maximus)	LICA	left internal carotid artery
LGN	lobular glomerulonephritis	LICD	lower intestinal Crohn's
LG-NHL	low-grade non-Hodgkin's		disease
	lymphoma	LICM	left intercostal margin
LGS	Lennox-Gastaut syndrome	Li_2CO_3	lithium carbonate
	low Gomco suction	LICS	left intercostal space
LGSIL	low grade squamous	Lido	lidocaine
	intraepithelial lesion	LIF	left iliac fossa
LGV	lymphagranuloma		left index finger
	venerum		leukemia-inhibiting factor
LH	left hand		liver (migration)
	left hyperphoria		inhibitory factor
	luteinizing hormone	LIFE	lung imaging fluorescence
LHA	left hepatic artery		endoscopy
LHC	left heart catheterization	LIG	ligament
LHF	left heart failure		lymphocyte immune
LHG	left hand grip		globulin

LIGHTS	phototherapy lights
LIH	left inguinal hernia
LIHA	low impulsiveness, high anxiety
LIJ	left internal jugular
LILA	low impulsiveness, low anxiety
LIMA	left internal mammary artery (graft)
LINDI	lithium-induced nephrogenic diabetes insipidus
LING	lingual
LIO	laser indirect ophthalmoscope
	left inferior oblique (muscle)
LIOU	laparoscopic intraoperative ultrasound
LIP	lithium-induced polydipsia
	lymphocytic interstitial pneumonia
LIPV	left inferior pulmonary vein
LIQ	liquid
	liquor
	lower inner quadrant
LIR	left iliac region
	left inferior rectus
LIS	left intercostal space
	locked-in syndrome
	lung injury score
	low intermittent suction
LISS	low ionic strength saline
LIT	literature
	liver injury test
LITA	left internal thoracic artery
LITH	lithotomy
LITHO	lithotripsy
LIV	left innominate vein
L-IVP	limited intravenous pyelogram
LIVB	live birth
LIVC	left inferior vena cava
LIVPRO	liver profile

LIWS	low intermittent wall suction
LJL	lateral joint line
LJM	limited joint mobility
LK	lamellar keratoplasty
	left kidney
LKA	Lazare-Klerman-Armour (Personality Inventory)
LKM-3	liver-kidney microsomal antibodies type 3
LKS	liver, kidneys, spleen
LKSB	liver, kidneys, spleen, and bladder
LKSNP	liver, kidneys, and spleen not palpable
$\begin{smallmatrix} L & & M \\ K & O & \\ S & & T \end{smallmatrix}$	liver, kidneys, and spleen negative, no masses, or tenderness
LL	large lymphocyte
	left lateral
	left leg
	left lower
	left lung
	lid lag
	long leg (brace or cast)
	lower lid
	lower lip
	lower lobe
	lumbar laminectomy
	lumbar length
	lymphocytic leukemia
	lymphoblastic lymphoma
L&L	lids and lashes
LL2	limb lead two
LLA	lids, lashes, and adnexa
	limulus lysate assay
LLAT	left lateral
LLB	last living breath
	left lateral bending
	left lateral border
	long leg brace
LLC	laparoscopic laser cholecystectomy
	long leg cast
LLBCD	left lower border of cardiac dullness
LLD	left lateral decubitus
	left length discrepancy
LLE	left lower extremity

	little league elbow	LMEE	left middle ear exploration
LLETZ	large-loop excision of the transformation zone	LMF	left middle finger
LLFG	long leg fiberglas (cast)		melphalan (L-PAM), methotrexate, and fluorouracil
LLG	left lateral gaze	L/min	liters per minute
LL-GXT	low-level graded exercise test	LML	left medial lateral
LLL	left lower lid		left middle lobe
	left lower lobe (lung)	LMLE	left mediolateral episiotomy
LLLE	lower lid left eye		
LLLNR	left lower lobe, no rales	LMM	lentigo maligna melanoma
LLO	Legionella-like organism	LMN	lower motor neuron
LLOD	lower lid, right eye	LMNL	lower motor neuron lesion
	lower limit of detection	LMP	last menstrual period
LLOS	lower lid, left eye		left mentoposterior
LLP	long leg plaster		low malignant potential
LLQ	left lower quadrant (abdomen)	LMR	left medial rectus
LLR	left lateral rectus	LMS	lateral medullary syndrome
LLRE	lower lid, right eye		
LLS	lazy leukocyte syndrome	LMT	left main trunk
LLSB	left lower sternal border		left mentotransverse
LLT	left lateral thigh	LMW	low molecular weight
LLWC	long leg walking cast	LMWD	low molecular weight dextran
LLX	left lower extremity		
LM	left main	LMWH	low molecular weight heparin
	light microscopy	LN	left nostril (nare)
	linguomesial		lymph nodes
	living male	LN₂	liquid nitrogen
	lung metastases	LNB	lymph node biopsy
L/M	liters per minute	LNCs	lymph node cells
LMA	laryngeal mask airway	LND	light-near dissociation
	left mentoanterior		lonidamine
	liver membrane autoantibody		lymph node dissection
LMB	Laurence-Moon-Biedl syndrome	LNE	lymph node enlargement
			lymph node excision
LMC	living male child	LNF	laparoscopic Nissen fundoplication
LMCA	left main coronary artery		
	left middle cerebral artery	LNG	levonorgestrel
LMCAT	left middle cerebral artery thrombosis	LNM	lymph node metastases
		LNMP	last normal menstrual period
LMCL	left midclavicular line		
LMD	local medical doctor	LNNB	Luria-Nebraska Neuropsychological Battery
	low molecular weight dextran		
		LO	lateral oblique (x-ray view)
LME	left mediolateral episiotomy		linguo-occlusal

	lumbar orthosis		left occiput posterior
LOA	late-onset agammaglobulinemia		level of pain
		LOQ	lower outer quadrant
	leave of absence	LORS-I	Level of Rehabilitation Scale-I
	left occiput anterior		
	looseness of associations	LOS	length of stay
	lysis of adhesions		loss of sight
LOAD	late-onset Alzheimer's disease	LOT	left occiput transverse
			Licensed Occupational Therapist
LOB	loss of balance		
LOC	laxative of choice	LOV	loss of vision
	level of care	LOZ	lozenge
	level of comfort	LP	light perception
	level of concern		linguopulpal
	level of consciousness		lipoprotein
	local		low protein
	loss of consciousness		lumbar puncture
LOCM	low-osmolality contrast media	L/P	lactate-pyruvate ratio
LOD	limit of detection	LP5	Life-Pak 5
	line of duty	LPA	left pulmonary artery
LOF	leaking of fluids	Lp(a)	lipoprotein (a)
	leave on floor	LPA%	left pulmonary artery oxygen saturation
LOFD	low outlet forceps delivery		
		L-PAM	melphalan
LOG	Logmar chart	LPC	laser photocoagulation
LOH	loss of heterozygosity		Licensed Professional Counselor
LOHF	late-onset hepatic failure		
LOIH	left oblique inguinal hernia	LPCC	Licensed Professional Certified Counselor
LOI	level of injury	LPc̄P	light perception with projection
	Leyton Obsessional Inventory	LPD	leiomyomatosis peritonealis disseminata
LOL	left occipitolateral		low potassium dextran
	little old lady		low protein diet
LOM	left otitis media		luteal phase defect
	limitation of motion		luteal phase deficiency
	little old man		lymphoproliferative disease
	loss of motion		
	low-osmolar (contrast) media	LPDA	left posterior descending artery
LOMSA	left otitis media, suppurative, acute	LPEP	left pre-ejection period
		LPF	liver plasma flow
LOMSC	left otitis media, suppurative, chronic		low-power field
			lymphocytosis-promoting factor
LoNa	low sodium		
LOO	length of operation	LPFB	left posterior fascicular block
LOP	laparoscopic orchiopexy		
	leave on pass		

LPH	left posterior hemiblock	LRCS	Licentiate of the Royal College of Surgeons
LPHB	left posterior hemiblock	LRD	limb reduction defects
LPI	laser peripheral iridectomy		living related donor living renal donor
LPICA	left posterior internal carotid artery	LRDT	living related donor transplant
LPIH	left-posterior-inferior hemiblock	LREH	low renin essential hypertension
LPL	left posterolateral lipoprotein lipase	LRF	left rectus femoris
LPLND	laparoscopic pelvic lymph node dissection	L&R gtt	Levophed® and Regitine® drip (infusion)
LPM	latent primary malignancy liters per minute	LRI	lower respiratory infection
LPN	Licensed Practical Nurse	LRLT	living-related liver transplantation
LPO	left posterior oblique light perception only	LRM	left radical mastectomy local regional metastases
LPPC	leukocyte-poor packed cells	LRMP	last regular menstrual period
LPPH	late postpartum hemorrhage	LRND	left radical neck dissection
LPS	last Pap smear lipopolysaccharide	LRO	long range objective
LP SHUNT	lumboperitoneal shunt	Lrot	left rotation
		LRQ	lower right quadrant
LP̄sP	light perception without projection	LROU	lateral rectus, both eyes
		LRS	lactated Ringer's solution
LPT	Licensed Physical Therapist	LRT	living renal transplant local radiation therapy lower respiratory tract
LPTN	Licensed Psychiatric Technical Nurse	LRTD	living relative transplant donor
LPV	left portal vein left pulmonary vein	LRTI	ligament reconstruction with tendon interposition lower respiratory tract infection
LQTS	long QT interval syndrome		
LR	labor room lactated Ringer's (injection) lateral rectus left-right light reflex	LRV	left renal vein log reduction value
		LRZ	lorazepam
		LS	left side legally separated Leigh's syndrome liver scan liver-spleen low salt lumbosacral
L&R	left and right		
L→R	left to right		
LR1A	labor room 1A		
LRA	left radial artery left renal artery		
LRC	lower rib cage		
LRCP	Licentiate of the Royal College of Physicians	L/S	lecithin-sphingomyelin ratio

L&S	ligation and stripping	L–Spar	Elspar (asparaginase)
L5-S1	lumbar fifth vertebra to sacral first vertebra	L-SPINE	lumbar spine
LSA	left sacrum anterior	LSR	left superior rectus
	lipid-bound sialic acid	L/S ratio	lecithin/sphingomyelin ratio
	lymphosarcoma	LSS	liver-spleen scan
LSB	left scapular border		lumbar spinal stenosis
	left sternal border	LST	left sacrum transverse
	local standby	LSTC	laparoscopic tubal coagulation
	lumbar spinal block		
	lumbar sympathetic block	LSTL	laparoscopic tubal ligation
LS BPS	laparoscopic bilateral partial salpingectomy	L's & T's	lines and tubes
		LSU	life support unit
LSC	last sexual contact	LSV	left subclavian vein
	late systolic click	LSVC	left superior vena cava
	left subclavian (artery) (vein)	LSW	left-side weakness
			Licensed Social Worker
	lichen simplex chronicus	LT	laboratory technician
LSCA	left scapuloanterior		left
LSCP	left scapuloposterior		left thigh
LSCS	lower segment cesarean section		left triceps
			leukotrienes
LSD	least significant difference		Levin tube
	low salt diet		light
	lysergide		light touch
LSE	local side effects		low transverse
LSF	low saturated fat		lumbar traction
LSFA	low saturated fatty acid (diet)		lung transplantation
			lunotriquetral
L-SIL	low-grade squamous intraepithelial lesions		lymphotoxin
		L&T	lettuce and tomato
LSK	liver, spleen, and kidneys	LT4	levothyroxine
LSKM	liver-spleen-kidney-megalgia	LTA	laryngotracheal applicator
			laryngeal tracheal anesthesia
LSL	left sacrolateral		
	left short leg (brace)		local tracheal anesthesia
LSLF	low sodium, low fat (diet)	LTAS	left transatrial septal
LSM	laser scanning microscope	LTB	laparoscopic tubal banding
	late systolic murmur		
	limited sampling model		laryngotracheo-bronchitis
	liver, spleen masses	LTB_4	leukotriene B_4
LSO	left salpingo-oophorectomy	LTC	left to count
			long-term care
	left superior oblique		long thick closed
	lumbosacral orthosis	LTC_4	leukotriene C_4
LSP	left sacrum posterior	LTC-101	long-term care form-101
	liver-specific (membrane) lipoprotein	LTCF	long-term care facility
		LTCS	low transverse cesarean section

LTD	largest tumor dimension	LUQ	left upper quadrant
	leg transfer device	LURD	living unrelated donor
LTFU	long-term follow-up	LUS	laparoscopic
LTG	lamotrigine		ultrasonography
	long-term goal		lower uterine segment
LTGA	left transposition of great	LUSB	left upper scapular border
	artery		left upper sternal border
LTH	luteotropic hormone	LUST	lower uterine segment
LTK	laser thermal keratoplasty		transverse
LTL	laparoscopic tubal ligation	LUT	lower urinary tract
LTM	long-term memory	LUTT	lower urinary tract tumor
LTOT	long-term oxygen therapy	LUX	left upper extremity
LTP	laser trabeculoplasty	LV	leave
	long-term plan		left ventricle
	long-term potentiation		leucovorin
LTR	long terminal repeats		live virus
	lower trunk rotation	LVA	left ventricular aneurysm
LTS	laparoscopic tubal	LVC	laser vision correction
	sterilization		low viscosity cement
	long-term survivors	LVAD	left ventricular assist
LTT	lactose tolerance test		device
	lymphocyte transforma-	LV Angio	left ventricular angiogram
	tion test	L-VAM	leuprolide acetate,
LTUI	low transverse uterine		vinblastine,
	incision		doxorubicin
LTV	long term variability		(Adriamycin), and
	Luche tumor virus		mitomycin
LTV+	long-term	LVAS	left ventricular assist
	variability–average to		system
	moderate	LVAT	left ventricular activation
LTV 0	long-term		time
	variability–absent	LVBP	left ventricle bypass pump
LTVC	long-term venous catheter	LVD	left ventricular dimension
LTZ	letrozole		left ventricular
LU	left upper		dysfunction
	left ureteral	LVDP	left ventricular diastolic
	living unit		pressure
	Lutheran	LVDT	linear variable differential
L & U	lower and upper		transformer
LUA	left upper arm	LVDV	left ventricular diastolic
LUD	left uterine displacement		volume
LUE	left upper extremity	LVE	left ventricular
Lues I	primary syphilis		enlargement
Lues II	secondary syphilis	LVEDP	left ventricular end
Lues III	tertiary syphilis		diastolic pressure
LUL	left upper lid	LVEDV	left ventricular end
	left upper lobe (lung)		diastolic volume
LUOB	left upper outer buttock	LVEF	left ventricular ejection
LUOQ	left upper outer quadrant		fraction

LVEP	left ventricular end pressure	LVSWI	left ventricular stroke work index
LVESVI	left ventricular end systolic volume index	LVV	left ventricular volume live varicella vaccine
LVET	left ventricular ejection time	LVW	left ventricular wall
		LVWI	left ventricular work index
LVF	left ventricular failure left visual field	LVWMA	left ventricular wall motion abnormality
LVFP	left ventricular filling pressure	LVWMI	left ventricular wall motion index
LVFU	leucovorin and fluorouracil	LVWT	left ventricular wall thickness
LVG	left ventrogluteal	LW	lacerating wound living will
LVH	left ventricular hypertrophy	L & W	Lee and White (coagulation) living and well
LVID	left ventricular internal diameter		
LVIDd	left ventricle internal dimension diastole	LWCT	Lee-White clotting time
		LWBS	left without being seen
LVIDs	left ventricle internal dimension systole	LWC	leave without consent
		LWOP	leave without pay
LVL	left vastus lateralis	LWOT	left without treatment
LVM	left ventricular mass	LWP	large whirlpool
LVMI	left ventricular mass index	LX	larynx local irradiation lower extremity
LVMM	left ventricular muscle mass	LXC	laxative of choice
		LXT	left exotropia
LVN	Licensed Visiting Nurse Licensed Vocational Nurse	LYCD	live yeast cell derivative
		LYEL	lost years of expected life
		LYG	lymphomatoid granulomatosis
LVO	left ventricular overactivity	LYM	lymphocytes
LVOP	left ventricular outflow tract	lymphs	lymphocytes
		LYS	large yellow soft (stools) lysine
LVP	large volume parenteral left ventricular pressure	lytes	electrolytes (Na, K, Cl, etc.)
LVPW	left ventricular posterior wall	LZ	landing zone
		LZP	lorazepam
LVR	leucovorin		
LVRT	liver volume replaced by tumor		
LVS	left ventricular strain		
LVS EMI	left ventricular subendocardial myocardial ischemia		**M**
LVSP	left ventricular systolic pressure		
LVSW	left ventricular stroke work	M	male manual

	marital
	married
	mass
	medial
	memory
	mesial
	meta
	meter (m)
	mild
	million
	minimum
	molar
	Monday
	monocytes
	mother
	mouth
	murmur
	muscle
	Mycobacterium
	Mycoplasma
	myopia
	myopic
	thousand
Ⓜ	murmur
M_1	first mitral sound
M1	left mastoid
M1 to M7	categories of acute nonlymphoblastic leukemia
M_2	second mitral sound
M^2	square meters (body surface)
M2	right mastoid
M-2	vincristine, carmustine, cyclophosphamide, melphalan, and prednisone
M_3	third mitral sound
M-3	medical student 3rd year
3M	mitomycin, mitoxantrone, and methotrexate
M-3+7	mitoxantrone and cytarabine
M-4	medical student 4th year
MA	machine
	Master of Arts
	mean arterial (blood pressure)

	medical assistance
	medical authorization
	megestrol acetate
	menstrual age
	mental age
	Mexican American
	microaneurysms
	Miller-Abbott (tube)
	milliamps
	monoclonal antibodies
	motorcycle accident
M/A	mood and/or affect
MA-1	Bennett volume ventilator
MAA	macroaggregates of albumin
MAB	maximum androgen blockade
Mab	monoclonal antibody
MABP	mean arterial blood pressure
MAC	macrocytic erythrocytes
	macrophage
	macula
	maximal allowable concentration
	membrane attack complex
	methotrexate, dactinomycin (Actinomycin D), and cyclophosphamide
	mid-arm circumference
	minimum alveolar concentration
	monitored anesthesia care
	multi-access catheter
	Mycobacterium avium complex
MACC	methotrexate, doxorubicin, (Adriamycin) cyclophosphamide, and lomustine
MACCC	Master Arts, Certified Clinical Competence
MACE	Malon antegrade continence enema
MACOP-B	methotrexate, doxorubicin, (Adriamycin)

	cyclophosphamide, vincristine (Oncovin), prednisone, and bleomycin		ifosfamide, and dacarbazine
MACRO	macrocytes	MAL	malignant
MACS	magnetic activated cell sorting		midaxillary line
		MALDI	matrix assisted laser desorption ionization
MACTAR	McMaster-Toronto Arthritis Patient Reference (Disability Questionnaire)	MALG	Minnesota antilympho-blast globulin
		malig	malignant
MAD	mind altering drugs moderate atopic dermatitis	MALT	mucosa-associated lymphoid tissue
		MALToma	lymphoma of mucosa-associated lymphoid tissue
MADD	Mothers Against Drunk Driving		
MADRS	Montgomery-Åsburg Depression Rating Scale	MAM	mammogram Mexican-American male monitored administration of medication
MAE	medical air evacuation moves all extremities		
		MAMC	mid-arm muscle circumference
MAES	moves all extremities slowly	Mammo	mammography
MAEEW	moves all extremities equally well	m-AMSA	amsacrine
		MAN	malignancy associated neutropenia
MAEW	moves all extremities well	Mand	mandibular
		MANE	Morrow Assessment of Nausea and Emesis
MAF	metabolic activity factor Mexican-American female	MANOVA	multivariate analysis of variance
MAFAs	movement-associated fetal (heart rate) accelerations	MAO	maximum acid output
		MAO-A	monoamine oxidase type A
MAFO	molded ankle/foot orthosis	MAO-B	monoamine oxidase type B
MAFP	maternal alpha-fetoprotein	MAOI	monoamine oxidase inhibitor
MAG	medication administration guideline (record)	MAOP	Mid-Atlantic Oncology Program
mag cit	magnesium citrate	MAP	magnesium, ammonium, and phosphate (Struvite stones) mean airway pressure mean arterial pressure Medical Assistance Program megaloblastic anemia of pregnancy mitomycin, doxorubicin
MAGP	meatal advancement glandulophaleoplasty		
mag sulf	magnesium sulfate		
MAHA	macroangiopathic hemolytic anemia		
MAI	maximal aggregation index minor acute illness *Mycobacterium avium-intracellulare*		
MAID	mesna, doxorubicin (Adriamycin),		

	(Adriamycin), and cisplatin (Platinol)	MAX A	maximum assistance (assist)
	muscle-action potential	MAxL	mid-axillary line
MAPI	Millon Adolescent Personality Inventory	MAYO	mayonnaise
MAPS	Make a Picture Story	MB	buccal margin
MAR	marital		mandible
	medication administration record		Mallory body
	mineral apposition rates		Medical Board
MARE	manual active-resistive exercise		medulloblastoma
			mesiobuccal
MARSA	methicillin- aminoglycoside- resistant *Staphylococ- cus aureus*		methylene blue
		M/B	mother/baby
		M-BACOD	methotrexate, calcium leucovorin, bleomycin, doxorubicin, (Adriamycin) cyclophosphamide, vincristine (Oncovin), and dexamethasone
MAS	macrophage activation syndrome		
	meconium aspiration syndrome	MBC	male breast cancer
	Memory Assessment Scale		maximum bladder capacity
	mobile arm support		maximum breathing capacity
MASA	mutant allele-specific amplification		metastatic breast cancer
MASER	microwave amplification (application) by stimulated emission of radiation		methotrexate, bleomycin, and cisplatin
			minimal bactericidal concentration
MASH POT	mashed potatoes	MB-CK	a creatinine kinase isoenzyme
MAST	mastectomy	MBD	metabolic bone disease
	medical antishock trousers		methylene blue dye
	Michigan Alcoholism Screening Test	MBEST	modulus blipped echo-planar single-pulse technique
	military antishock trousers		
MAT	manual arts therapy	MBD	minimal brain damage
	maternal		minimal brain dysfunction
	maternity	MBE	may be elevated
	mature		medium below elbow
	medication administration team	MBF	meat base formula
	multifocal atrial tachycardia		myocardial blood flow
		MBFC	medial brachial fascial compartment
MAU	microalbuminuria		
MAVR	mitral and aortic valve replacement	MBHI	Millon Behavioral Health Inventory
max	maxillary	MBI	methylene blue installation
	maximal		

MBL	menstrual blood loss	MCAD	medium-chain acyl-CoA dehydrogenase
MBM	mother's breast milk		
MBNW	multiple-breath nitrogen washout	MCAF	monocyte chemoattractant and activity factor
MBO	mesiobuccal occulsion	MCAO	middle cerebral artery occlusion
MBP	malignant brachial plexopathy		
	mannan-binding protein	MCAT	Medical College Admission Test
	mannose-binding protein	MCB	Medicines Control Board (United Kingdom's equivalent to the United States Food and Drug Administration)
	medullary bone pain		
	mesiobuccopulpal		
	myelin basic protein		
MBq	megabecquerels		
MBS	modified barium swallow		mid-cycle bleeding
MBT	maternal blood type		middle chamber bubbling
MC	male child	McB pt	McBurney's point
	medium-chain (triglycerides)	MCC	microcrystalline cellulose midstream clean-catch
	metacarpal		
	metatarso - cuneiform	MCCU	mobile coronary care unit
	mini-laparotomy cholecystectomy	MCD	minimal-change disease multicystic dysplasia
	mitoxantrone and cytarabine	MCDT	mast cell degranulation test
	mitral commissurotomy	MCFA	medium chain fatty acid
	mixed cellularity	mcg	microgram (μg)
	molluscum contagiosum	MCG	magnetocardiogram magnetocardiography
	monocomponent highly purified pork insulin		
		MCGN	minimal-change glomerular nephritis
	mouth care		
	myocarditis	MCH	mean corpuscular hemoglobin
m + c	morphine and cocaine		
MCA	Medicines Control Agency (United Kingdom)		microfibrillar collagen hemostat
			muscle contraction headache
	megestrol, cyclophospha-mide, and doxorubicin (Adriamycin)	MCHC	mean corpuscular hemoglobin concentration
	metacarpal amputation		
	micrometastases clonogenic assay	mCi	millicurie
	middle cerebral aneurysm	MCL	maximum comfort level
	middle cerebral artery		medial collateral ligament
	monoclonal antibodies		midclavicular line
	motorcycle accident		midcostal line
	multichannel analyzer		modified chest lead
	multiple congenital anomalies	mcL	microliter (1/1,000 of an mL)
2-MCA	2-methyl citric acid	MCLL	most comfortable listening level

MCLNS	mucocutaneous lymph node syndrome		major depression
MCMI	Millon Clinical Multiaxial Inventory		mammary dysplasia
			manic depression
			medical doctor
mcmol	micromoles		mediodorsal
MCN	minimal change nephropathy		mental deficiency
			mesiodistal
MCNS	minimal change nephrotic syndrome		movement disorder
			multiple dose
MCO	managed care organization		muscular dystrophy
			myocardial damage
MCP	mean carotid pressure	MD-50®	diatrizoate sodium injection 50%
	metacarpophalangeal joint	MDA	malondialdehyde
	metoclopramide		manual dilation of the anus
MCR	Medicare		methylenedioxyamphet- amine
	metabolic clearance rate		
	myocardial revasculariza- tion		micrometastases detection assay
MC=R	moderately constricted and equally reactive		motor discriminative acuity
MCS	microculture and sensitivity	MDAC	multiple-dose activated charcoal
	moderate constant suction	MDACC	MD Anderson Cancer Center
	multiple chemical sensitivity	MDA LDL	malondialdehydeconju- gated low-density lipoprotein
	myocardial contractile state		
MCSA	minimal cross-sectional area	MDC	medial dorsal cutaneous (nerve)
M-CSF	macrophage colony- stimulating factor	MDCM	mildly dilated congestive cardiomyopathy
MC-SR	moderately constricted and slightly reactive	MDD	major depressive disorder
			manic depressive disorder
MCT	manual cervical traction	MDE	major depressive episode
	mean circulation time	MDF	myocardial depressant factor
	medium chain triglyceride		
	medullary carcinoma of the thyroid	MDGF	macrophage-derived growth factor
MCTC	metrizamide computed tomography cisternogram	MDI	manic depressive illness
			metered dose inhaler
MCTD	mixed connective tissue disease		methylenedioxyindenes
			multiple daily injection
MCU	micturating cystourethro- gram		multiple dosage insulin
		MDIA	Mental Development Index, Adjusted
MCV	mean corpuscular volume		
MD	macula degeneration	MDII	multiple daily insulin injection
	maintenance dialysis		
	maintenance dose		

MDIS	metered-dose inhaler-spacer (device)		multiple dose vial
		MDY	month, date, and year
MDM	mid-diastolic murmur	ME	macula edema
	minor determinant mix (of penicillin)		manic episode
			medical events
MDMA	methylenedioxy-methamphetamine (ecstasy)		medical evidence
			medical examiner
			mestranol
MDNT	midnight		Methodist
MDO	mentally disordered offender		middle ear
			myalgic encephalomyelitis
MDP	methylene diphosphonate	M/E	myeloid-erythroid (ratio)
MDPH	Michigan Department of Public Health	M&E	Mecholyl and Eserine
		MEA-I	multiple endocrine adenomatosis type I
MDPI	maximum daily permissible intake		
		MEB	Medical Evaluation Board
MDR	Medical Device Reporting (regulation)		methylene blue
		MEC	meconium
	minimum daily requirement		middle ear canal(s)
		MeCCNU	semustine
	multi-drug resistance	MECG	maternal electrocardio-gram
MD=R	moderately dilated and equally reactive		
		MeCP	semustine (methyl CCNU) cyclophosphamide, and prednisone
MDRE	multiple-drug-resistant enterococci		
MDREF	multi-drug resistant enteric fever		
		MED	medial
MDRTB	multidrug-resistant tuberculosis		median erythrocyte diameter
MDS	maternal deprivation syndrome		medical
			medication
	Minimum Data Set		medicine
	myelodysplastic syndromes		medium
			medulloblastoma
MD-SR	moderately dilated and slightly reactive		minimal erythema dose
			minimum effective dose
MDSU	medical day stay unit	MEDAC	multiple endocrine deficiency Addison's disease (autoimmune) candidiasis
MDT	motion detection threshold		
	multidisciplinary team		
	multidrug therapy	MEDCO	Medcosonolator
MDTM	multidisciplinary team meeting	MEDEX	medication administration record
MDTP	multidisciplinary treatment plan	MED-LARS	Medical Literature Analysis and Retrieval System
MDU	maintenance dialysis unit		
MDUO	myocardial disease of unknown origin	MEDS	medications
		MEE	maintenance energy expenditure
MDV	Marek's disease virus		

	measured energy expenditure
	middle ear effusion
MEF	maximum expired flow rate
	middle ear fluid
MEFR	mid expiratory flow rate
MEFV	maximum expiratory flow-volume
MEG	magnetoencephalogram
	magnetoencephalography
Meg-CSF	megakaryocytic colony-stimulating factor
MEGX	monoethylglycinexylidide
MEI	medical economic index
MEIA	microparticle enzyme immunoassay
MEKC	micellar electrokinetic (capillary) chromatography
MEL	melatonin
MELAS	myopathy, encephalopathy, lactic acidosis, and stroke-like episodes (syndrome)
MEL B	melarsoprol
MEM	memory
	monocular estimate method (near retinoscopy)
MEN	meningeal
	meninges
	meningitis
MEN (II)	multiple endocrine neoplasia (type II)
MENS	mini-electrical nerve stimulator
MEO	malignant external otitis
MeOH	methyl alcohol
MEOS	microsomal ethanol oxidizing system
MEP	maximal expiratory pressure
	meperidine
mEq	milliequivalent
mEq/24 H	milliequivalents per 24 hours

mEq/L	milliequivalents per liter
MER	medical evidence of record
	methanol-extracted residue (of phenol-treated BCG)
M/E ratio	myeloid/erythroid ratio
MES	mesial
MET	medical emergency treatment
	metabolic
	metamyelocytes
	metastasis
	metronidazole
META	metamyelocytes
METH	methicillin
METHb	methemoglobin
methyl CCNU	semustine
methyl G	mitroguazone dihydrochloride
methyl GAG	mitroguazone dihydrochloride
METS	metabolic equivalents (multiples of resting oxygen uptake)
	metastases
METT	maximum exercise tolerance test
MEV	million electron volts
MEX	Mexican
MF	Malassezia folliculitis
	Malassezia furfur
	masculinity/femininity
	meat free
	mesial facial
	methotrexate, fluorouracil and calcium leucovorin
	midcavity forceps
	mid forceps
	mother and father
	mycosis fungoides
	myelofibrosis
	myocardial fibrosis
M & F	male and female
	mother and father
MFAT	multifocal atrial tachycardia

MFB	metallic foreign body		mast cell growth factor
	multiple-frequency		maternal grandfather
	bioimpedance	MGGM	maternal great
MFC	medial femoral condyle		grandmother
MFD	Memory for Designs	MGHL	middle glenohumeral
	midforceps delivery		ligament
	milk-free diet	mg/kg	milligram per kilogram
MFEM	maximal forced expiratory	mg/kg/d	milligram per kilogram
	maneuver		per day
MFFT	Matching Familiar	mg/kg/hr	milligram per kilogram
	Figures Test		per hour
MFH	malignant fibrous	MGM	maternal grandmother
	histiocytoma		milligram (mg is correct)
MFI	mean fluorescent intensity	MGN	membranous
MFR	mid-forceps rotation		glomerulonephritis
	myofascial release	MgO	magnesium oxide
MFS	Miller-Fisher syndrome	MG/OL	molecular genetics/oncol-
	mitral first sound		ogy laboratory
	monofixation syndrome	MGP	Marcus-Gunn's pupil
MFT	muscle function test	MGR	murmurs, gallops, or rubs
MFVNS	middle fossa vestibular	MGS	malignant glandular
	nerve section		schwannoma
MFVPT	Motor Free Visual	MgSO₄	magnesium sulfate
	Perception Test		(Epsom salt)
MFVR	minimal forearm vascular	MGT	management
	resistance	mgtt	minidrop (60 drops = 1
MG	Marcus Gunn		mL)
	Michaelis-Gutmann	MGUS	monoclonal gammopathy
	(bodies)		of undetermined
	milligram (mg)		significance
	myasthenia gravis	MGW	multiple gunshot
Mg	magnesium		wound
mG	milligauss	MGW	magnesium sulfate,
μg	microgram (1/1000 of a	enema	glycerin, and water
	milligram)		enema
M&G	myringotomy and	M-GXT	multi-stage graded
	grommets		exercise test
mg%	milligrams per 100	mGy	milligray (radiation unit)
	milliliters	MH	malignant hyperthermia
MGBG	mitoguazone		marital history
MGCT	malignant glandular cell		medical history
	tumor		menstrual history
MGD	meibomian gland		mental health
	dysfunction		moist heat
MGDF	megakaryocyte growth	MHA	Mental Health Assistant
	and development factor		(Associate)
mg/dl	milligrams per 100		methotrexate,
	milliliters		hydrocortisone, and
MGF	macrophage growth factor		cytarabine (ara-C)

	microangiopathic hemolytic anemia	MIBI	technetium 99m sestamibi (a myocardial perfusion agent, Cardiolite®)
	microhemagglutination		
MHA-TP	microhemagglutination-*Treponema pallidum*	MIBG	iobenguane sulfate I 123 (meta-iodobenzyl guanidine I 123)
MHB	maximum hospital benefits	MIC	maternal and infant care methacholine inhalation challenge
MHb	methemoglobin		medical intensive care
MHBSS	modified Hank's balanced salt solution		microscope microcytic erythrocytes
MHC	major histocompatibility complex		minimum inhibitory concentration
	mental health center (clinic)	MICA	mentally ill chemical abuser
	mental health counselor	MICE	mesna, ifosfamide,
M/hct	microhematocrit		carboplatin, and
mHg	millimeters of mercury		etoposide
MHH	mental health hold	MICN	mobile intensive care
MHI	Mental Health Index (information)		nurse
MHIP	mental health inpatient	MICR	methacholine inhalation challenge response
MH/MR	mental health and mental retardation	MICRO	microcytes
MHN	massive hepatic necrosis	MICU	medical intensive care
MHO	medical house officer		unit
MHRI	Mental Health Research Institute		mobile intensive care unit
MHS	major histocompatibility system	MID	mesioincisodistal minimal ineffective dose multi-infarct dementia
	malignant hyperthermia susceptible	MIDCAB	minimally invasive direct coronary artery bypass
MHT	mental health team	MID EPIS	midline episiotomy
	Mental Health Technician	Mid I	middle insomnia
MHTAP	microhemagglutination assay for antibody to *Treponema pallidum*	MIE	maximim inspiratory effort meconium ileus equivalent (cystic fibrosis)
MHW	medial heel wedge mental health worker		medical improvement expected
MHX	methohexital sodium	MIEI	medication-induced
MHxR	medical history review		esophageal injury
MHz	megahertz	MIF	Merthiolate®
MI	membrane intact		iodine-formalin
	mental illness		migration inhibitory factor
	mental institution	MIFR	mid-inspiratory flow rate
	mesial incisal	MIF	mid-inspiratory flow at
	mitral insufficiency	50%VC	50% of vital capacity
	myocardial infarction		
MIA	medically indigent adult missing in action		

MIG	measles immune globulin		moderate intermittent suction
MIH	migraine with interparoxysmal headache	MISC	miscarriage miscellaneous
MIL	military	M Isch	myocardial ischemia
	mesial incisal lingual (surface)	MISO	misonidazole
	mother-in-law	MISS	Modified Injury Severity Score (scale)
MIMCU	medical intermediate care unit	MIT	meconium in trachea miracidia immobilization test
MIN	mammary intraepithelial neoplasia	MITO-C	mitomycin
	mineral	mIU	milli-international unit
	minimum	MIW	mental inquest warrant
	minor	mix mon	mixed monitor
	minute (min)	MJ	marijuana
MIN A	minimal assistance (assist)		megajoule
MINE	mesna, ifosfamide, mitoxantrone (Novantrone), and etoposide	MJT	Mead Johnson tube
		μkat	microkatal (micro-moles/sec)
	medical improvement not expected	MKAB	may keep at bedside
		MKB	married, keeping baby
MIO	minimum identifiable odor	MK-CSF	megakaryocyte colony-stimulating factor
	monocular indirect ophthalmoscopy	MKI	mitotic-karyorrhectic index
MIP	maximum inspiratory pressure	MKM	microgram per kilogram per minute
	maximum-intensity projection	ML	malignant lymphoma middle lobe
	mean intrathoracic pressure	mL	midline milliliter
	mean intravascular pressure	M/L	monocyte to lymphocyte (ratio) mother-in-law
	medical improvement possible	MLA	mento-laeva anterior
	metacarpointerphalangeal	MLAP	mean left atrial pressure
MIRD	medical internal radiation dose	MLBW	moderately low birth weight
MIRP	myocardial infarction rehabilitation program	MLC	minimal lethal concentration mixed lymphocyte culture
MIRS	Medical Improvement Review Standard		multilevel care multilumen catheter
MIS	management information systems		myelomonocytic leukemia, chronic
	minimally invasive surgery	MLD	masking level difference metachromatic leukodystrophy
	mitral insufficiency		

	microlumbar diskectomy	MMD	malignant metastatic disease
	microsurgical lumbar diskectomy		myotonic muscular dystrophy
	minimal lethal dose	MMECT	multiple monitor electroconvulsive therapy
MLE	midline (medial) episiotomy		
MLF	median longitudinal fasciculus	MMEFR	maximal mid-expiratory flow rate
MLNS	minimal lesions nephrotic syndrome	MMF	mean maximum flow
	mucocutaneous lymph node syndrome (Kawasaki syndrome)		mycophenolate mofetil (CellCept)
		MMFR	maximal mid-expiratory flow rate
MLO	mesiolinguo-occlusal	mmHg	millimeters of mercury
MLP	mento-laeva posterior	MMK	Marshall-Marchetti-Krantz (cystourethropexy)
	mesiolinguopulpal		
MLPN	Medical Licensed Practical Nurse	MMM	mitoxantrone, methotrexate, and mitomycin
MLR	middle latency response		mucous membrane moist
	mixed lymphocyte reaction		myelofibrosis with myeloid metaplasia
	multiple logistic regression	MMMT	metastatic mixed müllerian tumor
MLT	mento-laeva transversa		
MLU	mean length of utterance	MMOA	maxillary mandibular odontectomy alveolectomy
MLV	monitored line voice		
MM	major medical (insurance)	mmol	millimole
	malignant melanoma	μmol	micromole
	Marshall-Marchetti	MMP	matrix metallopro-teinase
	medial malleolus		
	meningococcic meningitis		multiple medical problems
	mercaptopurine and methotrexate	MMP-8	metalloproteinase-8
	methadone maintenance	MMPI	matrix metalloproteinase inhibitor
	millimeter (mm)		
	mist mask		Minnesota Multiphasic Personality Inventory
	morbidity and mortality	MMPI-D	Minnesota Multiphasic Personality Inventory-Depression Scale
	motor meal		
	mucous membrane		
	multiple myeloma		
	muscle movement		
	myelomeningocele		
mM.	millimole (mmol)	6-MMPR	6-methylmercaptopurine riboside
mm	millimeter		
M&M	milk and molasses	MMR	measles, mumps, and rubella
	morbidity and mortality		
MMA	methylmalonic acid		midline malignant reticulosis
	methylmethacrylate		
MMC	mitomycin (mitomycin C)		

MMS	Mini-Mental State (examination)	MNTB	medial nucleus of the trapezoid body
	Mohs' micrographic surgery	MNZ	metronidazole
MMSE	Mini-Mental State Examination	MO	medial oblique (x-ray view)
MMT	malignant mesenchymal tumors		mesio-occlusal
	manual muscle test		mineral oil
	Mini Mental Test		month (mo)
	mixed müllerian tumors		months old
MMTP	Methadone Maintenance Treatment Program		morbidly obese
			mother
MMTV	malignant mesothelioma of the tunica vaginalis	Mo	molybdenum
		MOA	mechanism of action
	monomorphic ventricular tachycardia		metronidazole, omeprazole, and amoxicillin
	mouse mammary tumor virus	MoAb	monoclonal antibody
MMV	mandatory minute volume	MOB	medical office building
MMWR	*Morbidity and Mortality Weekly Report*	MOB-PT	mitomycin, vincristine (Oncovin), bleomycin, and cisplatin (Platinol)
MN	midnight		
	mononuclear	MOC	medial olivocochlear
Mn	manganese		Medical Officer on Call
M&N	morning and night		metronidazole, omeprazole, and clarithromycin
	Mydriacyl and Neo-Synephrine		
			mother of child
MNC	monomicrobial necrotizing cellulitis	MOCI	Maudsley Obsessive-Compulsive Inventory
	mononuclear leukocytes	MOD	maturity onset diabetes
M/NCV	motor nerve conduction velocity		medical officer of the day
			mesio-occlusodistal
MND	modified neck dissection		moderate
	motor neuron disease		mode of death
MNF	myelinated nerve fibers		moment of death
MNG	multinodular goiter		multiorgan dysfunction
MNM	mononeuritis multiplex	MOD A	moderate assistance (assist)
MNNB	Monas-Nitz Neuropsychological Battery	MODM	mature-onset diabetes mellitus
MNR	marrow neutrophil reserve	MODS	multiple organ dysfunction syndrome
MNSc	Master of Nursing Science	MODY	maturity onset diabetes of youth
MnSOD	manganese superoxide dismutase	MOE	movement of extremities
Mn SSEPS	median nerve somatosensory evoked potentials	MOF	mesial occlusal facial
			methoxyflurane
			methotrexate, vincristine

	(Oncovin), and fluorouracil	MOU	medical oncology unit memorandum of understanding
MOFS	multiple-organ failure syndrome	MOUS	multiple occurrences of unexplained symptoms
MoICU	mobile intensive care unit	MOV	minimum obstructive volume
MOJAC	mood orientation, judgement, affect, and content		multiple oral vitamin
MOM	milk of magnesia	MOW	Meals on Wheels
	mother	MP	melphalan and prednisone
	mucoid otitis media		menstrual period
MoM	multiples of the median		mercaptopurine
MOMP	major outer membrane protein		metacarpal phalangeal joint
MON	maximum observation nursery		moist park
	monitor		monitor pattern
MONO	infectious mononucleosis		monophasic
	monocyte		mouthpiece
	monospot		myocardial perfusion
mono, di	monochorionic, diamniotic	M & P	Millipore and phase
mono, mono	monochorionic, monoamniotic	4 MP	methylpyrazole (fomepizole)
MOP	medical outpatient	6-MP	mercaptopurine
8 MOP	methoxsalen	MPA	main pulmonary artery
MOPP	mechlorethamine, vincristine (Oncovin), procarbazine, and prednisone		medroxyprogesterone acetate
		MPa	megapascal
MOPV	monovalent oral poliovirus vaccine	MPAC	Memorial Pain Assessment Card
MOR	morphine	MPAP	mean pulmonary artery pressure
MOS	mirror optical system	MPAQ	McGill Pain Assessment Questionnaire
	Medical Outcome Study	MPB	male pattern baldness
	months		mephobarbital
mOsm	milliosmole	MPBFV	mean pulmonary-blood-flow velocity
MOSF	multiple organ system failure	MPBNS	modified Peyronie bladder neck suspension
MOS sf-20	Medical Outcomes Study, short form 20	MPC	meperidine, promethazine, and chlorpromazine
MOS sf-36	Medical Outcomes Study, short form, 36 items		mucopurulent cervicitis
mOsmol	milliosmole	MPCN	microscopically positive and culturally negative
MOT	motility examination	MPCU	medical progressive care unit
MOTS	mucosal oral therapeutic system	MPD	maximum permissable dose
MOTT	mycobacteria other than tubercle		methylphenidate

	moisture permeable		multiphasic screening
	dressing	MPSS	methylprednisolone
	multiple personality		sodium succinate
	disorder	MPT	multiple parameter
	myofascial pain		telemetry
	dysfunction (syndrome)	MPTRD	motor, pain, touch,
MPE	malignant pleural effusion		and reflex deficit
	mean prediction error	MPU	maternal pediatric unit
MPEC	multipolar	MPV	mean platelet volume
	electrocoagulation	MQ	memory quotient
MPF	methylparaben free	MR	Maddox rod
m-PFL	methotrexate, cisplatin		magnetic resonance
	(Platinol), fluorouracil,		manifest refraction
	and leucovorin		may repeat
MPGN	membranoproliferative		measles-rubella
	glomerulonephritis		medial rectus
MPH	Master of Public Health		medical record
	methylphenidate		mental retardation
	miles per hour		milliroentgen
MPI	Maudsley Personality		mitral regurgitation
	Inventory		moderate resistance
MPJ	metacarpophalangeal joint	M&R	measure and record
mpk	milligram per kilogram	MR × 1	may repeat times one
MPL	maximum permissable		(once)
	level	MRA	magnetic resonance
	mesiopulpolingual		angiography
MPL®	monophosphoryl lipid A		main renal artery
MPM	malignant pleural		medical record
	mesothelioma		administrator
	Mortality Prediction		medical research associate
	Model		midright atrium
MPN	monthly progress note		multivariate regression
	multiple primary		analysis
	neoplasms	mrad	millirad
MPO	male pattern obesity	MRAN	medical resident admitting
	myeloperoxidase		note
MPOA	medial preoptic area	MRAP	mean right atrial pressure
MPP	massive periretinal	MRAS	main renal artery stenosis
	proliferation	MRC	Master of Rehabilitation
MPQ	McGill Pain		Counseling
	Questionnaire	MRCA	magnetic resonance
MPPT	methylprednisolone pulse		coronary angiography
	therapy	MRCC	metastatic renal cell
MPR	massive periretinal		carcinoma
	retraction	MRCP	Member of the Royal
MPS	mean particle size		College of Physicians
	mononuclear phagocyte		mental retardation,
	system		cerebral palsy
	mucopolysaccharidosis	MRD	margin reflex distance

	Medical Records Department		tomographic angiography
	minimal residual disease	MRV®	mixed respiratory vaccine
MRDD	Mental Retardation and Development Disabilities	MS	mass spectroscopy
MRDM	malnutrition-related diabetes mellitus		Master of Science
			medical student
MRE	manual resistance exercise		mental status
MRFC	mouse rosette-forming cells		milk shake
			minimal support
MR FIT	Multiple Risk Factor Intervention Trial		mitral sounds
			mitral stenosis
MRG	murmurs, rubs, and gallops		moderately susceptible
			morning stiffness
MRH	Maddox rod hyperphoria		morphine sulfate
MRHD	maximum recommended human dose		motile sperm
			multiple sclerosis
MRHT	modified rhyme hearing test		muscle spasm
			muscle strength
MRI	magnetic resonance imaging		musculoskeletal
		M & S	microculture and sensitivity
M & R I & O	measure and record input and output	MS III	third-year medical student
MRL	minimal response level	MSA	Medical Savings Accounts
	moderate rubra lochia		membrane-stabilizing activity
MRLVD	maximum residue limits of veterinary drugs		microsomal autoantibodies
MRM	modified radical mastectomy		multiple system atrophy
		MSAF	meconium-stained amniotic fluid
MRN	medical resident's note		
mRNA	messenger ribonucleic acid	MSAFP	maternal serum alpha-fetoprotein
MROU	medial rectus, both eyes	MSAP	mean systemic arterial pressure
MRPN	medical resident progress note		
		MSAS	Memorial Symptom Assessment Scale – short form
MRS	magnetic resonance spectroscopy		
	methicillin-resistant *Staphylococcus aureus*	MSB	mainstem bronchus
		MSBOS	maximum surgical blood order schedule
MRSA	methicillin-resistant *Staphylococcus aureus*	MSC	major symptom complex
MRSE	methicillin-resistant *Staphylococcus epidermidis*		midsystolic click
			MS Contin®
		MSCA	McCarthy Scales of Children's Abilities
MRT	magnetic resonance tomography	MSCCC	Master Sciences, Certified Clinical Competence
	modified rhyme test		
MRTA	magnetic resonance	MSCU	medical special care unit

MSCWP	musculoskeletal chest wall pain	MSOF	multi-system organ failure
MSD	microsurgical diskectomy	MSPN	medical student progress notes
	mid-sleep disturbance		
MSDS	material safety data sheet	MSPU	medical short procedure unit
MSE	Mental Status Examination	MSQ	meters squared
Msec	milliseconds	MSR	muscle stretch reflexes
MSEL	myasthenic syndrome of Eaton-Lambert	MSRPP	Multidimensional Scale for Rating Psychiatric Patients
MSER	mean systolic ejection rate	MSS	Marital Satisfaction Scale
			mean sac size
	Mental Status Examination Record		minor surgery suite
MSF	meconium-stained fluid	MSSA	methicillin-susceptible *Staphylococcus aureus*
	megakaryocyte stimulating factor	MSS-CR	mean sac size and crown-rump length
MSG	methysergide	MSSU	mid-stream specimen of urine
	monosodium glutamate		
MSH	melanocyte-stimulating hormone	MST	mean survival time
			median survival time
MSHA	mannose-sensitive hemagglutinin		mental stress test
		MSTA®	mumps skin test antigen
MSI	magnetic source imaging	MSTI	multiple soft tissue injuries
	multiple subcortical infarction	MSU	maple syrup urine
	musculoskeletal impairment		midstream urine
MSIR®	morphine sulfate immediate release tablets	MSUD	maple-syrup urine disease
		MSUs	midstream specimens of urine
MSIS	Multiple Severity of Illness System	mSv	millisievert (radiation unit)
MSK	medullary sponge kidney	MSW	Master of Social Work
MSKCC	Memorial Sloan-Kettering Cancer Center		multiple stab wounds
		MT	empty
MSL	midsternal line		macular target
MSLT	multiple sleep latency test		malaria therapy
MSM	methsuximide		malignant teratoma
	mid-systolic murmur		Medical Technologist
MSN	Master of Science in Nursing		metatarsal
			middle turbinate
MSO	management services organization		monitor technician
			muscles and tendons
	mentally stable and oriented		muscle tone
			music therapy (Therapist)
	mental status, oriented		myringotomy tube(s)
MSO₄	morphine sulfate (this is a dangerous abbreviation)	M/T	masses of tenderness
			myringotomy with tubes
		M & T	*Monilia* and *Trichomonas*

166

	myringotomy and tubes		Therapeutic Recreation
MTA	Medical Technical Assistant		Specialist
		MTS	mesial temporal sclerosis
MTAD	tympanic membrane of the left ear	MTST	maximal treadmill stress test
MT/AK	music therapy/audiokinetics	MTT	mean transit time
			methylthiotetrazole
MTAS	tympanic membrane of the left ear	MTU	malignant teratoma undifferentiated
MTAU	tympanic membranes of both ears		methylthiouracil
		MTX	methotrexate
MTB	*Mycobacterium tuberculosis*	MTZ	mitoxantrone
		MU	million units
MTBC	Music Therapist-Board Certified		Murphy unit
		mU	milliunits
MTBE	methyl tert-butyl ether	MUA	manipulation under anesthesia
MTC	magnetization transfer contrast		
		MUAC	middle upper arm circumference
	medullary thyroid carcinoma		
		MUD	matched unrelated donor
	metoclopramide	MUE	medication use evaluation
	mitomycin	MUGA	multigated angiogram
MTD	maximal tolerated dose		multiple gated acquisition (scan)
	metastatic trophoblastic disease		
		MUGX	multiple gated acquisition exercise
	Monroe tidal drainage		
	Mycobacterium tuberculosis direct (test)	MULE	microcomputer upper limb exerciser
MTDI	maximum tolerable daily intake	MuLV	murine leukemia virus
		MUO	metastasis of unknown origin
MTE	multiple trace elements		
MTET	modified treadmill exercise testing	MUPAT	multiple-site perineal applicator technique
MTG	middle temporal gyrus (gyri)	MUSE®	Medicated Urethral System for Erection
	mid-thigh girth	mus-lig	musculoligamentous
MTI	malignant teratoma intermediate	MUU	mouse uterine units
		MV	mechanical ventilation
MTJ	mid-tarsal joint		millivolts
MTM	modified Thayer-Martin medium		minute volume
			mitoxantrone and etoposide
MTP	master treatment plan		
	medical termination of pregnancy		mitral valve
			mixed venous
	metatarsophalangeal		multivesicular
MTR͟	mother	MVA	malignant vertricular arrhythmias
MTR-O͟	no masses, tenderness, or rebound		manual vacuum aspiration
MTRS	Licensed Master		mitral valve area

	motor vehicle accident	MVS	mitral valve stenosis
M-VAC	methotrexate, vinblastine doxorubicin (Adriamycin), and cisplatin		motor, vascular, and sensory
MVAC	methotrexate, vinblastine doxorubicin (Adriamycin), and cisplatin	MVT	multiform ventricular tachycardia
			multivitamin
MVB	methotrexate and vinblastine	MVU	Montevideo units
	mixed venous blood	MVV	maximum ventilatory volume
MVC	maximal voluntary contraction		maximum voluntary ventilation
	motor vehicle collision		mixed vespid venom
MVc	mitral valve closure	MWB	minimal weight bearing
MVD	microvascular decompression	MWD	microwave diathermy
	microvessel density	M-W-F	Monday-Wednesday-Friday
	mitral valve disease	MWI	Medical Walk-In (Clinic)
	multivessel disease	MWS	Mickety-Wilson syndrome
MVE	mitral valve (leaflet) excursion	MWT	malpositioned wisdom teeth
	Murray Valley encephalitis	Mx	manifest refraction
MV Grad	mitral valve gradient		mastectomy
MVI	multiple vitamin injection		maxilla
MVI®	trade name for parenteral multivitamins		movement
			myringotomy
MVI 12®	trade name for parenteral multivitamins	My	myopia
		MYD	mydriatic
MVO	mixed venous oxygen saturation	myelo	myelocytes
			myelogram
MVO_2	myocardial oxygen consumption	MyG	myasthenia gravis
		MYOP	myopia
MVP	mean venous pressure	MYR	myringotomy
	mitral valve prolapse	MYS	medium yellow soft (stools)
MVPP	mechlorethamine, vinblastine, procarbazine, and prednisone	MZ	monozygotic
		MZL	marginal zone lymphocyte
		MZT	monozygotic twins
MVPS	mitral valve prolapse syndrome		
MVR	massive vitreous retraction		
	micro-vitreoretinal (blade)		
	mitral valve regurgitation		
	mitral valve replacement		
MVRI	mixed vaccine respiratory infections	N	nausea
			negative

N

		NAB	not at bedside
	Negro	NABS	normoactive bowel
	Neisseria		sounds
	nerve	NABX	needle aspiration biopsy
	neutrophil	NAC	acetylcysteine
	never		(N-acetylcysteine)
	newton		no acute changes
	nipple	NACD	no anatomical cause of
	nitrogen		death
	no	NaClO	sodium hypochlorite
	nodes	NaCl	sodium chloride (salt)
	nonalcoholic	NACT	neoadjuvant
	none		chemotherapy
	normal	NAD	nicotinamide adenine
	not		dinucleotide
	notified		no active disease
	noun		no acute distress
	NPH insulin		no apparent distress
N I thru	size of sample		no appreciable disease
N XII	first through twelfth		normal axis deviation
	cranial nerves		nothing abnormal
0.1 N	tenth-normal		detected
N₂	nitrogen	NADPH	nicotinamide adenine
5'-N	5'-nucleotidase		dinucleotide phosphate
Na	sodium	NADSIC	no apparent active disease
Na⁺	sodium		seen in chest
NA	Narcotics Anonymous	NaE	exchangeable sodium
	Native American	NaF	sodium fluoride
	Negro adult	NAF	nafcillin
	nicotinic acid		Negro adult female
	nonalcoholic		normal adult female
	normal axis		Notice of Adverse
	not admitted		Findings (FDA post-
	not applicable		audit letter)
	not available	NAG	narrow angle glaucoma
	nurse aide	NaHCO₃	sodium bicarbonate
	nurse's aid	NAI	no action indicated
	Nurse Anesthetist		no acute inflammation
	nursing assistant		non-accidental injury
N & A	normal and active	NaI	sodium iodide
NAA	neutron activation	NAION	non-arteritic ischemic
	analysis		optic neuropathy
	no apparent abnormalities	NAM	normal adult male
NAAC	no apparent anesthesia	NANB	non-A, non-B (hepatitis)
	(anesthetic)		(hepatitis C)
	complications	NANBH	non-A, non-B hepatitis
NAA/Cr	N-acetyl aspartate/creatine		(hepatitis C)
	ratio	NANC	nonadrenergic,
NAATPT	not available at the		noncholinergic
	present time		

NANDA	North American Nursing Diagnosis Association	NBF	not breast fed
		NBH	new bag (bottle) hung
NAP	narrative, assessment, and plan	NBHH	newborn helpful hints
		NBI	no bone injury
	nosocomial acquired pneumonia	NBICU	newborn intensive care unit
NAPA	N-acetyl procainamide	NBL/OM	neuroblastoma and opsoclonus-myoclonus
NAPD	no active pulmonary disease	NBM	no bowel movement
Na Pent	Pentothal Sodium®		normal bone marrow
NAR	no action required		normal bowel movement
	no adverse reaction		nothing by mouth
	non-ambulatory restraint	NBN	newborn nursery
	not at risk	NBP	needle biopsy of prostate
NARC	narcotic(s)		no bone pathology
NAS	nasal	NBQC	narrow base quad cane
	neonatal abstinence syndrome	NBR	no blood return
		NBS	newborn screen (serum thyroxine and phenylketonuria)
	no abnormality seen		
	no added salt		
NAS-NRC	National Academy of Sciences – National Research Council		no bacteria seen
			normal bowel sounds
		NBT	nitroblue tetrazolium reduction (tests)
NASTT	nonspecific abnormality of ST segment and T wave		
			normal breast tissue
NAT	N-acetyltransferase	NBTE	nonbacterial thrombotic endocarditis
	no action taken		
	no acute trauma	NBTNF	newborn, term, normal female
	non-accidental trauma		
	nonspecific abnormality of T wave	NBTNM	newborn, term, normal, male
Na⁹⁹ᵐTcO₄⁻	sodium pertechnetate Tc 99m	NBW	normal birth weight
		NC	nasal cannula
NAUC	normalized area under the curve		Negro child
			neurologic check
NAW	nasal antral window		no change
NB	nail bed		no charge
	needle biopsy		no complaints
	newborn		noncontributory
	nitrogen balance		normocephalic
	note well		nose clamp
NBC	newborn center		nose clips
	non-bed care		not classified
NBCCS	nevoid basal-cell carcinoma syndrome		not completed
			not cultured
NBD	neurologic bladder dysfunction	NCA	neurocirculatory asthenia
			no congenital abnormalities
	no brain damage	N/CAN	nasal cannula

NCAP	nasal continuous airway pressure	NCRC	non–child-resistant container
NCAS	zinostatin (neocarzinostatin)	NCS	nerve conduction studies
			no concentrated sweets
NC/AT	normocephalic atraumatic		zinostatin (neocarzinostatin)
NCB	natural childbirth		
	no code blue	NCT	neutron capture therapy
NCC	no concentrated carbohydrates		noncontact tonometry
			Nursing Care Technician
	nursing care card	NCV	nerve conduction velocity
NCCLS	National Committee for Clinical Laboratory Standards		nuclear venogram
		ND	nasal deformity
			nasoduodenal
NCCTG	North Central Cancer Treatment Group		natural death
			neck dissection
NCCU	neurosurgical continuous care unit		neonatal death
			neurological development
NCD	no congenital deformities		neurotic depression
	normal childhood diseases		Newcastle disease
	not considered disabling		no data
NCE	new chemical entity		no disease
NCEP	National Cholesterol Education Program		nondisabling
			non-distended
NCF	neutrophilic chemotactic factor		none detectable
			normal delivery
NCI	National Cancer Institute		normal development
NCIS	nursing care information sheet		nose drops
			not detect
NCJ	needle catheter jejunostomy		not diagnosed
			not done
NCL	neuronal ceroid lipofuscinosis		nothing done
			Nursing Doctorate
	nuclear cardiology laboratory	N&D	nodular and diffuse
		Nd	neodymium
NCM	nailfold capillary microscope	NDA	New Drug Application
			no data available
	nonclinical manager		no demonstrable antibodies
NCNC	normochromic, normocytic		no detectable activity
		NDC	National Drug Code
NCO	no complaints offered	NDD	no dialysis days
	non-commissioned officer	NDE	near-death experience
NCP	no caffeine or pepper	NDEA	no deviation of electrical axis
	nursing care plan		
NCPAP	nasal continuous positive airway pressure	NDF	neutral density filter (test)
			no disease found
NCPR	no cardiopulmonary resuscitation	NDI	National Death Index
			nephrogenic diabetes insipidus
nCR	nodular complete response		

NDIR	nondispersive infrared	NEI	National Eye Institute (NIH)
NDIRS	nondispersive infrared spectrometer	NEJM	*New England Journal of Medicine*
Nd/NT	nondistended, nontender	NEM	no evidence of malignancy
NDP	net dietary protein		
	Nurse Discharge Planner	NEMD	nonspecific esophageal motility disorder
NDR	neurotic depressive reaction		
		NENT	nasal endotracheal tube
	normal detrusor reflex	NEOH	neonatal high risk
NDS	Neurologic Disability Score	NEOM	neonatal medium risk
		NEP	no evidence of pathology
NDST	neurodevelopmental screening test	NEPD	no evidence of pulmonary disease
NDT	neurodevelopmental techniques	NEPHRO	nephrogram
		NER	no evidence of recurrence
	neurodevelopmental treatment	NERD	no evidence of recurrent disease
	noise detection threshold	NES	nonstandard electrolyte solution
NDV	Newcastle disease virus		
Nd:YAG	neodymium:yttrium-aluminum-garnet (laser)		not elsewhere specified
		NESP	novel erythropoiesis stimulating protein
NE	nausea and emesis		
	neurological examination	NET	choroidal or subretinal neovascularization
	never exposed		
	no effect		Internet
	no enlargement		naso-endotracheal tube
	norethindrone		neuroectodermal tumor
	norepinephrine	NETA	norethisterone acetate
	not elevated	NETT	nasal endotracheal tube
	not examined	NEX	nose to ear to xiphoid
NEAA	nonessential amino acids		number of excitations
NEAC	norethindrone acetate	NF	necrotizing fasciitis
NEB	hand-held nebulizer		Negro female
NEC	necrotizing entercolitis		neurofibromatosis
	noise equivalent counts		night frequency (of voiding)
	nonesterified cholesterol		
	not elsewhere classified		none found
NED	no evidence of disease		not found
NEEG	normal electroencephalo-gram		nursed fair
		NFA	Nerve Fiber Analyzer®
NEEP	negative end-expiratory pressure	NFALO	Nerve Fiber Analyzer laser oththalmoscope
NEF	negative expiratory force	NFAR	no further action required
NEFA	nonesterified fatty acids	NFD	no family doctor
NEFG	normal external female genitalia	NFFD	not fit for duty
		NFI	no-fault insurance
NEFT	nasoenteric feeding tube		no further information
NEG	negative	NFL	nerve fiber layer
	neglect		

NFLX	norfloxacin	NHLBI	National Heart, Lung, and Blood Institute (NIH)
NFP	natural family planning		
	no family physician	NHO	notify house officer
	not for publication	NHP	Nottingham Health Profile
NFT	no further treatment		nursing home placement
NFTD	normal full-term delivery	NHS	National Health Service (UK)
NFTs	neurofibrillary tangles		
NFTSD	normal full-term spontaneous delivery	NHT	nursing home transfer
		NHTR	nonhemolytic transfusion reaction
NFTT	nonorganic failure to thrive	NHW	non-healing wound
NFW	nursed fairly well	NI	neurological improvement
NG	nanogram		no improvement
	nasogastric		no information
	night guard		none indicated
	nitroglycerin		not identified
	no growth		not isolated
	norgestrel	NIA	no information available
NGB	neurogenic bladder	NIAID	National Institute of Allergy and Infectious Diseases (NIH)
NGF	nerve growth factor		
n giv	not given		
NGJ	nasogastro-jejunostomy	NIAL	not in active labor
NGM	norgestimate	NICC	neonatal intensive care center
NGOs	non-governmental organizations		
		NICHHD	National Institute of Child Health and Human Development (NIH)
NGR	nasogastric replacement		
NGRI	not guilty by reason of insanity		
		NICS	non-invasive carotid studies
NGSF	nothing grown so far		
NGT	nasogastric tube	NICU	neonatal intensive care unit
	normal glucose tolerance		
NgTD	negative to date		neurosurgical intensive care unit
NGU	nongonococcal urethritis		
NH	nursing home	NID	no identifiable disease
NHB	non-heart beating (donor)		not in distress
NHC	neighborhood health center	NIDA five	National Institute on Drug Abuse screen for cannabinoids, cocaine metabolite, amphetamine/metham-phetamine, opiates, and phencyclidine
	neonatal hypocalcemia		
	nursing home care		
NHCU	nursing home care unit		
NH₃	ammonia		
NH₄Cl	ammonium chloride		
NHCU	nursing home care unit	NIDD	non–insulin-dependent diabetes
NHD	normal hair distribution		
NHL	nodular histiocytic lymphoma	NIDDM	non–insulin-dependent diabetes mellitus
		NIF	negative inspiratory force
	non-Hodgkin's lymphomas		not in file
nHL	normalized hearing level	NIFS	non-invasive flow studies

173

NIG	NSAIA (non-steroidal anti-inflammatory agent) induced gastropathy	nkat	nanokatal (nanomole/sec)
NIH	National Institutes of Health	NKB	no known basis
			not keeping baby
NIHD	noise-induced hearing damage	NKC	nonketotic coma
		NKDA	no known drug allergies
NIHL	noise-induced hearing loss	NKFA	no known food allergies
NIL	not in labor	NKH	nonketotic hyperglycemia
NIMAs	non-inherited maternal antigens	NKHA	nonketotic hyperosmolar acidosis
NIMHDIS	National Institute for Mental Health Diagnostic Interview Schedule	NKHHC	nonketotic hyperglycemic-hyperosmolar coma
		NKHOC	nonketotic hyperosmolar coma
NINDS	National Institute of Neurological Disorders and Stroke (NIH)	NKHS	nonketotic hyperosmolar syndrome
		NKMA	no known medication (medical) allergies
NINU	neuro intermediate nursing unit	NL	nasolacrimal
			non-latex
NINVS	non-invasive neurovascular studies		normal
		NLB	needle liver biopsy
NIOPCs	no intraoperative complications	NLC	nocturnal leg cramps
		NLC & C	normal libido, coitus, and climax
NIOSH	National Institute of Occupational Safety and Health (NIH)	NLD	nasolacrimal duct necrobiosis lipoidica diabeticorum no local doctor
NIP	no infection present		
	no inflammation present	NLDO	nasolacrimal duct obstruction
NIPAs	non-inherited paternal antigens	NLE	neonatal lupus erythematosus nursing late entry
NIPPV	noninvasive positive-pressure ventilation		
		NLF	nasolabial fold
NIP/S	non-invasive programming stimulation	NLFGNR	non-lactose fermenting gram-negative rod
NITD	neuroleptic-induced tardive dyskinesia	NLM	National Library of Medicine no limitation of motion
Nitro	nitroglycerin (this is a dangerous abbreviation) sodium nitroprusside (this is a dangerous abreviation)		
		NLMC	nocturnal leg muscle cramp
		NLN	no longer needed
		NLO	nasolacrimal occlusion
NIVLS	non-invasive vascular laboratory studies	NLP	no light perception nodular liquifying panniculitis
NJ	nasojejunal		
NK	natural killer (cells)	NLS	neonatal lupus syndrome
	not known	NLT	not later than
NKA	no known allergies		not less than

NM	Negro male	NMSIDS	near-miss sudden infant
	neuromuscular		death syndrome
	nodular melanoma	NMT	nebulized mist treatment
	nonmalignant		no more than
	not measurable	NMTB	neuromuscular
	not measured		transmission blockade
	not mentioned	NMTCB	Nuclear Medicine
	nuclear medicine		Technology
	nurse manager		Certification Board
N & M	nerves and muscles	NMT(R)	Nuclear Medicine
	night and morning		Technologist Registered
NMBA	neuromuscular blocking	NN	narrative notes
	agent		Navajo neuropathy
NMD	neuromuscular disorders		neonatal
	Normosol M and 5%		neural network
	Dextrose®		normal nursery
NME	new molecular entity		nurses' notes
NMF	neuromuscular facilitation	N/N	negative/negative
NMH	neurally mediated	NNB	normal newborn
	hypotension	NNBC	node-negative breast
NMHH	no medical health history		cancer
NMI	no manifest improvement	NND	neonatal death
	no mental illness	NNE	neonatal necrotizing
	no middle initial		enterocolitis
	no more information	NNM	Nicolle-Novy-MacNeal
	normal male infant		(media)
NMJ	neuromuscular junction	NNL	no new laboratory (test
NMKB	not married, keeping baby		orders)
NMM	nodular malignant	NNN	normal newborn nursery
	melanoma	NNO	no new orders
NMN	no middle name	NNP	Neonatal Nurse
NMNKB	not married, not keeping		Practitioner
	baby	N:NPK	grams of nitrogen to
nmol	nanomole		non-protein kilocalories
NMOH	no medical ocular history	NNR	not necessary to return
NMP	normal menstrual period	NNRTI	non-nucleoside reverse
NMR	nuclear magnetic		transcriptase inhibitor
	resonance (same as	NNS	neonatal screen
	magnetic resonance		(hematocrit, total
	imaging)		bilirubin, and total
NMRS	nuclear magnetic		protein)
	resonance spectroscopy		nicotine nasal spray
NMRT (R)	Nuclear Medicine Radio-		nonnutritive sucking
	logic Technologist	NNT	number needed to treat
	(Registered)	NNU	net nitrogen utilization
NMS	neuroleptic malignant	NO	nasal oxygen
	syndrome		nitric oxide
NMSE	normalized mean square		nitroglycerin ointment
	root		none obtained

	nonobese		ophthalmopathy: no
	number (no.)		signs or symptoms,
	nursing office		only signs, soft tissue
N₂O	nitrous oxide		involvement with
NOAEL	no observed adverse		symptoms and signs,
	effect level		proptosis, extraocular
N₂O:O₂	nitrous oxide to oxygen		muscle involvement,
	ratio		corneal involvement,
noc.	night		and sight loss (visual
noct	nocturnal		acuity)
NOD	nonobese diabetic	NOT	nocturnal oxygen therapy
	notice of disagreement	NOU	not on unit
	notify of death	NOV	human insulin, regular 30
NOFT	non-organic failure to	70/30	units/mL with human
	thrive		insulin isophane
NOFTT	non-organic failure to		suspension 70 units/mL
	thrive		(Novolin® 70/30)
NOK	next of kin	NOV L	human insulin zinc sus-
NOL	not on label		pension (Novolin® L)
NOM	nonsuppurative otitis	NOV N	human insulin isophane
	media		suspension (Novolin®
NOMI	nonocclusive mesenteric		N)
	infarction	NOV R	human insulin regular
NOMS	not on my shift		(Novolin® R)
NONMEM	non-linear mixed-effects	NP	nasal prongs
	model		nasopharyngeal
non pal	not palpable		near point
non-REM	non-rapid eye movement		neutrogenic precautions
	(sleep)		neurophysin
non rep	do not repeat		neuropsychiatric
NON VIZ	not visualized		newly presented
NOOB	not out of bed		nonpalpable
NOP	not on patient		no pain
NOR	norethynodrel		not performed
	normal		not pregnant
	nortriptyline		not present
NOR-EPI	norepinephrine		nuclear pharmacist
norm	normal		nuclear pharmacy
NOS	nitric oxide synthase		nursed poorly
	no organisms seen		nurse practitioner
	not on staff	NPA	nasal pharyngeal airway
	not otherwise specified		near point of
NOSI	nitric oxide synthase		accommodation
	inhibitors		no previous admission
NOSIE	Nurse's Observation Scale	NPAT	nonparoxysmal atrial
	(Schedule) for Inpatient		tachycardia
	Evaluation	NPC	near point convergences
NOSPECS	categories for classifying		nodal premature
	eye changes in Graves'		contractions

	nonpatient contact		producing *Neisseria*
	nonproductive cough		*gonorrhoeae*
	nonprotein calorie	NPR	normal pulse rate
	no prenatal care		nothing per rectum
	no previous complaint(s)	NPS	new patient set-up
NPCC	non-protein carbohydrate	NPSA	nonphysician surgical
	calories		assistant
NPCPAP	nasopharyngeal	NPSD	non-potassium-sparing
	continuous positive		diuretics
	airway pressure	NPSG	nocturnal
NPD	Niemann-Pick disease		polysomnography
	nonprescription drugs	NPT	near-patient tests
	no pathological diagnosis		neopyrithiamin
NPDL	nodular poorly		hydrochloride
	differentiated		nocturnal penile
	lymphocytic		tumescence
NPDR	nonproliferative diabetic		no prior tracings
	retinopathy		normal pressure and
NPE	neuropsychologic		temperature
	examination	NPU	net protein utilization
	no palpable enlargement	NPV	negative predictive value
	normal pelvic		nothing per vagina
	examination	NQECN	non-queratinizing
NPEM	nocturnal penile erection		epidermoid carcinoma
	monitoring	NQMI	non-Q wave myocardial
NPF	nasopharyngeal fiberscope		infarction
	no predisposing factor	NQWMI	non-Q wave myocardial
NPH	isophane insulin (neutral		infarction
	protein Hagedorn)	NR	do not repeat
	no previous history		newly reformulated
	normal pressure		nonreactive
	hydrocephalus		nonrebreathing
NPG	nonpregnant		no refills
NPhx	nasopharynx		no report
NPI	no present illness		no response
NPJT	nonparoxysmal junctional		no return
	tachycardia		normal range
NPLSM	neoplasm		normal reaction
NPK	non-protein kilocalories		not reached
NPM	nothing per mouth		not reacting
NPN	nonprotein nitrogen		not remarkable
NPNC	no prenatal care		not resolved
NPO	nothing by mouth		number
NPOC	nonpurgeable organic	NRAF	nonrheumatic atrial
	carbon		fibrillation
NPOD	Neuropsychiatric Officer	NRB	Noninstitutional Review
	of the Day		Board
NPP	normal postpartum		non-rebreather
NPPNG	nonpenicillinase-	NRBC	normal red blood cell

	nucleated red blood cell		nylon suture
	non-rebreathing system	NSA	normal serum albumin
NRBS			(albumin, human)
NRC	National Research		no salt added
	Council		no significant
	normal retinal		abnormalities
	correspondence	NSAA	nonsteroidal antiandrogen
	Nuclear Regulatory	NSABP	National Surgical
	Commission		Adjuvant Breast Project
NREM	nonrapid eye movement	NSAD	no signs of acute disease
NREMS	nonrapid eye movement	NSAIA	non-steroidal
	sleep		anti-inflammatory agent
NRF	normal renal function	NSAID	non-steroidal
NRI	nerve root involvement		anti-inflammatory drug
	nerve root irritation	NSBGP	non-specific bowel gas
	no recent illnesses		pattern
N-RLX	non-relaxed	NSC	no significant change
NRM	non rebreathing mask		nonservice-connected
	no regular medicines	NSCC	non-small cell carcinoma
	normal range of motion	NSCD	nonservice-connected
	normal retinal movement		disability
NRN	no return necessary	NSCFPT	no significant change
NRO	neurology		from previous tracing
NROM	normal range of motion	NSCLC	non–small-cell lung
NRP	non-reassuring patterns		cancer
NRPR	non-breathing pressure	NSCST	nipple stimulation
	relieving		contraction stress test
NRS	Neurobehavioral Rating	NSD	nasal septal deviation
	Scale		no significant disease
NRT	neuromuscular		(difference, defect,
	reeducation techniques		deviation)
	nicotine-replacement		nominal standard dose
	therapy		normal spontaneous
NS	nephrotic syndrome		delivery
	neurological signs	NSDA	non-steroid dependent
	neurosurgery		asthmatic
	nipple stimulation	NSDU	neonatal stepdown unit
	nodular sclerosis	NSE	neuron-specific enolase
	no-show		normal saline enema
	nonsmoker		(0.9% sodium chloride)
	normal saline solution	N s̄ E	nausea without emesis
	(0.9% sodium chloride	NSF	no significant findings
	solution)	NSFTD	normal spontaneous
	normospermic		full-term delivery
	no sample	NSG	nursing
	not seen	NSGCT	nonseminomatous germ-
	not significant		cell tumors
	nuclear sclerosis	NSGCTT	non-seminomatous germ-
	nursing service		cell tumor of the testis
	nutritive sucking		

NSGT	non-seminomatous germ-cell tumor	NSTT	nonseminomatous testicular tumors
NSHD	nodular sclerosing Hodgkin's disease	NSU	neurosurgical unit nonspecific urethritis
NSI	negative self-image no signs of infection no signs of inflammation	NSV	nonspecific vaginitis
		NSVD	normal spontaneous vaginal delivery
NSICU	neurosurgery intensive care unit	NSVT	non-sustained ventricular tachycardia
NSILA	nonsuppressible insulin-like activity	NSX	neurosurgical examination
		NSY	nursery
NSN	nephrotoxic serum nephritis	NT	nasotracheal next time
NSO	Neosporin® ointment		Nordic Track®
NSP	neck and shoulder pain		normal temperature
NSPs	non-starch polysaccharides		normotensive nortriptyline
NSPVT	nonsustained polymorphic ventricular tachycardia		not tender not tested nourishment taken
NSR	nasoseptal repair nonspecific reaction normal sinus rhythm not seen regularly		nursing technician
		N&T	nose and throat
		N Tachy	nodal tachycardia
NSRP	nerve-sparing radical prostatectomy	NTBR	not to be resuscitated
		NTC	neurotrauma center
NSS	neurological signs stable normal size and shape not statistically significant nutritional support service sodium chloride 0.9% (normal saline solution)	NTCS	no tumor cells seen
		NTD	negative to date neural-tube defects
		NTE	not to exceed neutral thermal environment
1/2 NSS	sodium chloride 0.45% (1/2 normal saline solution)	NTF	normal throat flora
		NTG	nitroglycerin nontoxic goiter nontreatment group normal tension glaucoma
NSSL	normal size, shape, and location		
NSSP	normal size, shape, and position	NTGO	nitroglycerin ointment
NSSTT	nonspecific ST and T (wave)	NTI	no treatment indicated
		NTIS	National Technical Information Service (U.S. Department of Commerce)
NSST-TWCs	nonspecific ST-T wave changes		
NST	non-stress test not sooner than nutritional support team	NTL	nortriptyline no time limit
		NTM	nocturnal tumescence monitor nontuberculous mycobacterium
NSTD	non-sexually transmitted disease		
NSTI	necrotizing soft-tissue infection		

NTMB	nontuberculous myobacteria		neurovesicle dysfunction
			normal vaginal delivery
NTMI	non-transmural myocardial infarction		no venereal disease
			no venous distention
NTND	not tender, not distended		nonvalvular disease
NTP	narcotic treatment program	NVDC	nausea, vomiting, diarrhea, and constipation
	Nitropaste® (nitroglycerin ointment)	NVE	native
	normal temperature and pressure		native valve endocarditis neovascularization elsewhere
	sodium nitroprusside	NVG	neovascular glaucoma
NTS	nasotracheal suction		neoviridogrisein
	nucleus tractus solitarii	NVL	neurovascular laboratory
NTT	nasotracheal tube	NVP	nevirapine (Viramune)
NTU	nephelometric turbidity units	NVS	neurological vital signs neurovascular status
NTX	naltrexone	NVSS	normal variant short stature
NTZ	nitazoxanide		
NTZ Long-acting®	oxymetazoline nasal spray	NW	naked weight nasal wash
NU	name unknown		not weighed
NUD	nonulcer dyspepsia	NWB	non-weight bearing
NUG	necrotizing ulcerative gingivitis	NWBL	non-weight bearing, left
nullip	nullipara	NWBR	non-weight bearing, right
NV	naked vision	NWC	number of words chosen
	nausea and vomiting	NWD	neuroleptic withdrawal normal well developed
	near vision	NWTS	National Wilms' Tumor Study (rating scale)
	negative variation		
	neovascularization	Nx	nephrectomy
	neurovascular		next
	next visit	NYD	not yet diagnosed
	nonvenereal	NYHA	New York Heart Association (classification of heart disease)
	nonveteran		
	normal value		
	not vaccinated		
	not verified	nyst	nystagmus
N&V	nausea and vomiting	NZ	enzyme
NVA	near visual acuity		
NVAF	nonvalvular atrial fibrillation		
NVB	Navelbine (vinorelbine tartrate)		
NVC	neurovascular checks		
NVD	nausea, vomiting, and diarrhea		
	neck vein distention	O	eye
	neovascularization of the (optic) disk		objective findings

O

180

	obvious	OAS	oral allergy syndrome
	occlusal		organic anxiety syndrome
	often		outpatient assessment service
	open		overall survival
	oral	OASI	Old Age and Survivors Insurance
	ortho		
	other	OASO	overactive superior oblique
	oxygen		
	pint	OASR	overactive superior rectus
	zero	OAW	oral airway
$\bar{o}$	negative	OB	obese
	no		obesity
	none		obstetrics
	pint		occult blood
	without		osteoblast
Ⓞ	orally (by mouth)	OB-A	obstetrics-aborted
$_1O_2$	singlet oxygen	OB-Del	obstetrics-delivered
O_2	both eyes	OBE	out-of-body experience
	oxygen	OBE-CALP	placebo capsule or tablet
O_2^-	superoxide		
O_3	ozone	OBG	obstetrics and gynecology
OA	occiput anterior	Ob-Gyn	obstetrics and gynecology
	old age	Obj	objective
	on admission	obl	oblique
	on arrival	OB marg	obtuse marginal
	ophthalmic artery	OB-ND	obstetrics-not delivered
	oral airway	OBP	office blood pressure
	oral alimentation	OBRR	obstetric recovery room
	osteoarthritis	OBS	obstetrical service
	Overeaters Anonymous		organic brain syndrome
O & A	observation and assessment	OBT	obtained
	odontectomy and alveoloplasty	OBTM	omeprazole, bismuth subcitrate, tetracycline, and metronidazole
OAA	Old Age Assistance		
OAC	oral anticoagulant(s)	OBUS	obstetrical ultrasound
	overaction	OBW	open bed warmer
OAD	obstructive airway disease	OC	obstetrical conjugate
	occlusive arterial disease		office call
	overall diameter		on call
OAE	otoacoustic emissions		only child
OAF	oral anal fistula		open cholecystectomy
	osteoclast activating factor		oral care
			oral contraceptive
OAG	open angle glaucoma		osteocalcin
OAP	old age pension		osteoclast
OASDHI	Old Age, Survivors, Disability, and Health Insurance	O & C	onset and course
		OCA	oculocutaneous albinism
			open care area

	oral contraceptive agent	OCVM	occult cerebrovascular
OCAD	occlusive carotid artery		malformations
	disease	OD	Doctor of Optometry
OCC	occasionally		Officer-of-the-Day
	occlusal		once daily (this is a
	old chart called		dangerous abbreviation
OCCC	open chest cardiac		as it is read as right
	compression		eye)
occl	occlusion		on duty
OCCM	open chest cardiac		optic disk
	massage		oral-duodenal
OCC PR	open-chest cardiopulmo-		outdoor
	nary resuscitation		outside diameter
OCC Th	occupational therapy		ovarian dysgerminoma
Occup Rx	occupational therapy		overdose
OCD	obsessive-compulsive		right eye
	disorder	Δ OD 450	deviation of optical
	osteochondritis dissecans		density at 450
OCG	oral cholecystogram	ODA	occipitodextra anterior
OCI	Obsessive-Compulsive		once-daily aminoglyco-
	Inventory		side
OCL®	oral colonic lavage		osmotic driving agent
OCN	Oncology Certified Nurse	ODAC	on demand analgesia
	obsessive compulsive		computer
	neurosis	ODAT	one day at a time
OCNS	Obsessive-Compulsive	ODC	oral disease control
	Neurosis Scale		ornithine decarboxylase
O-CNV	occult choroidal		outpatient diagnostic
	neovascularization		center
OCOR	on-call to operating	ODCH	ordinary diseases of
	room		childhood
OCP	ocular cicatricial	ODD	opposition defiance
	pemphigoid		disorder
	oral contraceptive pills	OD'd	overdosed
	ova, cysts, parasites	ODed	overdosed
OCR	oculocephalic reflex	ODM	occlusion dose monitor
	optical character		ophthalmodynamometry
	recognition	ODN	optokinetic nystagmus
OCS	Obsessive-Compulsive	ODP	occipitodextra posterior
	Scale		offspring of diabetic
	oral cancer screening		parents
11-OCS	11-oxycorticosteroid	OD/P	right eye patched
OCT	optical coherence	ODQ	on direct questioning
	tomograph	ODS	organized delivery system
	(tomography)	ODSU	oncology day stay unit
	ornithine carbamyl		One Day Surgery Unit
	transferase	ODT	occipitodextra transerve
	oxytocin challenge test	OE	on examination
OCU	observation care unit		orthopedic examination

	otitis externa	25(OH)D₃	25-hydroxy vitamin D
O-E	standard observed minus		(calcifediol, Calderol)
	expected	OHF	old healed fracture
O&E	observation and		Omsk hemorrhagic fever
	examination		overhead frame
OEC	outer ear canal	OHFA	hydroxy fatty acid
O₂EI	oxygen extraction index	OHFT	overhead frame and
OENT	oral endotracheal tube		trapeze
OER	oxygen extraction ratios	OHG	oral hypoglycemic
O₂ER	oxygen extraction ratio	OHI	oral hygiene instructions
OET	oral esophageal tube	OHIAA	hydroxyindolacetic acid
OETT	oral endotracheal tube	OHL	oral hairy leukoplakia
OF	occipital-frontal	OHNS	Otolaryngology, Head, and
	optic fundi		Neck Surgery (Dept.)
	osteitis fibrosa	OHP	obese hypertensive patient
OFC	occipital-frontal		oxygen under hyperbaric
	circumference		pressure
	orbitofacial cleft	OHRP	open-heart rehabilitation
OFLOX	ofloxacin		program
OFLX	ofloxacin	OHRR	open-heart recovery room
OFM	open face mask	OHS	occupational health
OFNE	oxygenated fluorocarbon		service
	nutrient emulsion		ocular hypoperfusion
OFPF	optic fundi and peripheral		syndrome
	fields		open-heart surgery
OFTT	organic failure to thrive	OHSS	ovarian hyperstimulation
OG	Obstetrics-Gynecology		syndrome
	orogastric (feeding)	OHT	ocular hypertension
	outcome goal (long-term		overhead trapeze
	goal)	OHTN	ocular hypertension
OGC	oculogyric crisis	OHTx	orthotopic heart
OGCT	ovarian germ cell tumor		transplantation
OGT	orogastric tube	OI	opportunistic infection
OGTT	oral glucose tolerance test		osteogenesis imperfecta
OH	occupational history		otitis interna
	ocular history	OIF	oil-immersion field
	on hand	OIG	Office of the Inspector
	open-heart		General
	oral hygiene	OIH	orthoiodohippurate
	orthostatic hypotension	OIHA	orthoiodohippuric acid
	outside hospital	OINT	ointment
17-OH	17-hydroxycorticosteroids	OIT	ovarian immature
OHA	oral hypoglycemic agents		teratoma
OHC	outer hair cell (in	OIU	optical internal
	cochlea)		urethrotomy
OH Cbl	hydroxycobalamine	OJ	orange juice (this is a
17-OHCS	17-hydroxycorticosteroids		dangerous abbreviation
OHD	hydroxy vitamin D		as it is read as OS-left
	organic heart disease		eye)

	orthoplast jacket	OMB	obtuse marginal branch
OK	all right	OMB_1	first obtuse marginal
	approved		branch
	correct	OMB_2	second obtuse marginal
OKAN	optokinetic after		branch
	nystagmus	OMC	open mitral
OKN	optokinetic nystagmus		commissuortomy
OKT	Ortho Kung T cell,	OMCA	otitis media, catarrhalis,
	designation for a series		acute
	of antigens	OMCC	otitis media, catarrhalis,
OL	left eye		chronic
	open label (study)	OMD	organic mental disorder
OLA	occiput left anterior	OME	Office of Medical
	occipitolaevoanterior		Examiner
OLB	open liver biopsy		otitis media with effusion
OLD	obstructive lung disease	7-OMEN	menogaril
OLF	ouabain-like factor	OMFS	oral and maxillofacial
OLM	ocular larva migrans		surgery
	ophthalmic laser	OMG	ocular myasthenia gravis
	microendoscope	OMI	old myocardial infarct
OLNM	occult lymph node	OMP	oculomotor (third nerve)
	metastases		palsy
OLP	abnormal lipoprotein	OMPA	otitis media, purulent,
OLR	otology, laryngology, and		acute
	rhinology	OMPC	otitis media, purulent,
OLT	occipitolaevoposterior		chronic
	orthotopic liver	OMR	operative mortality rate
	transplantation	OMS	oral morphine sulfate
OLTx	orthotopic liver		organic mental syndrome
	transplantation		organic mood syndrome
OM	every morning (this is a	OMSA	otitis media secretory (or
	dangerous abbreviation)		suppurative) acute
	obtuse marginal	OMSC	otitis media secretory (or
	ocular melanoma		suppurative) chronic
	oral motor	OMT	oral mucosal transudate
	oral mucositis	OMVC	open mitral valve
	osteomalacia		commissurotomy
	osteomyelitis	OMVI	operating motor vehicle
	otitis media		intoxicated
O_2M	oxygen mask	ON	every night (this is a
OM_1	first obtuse marginal		dangerous abbreviation)
	(branch)		optic nerve
OM_2	second obtuse marginal		optic neurophathy
	(branch)		oronasal
OMA	older maternal age		Ortho-Novum®
OMAC	otitis media, acute,		overnight
	catarrhal	ONC	over-the-needle catheter
OMAS	otitis media, acute,		vincristine (Oncovin)
	suppurating	OND	ondansetron

	other neurologic disorder(s)		open
			operation
ONH	optic nerve head		oropharynx
	optic nerve hypoplasia		oscillatory potentials
ON RR	overnight recovery room		osteoporosis
ONSD	optic nerve sheath decompression		outpatient
		O&P	ova and parasites (stool examination)
ONSF	optic nerve sheath fenestration	OPA	outpatient anesthesia
ONTR	orders not to resuscitate		oral pharyngeal airway
OO	ophthalmic ointment	OPAT	outpatient parenteral antibiotic therapy
	oral order	OPB	outpatient basis
	other	OPC	operable pancreatic carcinoma
	out of		
o/o	on account of		oropharyngeal candidiasis
O&O	off and on		outpatient care
OOB	out of bed		outpatient catheterization
OOBL	out of bilirubin light		outpatient clinic
OOBBRP	out of bed with bathroom privileges	OPCA	olivopontocerebellar atrophy
OOC	onset of contractions	op cit	in the work cited
	out of cast	OPD	outpatient department
	out of control	O'p'-DDD	mitotane
OO Con	out of control	OPE	outpatient evaluation
OOD	outer orbital diameter	OPEN	vincristine (Oncovin), prednisone, etoposide, and mitoxantrone (Novantrone)
	out of doors		
OOH&NS	ophthalmology, otorhinolaryngology, and head and neck surgery		
		OPG	ocular plethysmography
OOI	out of isolette	OPL	other party liability
OOL	onset of labor	OPM	occult primary malignancy
OOLR	ophthalmology, otology, laryngology, and rhinology	OPN	osteopontin
		OPO	organ procurement organizations
OOM	onset of menarche		
OOP	out of pelvis	OPOC	oral pharynx, oral cavity
	out of plaster	OPP	opposite
	out on pass	OPPG	oculopneumoplethysmography
OOPS	out of program status		
OOR	out of room	OPPOS	opposition
OORW	out of radiant warmer	OPRDU	outpatient renal dialysis unit
OOS	out of sequence		
	out of splint	OPS	Objective Pain Scores
	out of stock		operations
OOT	out of town		outpatient surgery
OOW	out of wedlock	O PSY	open psychiatry
OP	oblique presentation	OPT	optimum
	occiput posterior		outpatient treatment

OPT c CA	Ohio pediatric tent with compressed air
OPT c O₂	Ohio pediatric tent with oxygen
OPT-NSC	outpatient treatment, non-service connected
OPT-SC	outpatient treatment, service-connected
OPV	oral polio vaccine
	outpatient visit
OR	odds ratio
	oil retention
	open reduction
	operating room
	Orthodox
	own recognizance
ORA	occiput right anterior
ORCH	orchiectomy
ORD	orderly
OREF	open reduction, external fixation
OR&F	open reduction and fixation
ORIF	open reduction internal fixation
ORL	otorhinolaryngology
ORMF	open reduction metallic fixation
ORN	operating room nurse
	osteoradionecrosis
OROS	ostomotic release oral system
ORP	occiput right posterior
ORS	olfactory reference syndrome
	oral rehydration salts
ORT	operating room technician
	oral rehydration therapy
	Registered Occupational Therapist
OR X1	oriented to time
OR X2	oriented to time and place
OR X3	oriented to time, place, and person
OR X4	oriented to time, place, person, and objects (watch, pen, book)
OS	left eye
	mouth (this is a dangerous abbreviation as it is read as left eye)
	occipitosacral
	oligospermic
	opening snap
	ophthalmic solution (this is a dangerous abbreviation as it is read as left eye)
	oral surgery
	osmium
	osteosarcoma
	overall survival
OSA	obstructive sleep apnea
OSAS	obstructive sleep apnea syndrome
OSCE	Objective Structured Clinical Examination
OSD	overseas duty
	overside drainage
OSESC	opening snap ejection systolic click
OSFT	outstretched fingertips
OSH	outside hospital
OSHA	Occupational Safety & Health Administration
OSM S	osmolarity serum
OSM U	osmolarity urine
OSN	off service note
OSP	outside pass
OS/P	left eye patched
OSS	osseous
	over-shoulder strap
OT	occiput transverse
	occupational therapy
	old tuberculin
	oral transmucosal
	orotracheal
	oxytocin
O/T	oral temperature
OTA	open to air
OTC	ornithine transcarbamoylase
	Orthopedic Technician, Certified
	over the counter (sold without prescription)
OTD	optimal therapeutic dose
	organ tolerance dose

	out the door	OXM	pulse oximeter
OTH	other	Oxy-5®	benzoyl peroxide
OTHS	occupational therapy home service	OXZ	oxazepam
		OZ	optical zone
OTO	one time only		ounce
	otolaryngology		
	otology		
OTR	Occupational Therapist, Registered		
OTRL	Occupational Therapist, Registered Licensed		

OT/RT	occupational therapy/ recreational therapy		
OTS	orotracheal suction		
OTT	orotracheal tube		
OTW	off-the-wall		
OU	both eyes	P	para
OULQ	outer upper left quadrant		peripheral
OU/P	both eyes patched		phosphorus
OURQ	outer upper right quadrant		pint
OV	office visit		plan
	ovary		poor
	ovum		protein
OVAL	ovalocytes		Protestant
OVF	Octopus® visual field		pulse
OVR	Office of Vocational Rehabilitation		pupil
OVS	obstructive voiding	$\bar{p}$	after
	symptoms (syndrome)	/P	partial lower denture
OW	once weekly (this is a	P/	partial upper denture
	dangerous abbreviation)	P_2	pulmonic second heart sound
	open wound	P20	Ocusert® P20
	outer wall	P40	Ocusert® P40
	out of wedlock	^{32}P	radioactive phosphorus
O/W	oil in water	PA	paranoid
	otherwise		periapical (x-ray)
OWNK	out of wedlock not keeping		pernicious anemia
			phenol alcohol
OWT	zero work tolerance		Physician Assistant
OX	oximeter		pineapple
O×1	oriented to time		posterior-anterior
O×2	oriented to time and place		(posteroanterior) (x-ray)
O×3	oriented to time, place,		presents again
	and person		professional association
O×4	oriented to time, place,		*Pseudomonas aeruginosa*
	person, and objects		psychiatric aide
Oxi	oximeter (oximetry)		psychoanalysis
Ox-LDL	oxidized low-density		pulmonary artery
	lipoprotein	Pa	pascal

P&A	percussion and auscultation	PAC-V	cisplatin (Platinol), doxorubicin (Adriamycin), and cyclophosphamide
	phenol and alcohol (procedure for permanent removal of toenail)	PACU	postanesthesia care unit
		PAD	pelvic adhesive disease
	position and alignment		peripheral artery disease
$P_2>A_2$	pulmonic second heart sound greater than aortic second heart sound		pharmacologic atrial defibrillator
			preliminary anatomic diagnosis
			preoperative autologous donation
PAB	premature atrial beat		
	pulmonary artery banding		primary affective disorder
PABA	aminobenzoic acid (para-aminobenzoic acid)	PADP	pulmonary arterial diastolic pressure
PAC	cisplatin (Platinol), doxorubicin (Adriamycin), and cylcophosphamide		pulmonary artery diastolic pressure
		PAE	postanoxic encephalopathy
	phenacemide		postantibiotic effect
	Physical Assessment Center		pre-admission evaluation
	Physician Assistant, Certified		progressive assistive exercise
	picture archiving communication (system)	PAEDP	pulmonary artery and end-diastole pressure
	Port-a-cath®	PAF	paroxysmal atrial fibrillation
	premature atrial contraction		platelet activating factor
	prophylactic anticonvulsants	PA&F	percussion, auscultation, and fremitus
	pulmonary artery catheter	PAGA	premature appropriate for gestational age
PACATH	pulmonary artery catheter	PAGE	polyacrylamide gel electrophoresis
PACH	pipers to after coming head	PAH	para-aminohippurate
$PACO_2$	partial pressure (tension) of carbon dioxide, alveolar		phenylalanine hydroxylase
			pulmonary arterial hypertension
$PaCO_2$	partial pressure (tension) of carbon dioxide, artery	PAI	plasminogen activator inhibitor
PACS	picture archiving and communications systems		platelet accumulation index
		PAIDS	pediatric acquired immunodeficiency syndrome
PACT	prism and alternate cover test	PAIVS	pulmonary atresia with intact ventricle septum
	Program of Assertive Community Treatment	PAL	posterior axillary line

	posteroanterior and lateral		pulmonary alveolar proteinosis
Pa Line	pulmonary artery line		pulmonary artery pressure
PALN	para-aortic lymph node	Pap smear	Papanicolaou smear
PALS	pediatric advanced life support	PA/PS	pulmonary atresia/ pulmonary stenosis
	periarterial lymphatic sheath	PAPVC	partial anomalous pulmonary venous connection
PAM	penicillin aluminum monostearate	PAPVR	partial anomalous pulmonary venous return
	potential acuity meter	PAR	parafin
	primary acquired melanosis		parallel
	primary amebic meningoencephalitis		perennial allergic rhinitis
2-PAM	pralidoxime		platelet aggregate ratio
PAMP	pulmonary arterial (artery) mean pressure		postanesthetic recovery
			procedures, alternatives, and risks
PAN	pancreas		pulmonary arteriolar resistance
	pancreatic	PARA	number of pregnancies producing viable offspring
	pancuronium		paraplegic
	panoral x-ray examination		parathyroid
	periodic alternating nystagmus	PARA 1	having borne one child
	polyacrylonitrile (filter)	PARC	perennial allergic rhinoconjunctivitis
	polyarteritis nodosa		
PANENDO	panendoscopy	PAROM	passive assistance range of motion
PANESS	physical and neurological examination for soft signs	PARR	postanesthesia recovery room
PANSS	Positive and Negative Syndrome Scale	PARS	postanesthesia recovery score
PAO	peripheral arterial occlusion	PARU	postanesthetic recovery unit
PAO₂	alveolar oxygen pressure (tension)	PAS	aminosalicylic acid (para-aminosalicylic acid)
PaO₂	arterial oxygen pressure (tension)		periodic acid-Schiff (reagent)
PAO	peak acid output		peripheral anterior synechia
PAOD	peripheral arterial occlusive disease		physician-assisted suicide
PAOP	pulmonary artery occlusion pressure		pneumatic antiembolic stocking
PAP	passive aggressive personality		postanesthesia score
	peroxidase-anti-peroxidase		premature auricular systole
	primary atypical pneumonia		
	prostatic acid phosphatase		

	Professional Activities Study			phenobarbital
	pulmonary artery stenosis	p/b		post-burn
	pulsatile antiembolism system (stockings)	P&B		pain and burning
				phenobarbital and belladonna
PASA	aminosalicylic acid (para-aminosalicylic acid)	PBA		percutaneous bladder aspiration
PA/S/D	pulmonary artery systolic/diastolic	PBAL		protected bronchoalveolar lavage
Pas Ex	passive exercise	PbB		whole blood lead
PASG	pneumatic antishock garment	PBC		point of basal convergence
				pre-bed care
PASI	Psoriasis Area and Severity Index			primary biliary cirrhosis
PASK	peripheral anterior stromal keratopathy	PBD		percutaneous biliary drainage
				postburn day
PASP	pulmonary artery systolic pressure			proliferative breast disease
PAT	paroxysmal atrial tachycardia	PBE		partial breech extraction
				power building exercise
	patella	PBF		placental blood flow
	patient			pulmonary blood flow
	percent acceleration time	PBG		porphobilinogen
	platelet aggregation test	PBI		protein-bound iodine
	preadmission testing	PBK		pseudophakic bullous keratopathy
	pregnancy at term	PBL		peripheral blood lymphocyte
PATH	pituitary adrenotropic hormone			primary brain lymphoma
	pathology	PBLC		premature birth live child
PATS	payment at time of service	PBM		pharmacy benefit management (manager)
PAV	Pavulon (pancuronium bromide)	PBMC		peripheral blood mononuclear cell
PAVM	pulmonary arteriovenous malformation	PBMNC		peripheral blood mononuclear cell
PAWP	pulmonary artery wedge pressure	PBN		polymyxin B sulfate, bacitracin, and neomycin
PAX	periapical x-ray	PB:ND		problem: nursing diagnosis
PB	barometric pressure	PBO		placebo
	British Pharmacopeia	PBP		protein-bound polysaccharide
	parafin bath	PBPC		peripheral blood progenitor cell
	power building			
	powder board	PBPCT		peripheral blood progenitor cell transplant
	premature beat			
	Presbyterian			
	protein-bound			
	pudendal block			
Pb	lead			

PBPI	penile-brachial pulse index		placebo
			postcoital bleeding
PBS	phosphate-buffered saline		prepared childbirth
PBSC	peripheral blood stem cells		*Pseudomonas cepacia* bacteremia
PBT₄	protein-bound thyroxine	PCBH	personal care boarding home
PBV	percutaneous balloon valvuloplasty	PCBMN	palmar cutaneous branch of the median nerve
PBZ	phenoxybenzamine	PCBs	polychlorinated biphenyls
	phenylbutazone	PCBUN	palmar cutaneous branch
	pyribenzamine		of the ulnar nerve
ΦBZ	phenylbutazone	PCC	patient care coordinator
PC	after meals		petrous carotid canal
	cisplatin (Platinol) and cyclophosphamide		pheochromocytoma
			pneumatosis cystoides coli
	packed cells		poison control center
	pancreatic carcinoma		progressive cardiac care
	pathologic consultation	PCCC	pediatric critical care
	platelet concentrate		center
	poor condition	PCCU	postcoronary care unit
	popliteal cyst	PCD	pacer-cardioverter-
	posterior chamber		defibrillator
	premature contractions		plasma cell dyscrasias
	present complaint		postmortem cesarean
	productive cough		delivery
	professional corporation		programmed cell death
	psychiatric counselor	PCE	physical capacities
	pubococcygeus (muscle)		evaluation
PCA	passive cutaneous anaphylaxis		potentially compensable event
	patient care assistant (aide)	PCE®	erythromycin particles in tablets
	patient controlled analgesia	PCEA	patient-controlled epidural analgesia
	penicillamine	PCF	pharyngeal conjunctival
	porous coated anatomic (joint replacement)		fever
		PCFT	platelet complement
	post ciliary artery		fixation test
	postconceptional age	PCG	phonocardiogram
	posterior cerebral artery		pubococcygeus (muscle)
	posterior communicating artery	PCGG	percutaneous coagulation of gasserian ganglion
	procainamide	PCH	paroxysmal cold
	procoagulation activity		hemoglobinuria
	prostate cancer		personal care home
PCAC	Physical Care Assessment Center	PC&HS	after meals and at bedtime
PCB	pancuronium bromide		
	para cervical block		

PCI	prophylactic cranial irradiation		prochlorperazine
			pulmonary capillary pressure
PCIOL	posterior chamber intraocular lens	PCR	polymerase chain reaction
PCKD	polycystic kidney disease		protein catabolic rate
PCL	pacing cycle length	PCr	plasma creatinine
	posterior chamber lens	PCRA	pure red-cell aplasia
	posterior cruciate ligament	PCR/PSA	polymerase chain reaction analysis of prostate-specific antigen
	proximal collateral ligament	PCS	patient care system
PCLI	plasma cell labeling index		portable cervical spine
PCLN	psychiatric consultation liaison nurse		portacaval shunt
			postconcussion syndrome
PCLR	paid claims loss ratio	P c/s	primary cesarean section
PCM	primary cutaneous melanoma	PCT	percent
			porphyria cutanea tarda
	protein-calorie malnutrition		post coital test
PCMX	chloroxylenol		posterior chest tube
PCN	penicillin		progestin challenge test
	percutaneous nephrostomy	PCU	palliative care unit
	primary care nursing		primary care unit
PCNA	proliferating cell nuclear antigen		progressive care unit
			protective care unit
PCNL	percutaneous nephrostolithotomy	PCV	packed cell volume
PCNSL	primary central nervous system lymphoma	PCVC	percutaneous central venous catheter
PCNT	percutaneous nephrostomy tube	PCWP	pulmonary capillary wedge pressure
PCO	patient complains of	PCX	paracervical
	polycystic ovary	PCXR	portable chest radiograph
	posterior capsular opacification	PCZ	procarbazine
			prochlorperazine
PCO_2	partial pressure (tension) of carbon dioxide, artery	PD	interpupillary distance
			Paget's disease
			panic disorder
			Parkinson's disease
PCOD	polycystic ovarian disease		percutaneous drain
P COMM A	posterior communicating artery		peritoneal dialysis
			personality disorder
PCOS	polycystic ovary syndrome		pharmacodynamics
			poorly differentiated
PCP	patient care plan		postural drainage
	phencyclidine		prism diopter
	Pneumocystis carinii pneumonia		progressive disease
			pupillary distance
	primary care person	P/D	packs per day (cigarettes)
	primary care physician	2PD	two point discriminatory test

192

^{103}Pd	palladium 103	PDL-N	poorly differentiated lymphocytic-nodular
PDA	parenteral drug abuser		
	patent ductus arteriosus	PDMC	premature dead male child
	poorly differentiated adenocarcinoma		
		PDN	Paget's disease of the nipple
	posterior descending (coronary) artery		
			prednisone
PDAF	platelet-derived angiogenesis factor		private duty nurse
		PDP	peak diastolic pressure
PDB	preperitoneal distention balloon	PD & P	postural drainage and percussion
PDC	patient denies complaints	PDPH	postdural puncture headache
	poorly differentiated carcinoma	PDQ	pretty damn quick (at once)
	private diagnostic clinic	PDR	patients' dining room
PD&C	postural drainage and clapping		*Physician's Desk Reference*
PDCA	Plan-Do-Check-Act (process improvement)		postdelivery room
			proliferative diabetic retinopathy
PDD	cisplatin		prospective drug review
	premenstrual dysphoric disorder	PDRcVH	proliferative diabetic retinopathy with vitreous hemorrhage
	primary degenerative dementia		
		PDRP	proliferative diabetic retinopathy
PDE	paroxysmal dyspnea on exertion	PDS	pain dysfunction syndrome
	pulsed Doppler echocardiography		polydioxanone suture
PDEGF	platelet-derived epidermal growth factor		Progressive Deterioration Scale
PDFC	premature dead female child	PDT	percutaneous dilatational tracheostomy
PDGF	platelet-derived growth factor		photodynamic therapy
			post-disaster trauma
PDGXT	predischarge graded exercise test	PDU	pulsed Doppler ultrasonography
PDH	past dental history	PDW	platelet distribution width
	pyruvate dehydrogenase	pDXA	peripheral dual energy x-ray absorptiometry
PDI	Pain Disability Index		
PDIGC	patient dismissed in good condition	PE	cisplatin and etoposide
			pedal edema
PDL	periodontal ligament		pelvic examination
	poorly differentiated lymphocytic		physical education (gym)
			physical examination
	postures of daily living		physical exercise
	progressively diffused leukoencephalopathy		plasma exchange
PDL-D	poorly differentiated lymphocytic-diffuse		pleural effusion

	polyethylene	PEFSR	partial expiratory flow static recoil curve
	preeclampsia		
	premature ejaculation	PEG	percutaneous endoscopic gastrostomy
	pressure equalization		
	pulmonary edema		pneumoencephalogram
	pulmonary embolism		polyethylene glycol
P₁E₁®	epinephrine 1%, pilocarpine 1% ophthalmic solution	PEG-ELS	polyethylene glycol and iso-osmolar electrolyte solution
P&E	prep and enema	PEGG	Parent Education and Guidance Group
PEA	pelvic examination under anesthesia		
	pre-emptive analgesia	PEG-J	percutaneous endoscopic gastrojejunostomy
	pulseless electrical activity	PEG-SOD	polyethylene glycol-conjugated superoxide dismutase (pegorgotein)
PEARL	pupils equal accommodation, reactive to light	PEI	percutaneous ethanol injection
	pupils equal and reactive to light	PEJ	percutaneous endoscopic jejunostomy
PEARLA	pupils equal and react to light and accommodation	PEK	punctate epithelial keratopathy
PEB	cisplatin, etoposide, and bleomycin	PEL	permissible exposure limits
PEC	pulmonary ejection click	PELV	pelvimetry
PECCE	planned extracapsular cataract extraction	PEM	prescription event monitoring
PECHR	peripheral exudative choroidal hemorrhagic retinopathy		protein-energy malnutrition
PECHO	prostatic echogram	PEMA	phenylethylmalonamide
PECO₂	mixed expired carbon dioxide tension	PEMS	physical, emotional, mental, and safety
PED	paroxysmal exertion-induced dyskinesia	PEN	parenteral and enteral nutrition
	pediatrics	PENS	percutaneous epidural nerve stimulator
	pigment epithelial detachments	PEO	progressive external ophthalmoplegia
PEDD	proton-electron dipole-dipole	PEP	patient education program
PEDI-DEG	pediatric deglycerolized red blood cells		pharmacologic erection program
Peds	pediatrics		pre-ejection period
PEE	punctate epithelial erosion		protein electrophoresis
PEEP	positive end-expiratory pressure	PEPI	pre-ejection period index
PEF	peak expiratory flow	PER	by
			pediatric emergency room
			protein efficiency ratio
PEFR	peak expiratory flow rate	PERC	perceptual

	percutaneous		preservative free
PERF	perfect		prostatic fluid
	perforation		push fluids
Peri Care	perineum care	PF3	platelet factor 3
PERIO	periodontal disease	PF4	repligen
	periodontitis	16PF	The Sixteen Personality
peri-pads	perineal pads		Factors test
PERL	pupils equal, reactive to	PFA	foscarnet (phosphonofor-
	light		matic acid)
PERLA	pupils equally reactive to		pure free acid
	light and accommoda-	PFB	potential for breakdown
	tion	PFC	patient focused care
per os	by mouth (this is a		perfluorochemical
	dangerous abbreviation		permanent flexure
	as it is read as left		contracture
	eye)		persistent fetal circulation
PERR	pattern evoked retinal	$\overline{P}$ FEEDS	after feedings
	response	PFFD	proximal femoral focal
PERRL	pupils equal, round, and		deficiency (defect)
	reactive to light	PFFFP	Pall filtered fresh frozen
PERRLA	pupils equal, round,		plasma
	reactive to light and	PFGE	pulsed field gel
	accommodation		electrophoresis
PERRRLA	pupils equal, round,	PfHRP-2	*Plasmodium falciparum*
	regular, react to light		histidine-rich protein 2
	and accommodation	PFI	progression-free interval
PERT	program evaluation and	PFJ	patellofemoral joint
	review technique	PFJS	patellofemoral joint
PES	pre-excitation syndrome		syndrome
	programmed electrical	PFL	cisplatin (Platinol),
	stimulation		fluorouracil, and
	pseudoexfoliation		leucovorin
	syndrome	PFL+IFN	cisplatin (Platinol),
peSPL	peak equivalent sound		fluorouracil,
	pressure level		leucovorin, and
PET	poor exercise tolerance		interferon alfa 2b
	positron-emission	PFM	primary fibromyalgia
	tomography		porcelain fused to metal
	pre-eclamptic toxemia	PFO	patent foramen ovule
	pressure equalizing tubes	PFPC	Pall filtered packed cells
PETN	pentaerythritol tetranitrate	PFR	parotid flow rate
PEx	physical examination		peak flow rate
PEX# 3	plasma exchange number	PFRC	plasma-free red cells
	three	PFROM	pain-free range of motion
PF	patellofemoral	PFS	patellar femoral syndrome
	peak flow		prefilled syringe
	peripheral fields		progression-free survival
	plantar flexion		pulmonary function
	power factor		studies (study)

PFT	parafascicular thalamotomy	PGP	paternal grandparent
	pulmonary function test	PGR	pulse generated runoff
PFU	plaque-forming unit	PgR	progesterone receptor
PFW	pHisoHex® face wash	P-graph	penile plethysmograph
PFWB	Pall filtered whole blood	PGS	Persian Gulf syndrome
PG	paged in hospital	PGT	play-group therapy
	paregoric	P±GTC	partial seizures with or
	performance goal (short-term goal)		without generalized tonic-clonic seizures
	phosphatidylglycerol	PGU	postgonococcal urethritis
	picogram (pg)	PGW	person gametocyte week
	placental grade (biophysical profile)	PGY-1	post-graduate year one (first year resident)
	polygalacturonate	pH	hydrogen ion concentration
	pregnant	PH	past history
	prostaglandin		personal history
	pyoderma gangrenosum		pinhole
PGA	prostaglandin A		poor health
	prothrombin time, gamma-glutamyl transpeptidase activity, and serum apolipoprotein AI concentration		pubic hair
			public health
			pulmonary hypertension
		P&H	physical and history
		Ph[1]	Philadelphia chromosome
		PHA	arterial pH
PGCs	primordial germ cells		passive hemagglutinating
PGE	posterior gastroenterostomy		peripheral hyperalimentation
	proximal gastric exclusion		phenylalanine
PGE₁	alprostadil (prostaglandin E₁)		phytohemagglutinin antigen
PGE₂	dinoprostone (prostaglandin E₂)		postoperative holding area
		PHACO	phacoemulsification
PGF	paternal grandfather	PHACO OD	phacoemulsification of the right eye
PGF₂α	dinoprost (prostaglandin F₂α)		
		PHACO OS	phacoemulsification of the left eye
PGGF	paternal great-grandfather		
PGGM	paternal great-grandmother	PHAL	peripheral hyperalimentation
PGH	pituitary growth hormones	PHAR	pharmacist
PGI	potassium, glucose, and insulin		pharmacy
			pharynx
PGI₂	epoprostenol (Prostacyclin)	Pharm	Pharmacy
		PharmD	Doctor of Pharmacy
PGL	persistent generalized lymphadenopathy	PHb	pyridoxylated hemoglobin
		PHC	post hospital care
	primary gastric lymphoma		primary hepatocellular carcinoma
PGM	paternal grandmother		
	phosphoglucomutase		primary health care

PHCA	profound hypothermic cardiac arrest	PHS	partial hospitalization program
PHD	paroxysmal hypnogenic dyskinesia		US Public Health Service
	Public Health Department	PHT	phenytoin
PhD	Doctor of Philosophy		portal hypertension
PHE	periodic health examination		primary hyperthyroidism
PHEN-FEN	phentermine and fenfluramine		pulmonary hypertension
		PHVA	pinhole visual acuity
PHEO	pheochromocytoma	PHx	past history
PHF	paired helical filament	Phx	pharynx
PHH	posthemorrhagic hydrocephalus	PI	package insert
			pallidal index
PHI	phosphohexose isomerase		pancreatic insufficiency
	prehospital index		Pearl Index
PHIS	posthead injury syndrome		peripheral iridectomy
PHL	Philadelphia (chromosome)		persistent illness
			physically impaired
PHLS	Public Health Laboratory Service (United Kingdom)		poison ivy
			postinjury
			premature infant
PHMB	polyhexamethylene biguanide		present illness
			principal investigator
PHN	postherpetic neuralgia		pulmonary infarction
	public health nurse	PI-3	parainfluenza 3 virus
	Puritan® heated nebulizer	P & I	probe and irrigation
PHNC	public health nurse coordinator	PIAT	Peabody Individual Achievement Test
PHNI	pinhole no improvement	PIC	peripherally inserted catheter
PHO	Physician/Hospital Organization		post intercourse
PHOB	phobic anxiety	PICA	Porch Index of Communicative Ability
PHP	pooled human plasma		posterior inferior cerebellar artery
	postheparin plasma		
	prepaid health plan		posterior inferior communicating artery
	pseudohypoparathy-roidism		
PHPT	primary hyperparathy-roidism	PICC	peripherally inserted central catheter
		PICT	pancreatic islet cell transplantation
PHPV	persistent hyperplastic primary vitreous	PICU	pediatric intensive care unit
PHR	peak heart rate		psychiatric intensive care unit
PhRMA	Pharmaceutical Research and Manufacturers of America (Formerly the Pharmaceutical Manufacturers Association)	PICVC	peripherally inserted central venous catheter
		PID	pelvic inflammatory disease

	prolapsed intervertebral disk		postinfusion phlebitis
	proportional-integral-derivative (controller)		proximal interphalangeal (joint)
PIE	pulmonary infiltration with eosinophilia		pulmonary insufficiency of the premature
	pulmonary interstitial emphysema	PIPB	performance index phonetic balance
PIEE	pulsed irrigation for enhanced evacuation	PIPIDA	N-para-isopropyl-acetanilide-iminodiacetic acid
PIF	peak inspiratory flow	PIPJ	proximal interphalangeal joint
PIFG	poor intrauterine fetal growth	PIP/TZ	piperacillin-tazobactam (Zosyn)
PIG	pertussis immune globulin	PIQ	Performance Intelligence Quotient (part of Wechsler tests)
PIGI	pregnancy-induced glucose intolerance
PIGN	postinfectious glomerulonephritis	PIS	pregnancy interruption service
PIH	pregnancy induced hypertension	PISA	phase invariant signature algorithm
	preventricular intraventricular hemorrhage		proximal isovelocity surface area
	prolactin inhibiting hormone	PIT	patellar inhibition test
			Pitocin® (oxytocin)
PIIID	peripheral indwelling intermediate infusion device		Pitressin® (vasopressin) (this is a dangerous abbreviation)
PIIIP	aminoterminal type three procollagen propeptide		pituitary
			pulsed inotrope therapy
PIIS	posterior inferior iliac spine	PITP	pseudo-idiopathic thrombocytopenic purpura
PIMIA	potentiometric ionophore mediated immunoassay	PITR	plasma iron turnover rate
PIMS	programmable implantable medication system	PIV	peripheral intravenous
		PIVD	protruded intervertebral disk
PIN	personal identification number	PIVH	periventricular-intraventricular hemorrhage
	prostatic intraepithelial neoplasia	PIVKA	proteins induced in vitamin K absence
PIO	pemoline
PIO₂	partial pressure of inspired oxygen	PIWT	partially impacted wisdom teeth
PIOK	poikilocytosis	PJ	procelin jacket (crown)
PI-PB	performance intensity-phonemically balanced	PJB	premature junctional beat
		PJC	premature junctional contractions
PIP	peak inspiratory pressure	PJRT	permanent form of

	junctional reciprocating tachycardia	PLBO	placebo
PJS	peritoneojugular shunt	PLC	pityriasis lichenoides chronica
	Peutz-Jeghers syndrome		
PJT	paroxysmal junctional tachycardia	PLD	partial lower denture
			percutaneous laser diskectomy
PJVT	paroxysmal junctional-ventricular tachycardia	PLDD	percutaneous laser disk decompression
PK	penetrating keratoplasty	PLE	polymorphic light eruption
	pharmacokinetics		
	plasma potassium		protein-losing enteropathy
	pyruvate kinase	PLED	periodic lateralizing epileptiform discharge
PKB	prone knee bend		
PKC	protein kinase C	PLEVA	pityriasis lichenoides et varioliformis acuta
PKD	polycystic kidney disease		
PKP	penetrating keratoplasty	PLFC	premature living female child
PKR	phased knee rehabilitation		
PK Test	Prausnitz-Küstner transfer test	PLH	paroxysmal localized hyperhidrosis
PKU	phenylketonuria	PLIF	posterior lumbar interbody fusion
pk yrs	pack-years (smoking one pack of cigarettes a day for one year is termed 1 pack-year of smoking, thus 2 packs a day for 20 years would be 40 pack-years)	PLL	prolymphocytic leukemia
		PLM	Plasma-Lyte M®
			polarized-light microscope
			product-line manager
		PLMC	premature living male child
		PLMS	periodic limb movements during sleep
PL	light perception	PLN	pelvic lymph node
	palmaris longus		popliteal lymph node
	place	PLND	pelvic lymph node dissection
	placebo		
	plantar	PLOSA	physiologic low stress angioplasty
	transpulmonary pressure		
PLA	Plasma-Lyte A®	PLP	partial laryngopharyngec-tomy
	potentially lethal arrhythmia		
			phantom limb pain
	Product License Application		protolipid protein
		PLPH	post-lumbar puncture headache
	pulpolinguoxial		
PLAD	proximal left anterior descending (artery)	PLR	pupillary light reflex
		PLS	plastic surgery
PLAP	placental alkaline phosphatase		Preschool Language Scale
			primary lateral sclerosis
PLAT C	platelet concentration	PLSO	posterior leafspring orthosis
PLAT P	platelet pheresis		
PLAX	parasternal long axis	PLST	progressively lowered stress threshold
PLB	posterolateral branch		
	phospholamban		

PLSURG	plastic surgery		primary myocardial disease
PLT	platelet		primidone
PLT EST	platelet estimate		private medical doctor
PLTF	plaintiff		progressive muscular dystrophy
plts	platelets		
PLUG	plug the lung until it grows	PMDD	premenstrual dysphoric disorder
PLV	posterior left ventricular	PM/DM	polymyositis and dermatomyositis
PLX	plexus		
PLYO	plyometric	PME	polymorphonuclear esosinophil (leukocytes)
PM	afternoon		
	evening		postmenopausal estrogen
	pacemaker	PMEALS	after meals
	particulate matter	PMEC	pseudomembranous enterocolitis
	petit mal		
	physical medicine	PMF	progressive massive fibrosis
	pneumomediastinum		
	poliomyelitis		pupils mid-position, fixed
	polymyositis		
	poor metabolizers	PMH	past medical history
	post menopausal	PMI	Pain Management Index
	post mortem		past medical illness
	presents mainly		patient medication instructions
	pretibial myxedema		
	primary motivation		plea of mental incompetence
	prostatic massage		
	pulpomesial		point of maximal impulse
PMA	Pharmaceutical Manufacturers Association (see PhRMA)		posterior myocardial infarction
		PML	polymorphonuclear leukocytes
	premarket approval		posterior mitral leaflet
	premenstrual asthma		premature labor
	Prinzmetal's angina		progressive multifocal leukoencephalopathy
PMAA	Premarket Approval Application (medical devices)		
		PMMA	polymethyl methacrylate
PMB	polymorphonuclear basophil (leukocytes)	PMMF	pectoralis major myocutaneous flap
	polymyxin B	PMN	polymodal nociceptors
	postmenopausal bleeding		polymorphonuclear leukocyte
PMC	premature mitral closure		
	pseudomembranous colitis		Premarket Notification (medical devices)
PMCP	para-monochlorophenol		
	perinatal mortality counseling program	PMNN	polymorphonuclear neutrophil
PMCT	perinatal mortality counseling team	PMO	postmenopausal osteoporosis
PMD	perceptual motor development	pmol	picomole

PMP	pain management program	PN₂	partial pressure of nitrogen
	previous menstrual period	PNA	Pediatric Nurse Associate
	psychotropic medication plan		polynitroxyl albumin
PMPM	per member, per month	PNa	plasma sodium
PMPO	postmenopausal palpable ovary	PNAB	percutaneous needle aspiration biopsy
PMR	pacemaker rhythm	PNAS	prudent no added salt
	polymorphic reticulosis	PNB	percutaneous needle biopsy
	polymyalgia rheumatica		premature newborn
	prior medical record		premature nodal beat
	progressive muscle relaxation		prostate needle biopsy
PM&R	physical medicine and rehabilitation	PNC	penicillin
			peripheral nerve conduction
PMS	periodic movements of sleep		premature nodal contraction
	poor miserable soul		prenatal care
	post-marketing surveillance		prenatal course
	postmenopausal syndrome		Psychiatric Nurse Clinician
	premenstrual syndrome	PND	paroxysmal nocturnal dyspnea
PMT	point of maximum tenderness		pelvic node dissection
	premenstrual tension		postnasal drip
PMTS	premenstrual tension syndrome		pregnancy, not delivered
PMV	prolapse of mitral valve	PNE	peripheral neuroepithelioma
PMW	pacemaker wires		primary nocturnal enuresis
PN	parenteral nutrition	PNET	primitive neuroectodermal tumors
	percussion note	PNET-MB	primitive neuroectodermal tumors-medulloblastoma
	percutaneous nephrosonogram		
	percutaneous nucleotomy	PNEUMO	pneumothorax
	periarteritis nodosa	PNF	proprioceptive neuromuscular fasciculation reaction
	peripheral neuropathy		
	pneumonia		
	polyarteritis nodosa	PNH	paroxysmal nocturnal hemoglobinuria
	poorly nourished		
	positional nystagmus	PNI	peripheral nerve injury
	postnasal		prognostic nutrition index
	postnatal	PNKD	paroxysmal nonkinesigenic dyskinesia
	practical nurse		
	premie nipple		
	primary nurse	PNL	percutaneous nephrolithotomy
	progress note		
	pyelonephritis		
P & N	psychiatry and neurology		

PNMG	persistent neonatal myasthenia gravis	
PNNP	Perinatal Nurse Practitioner	
PNP	peak negative pressure Pediatric Nurse Practitioner	
	progressive nuclear palsy	
	purine nucleoside phosphorylase	
PNS	partial nonprogressing stroke	
	peripheral nerve stimulator	
	peripheral nervous system	
	practical nursing student	
PNT	percutaneous nephrostomy tube	
pnthx	pneumothorax	
PNU	protein nitrogen units	
PNV	postoperative nausea and vomiting	
	prenatal vitamins	
Pnx	pneumonectomy pneumothorax	
PO	by mouth (*per os*)	
	phone order	
	postoperative	
P&O	parasites and ova	
	prosthetics and orthotics	
P$_{O2}$	partial pressure (tension) of oxygen, artery	
PO$_4$	phosphate	
POA	pancreatic oncofetal antigen	
	power of attorney	
	primary optic atrophy	
POACH	prednisone, vincristine, doxorubicin, cyclophosphamide, and cytarabine	
POAG	primary open-angle glaucoma	
POB	phenoxybenzamine	
	place of birth	
POC	plans of care	
	point-of-care	
	position of comfort	

	postoperative care
	product of conception
POD	pacing on demand
	place of death
	Podiatry
	polycystic ovarian disease
PODx	preoperative diagnosis
POD 1	postoperative day one
POE	point (portal, port) of entry
	position of ease
POEMS	plasma cell dyscrasia with polyneuropathy, organomegaly, endocrinopathy, monoclonal protein (M-protein), and skin changes
POEx	postoperative exercise
POF	position of function
	physician's order form
	premature ovarian failure
P of I	proof of illness
POG	Pediatric Oncology Group
	Penthrane,® oxygen, and gas (nitrous oxide)
	products of gestation
POH	personal oral hygiene
	presumed ocular histoplasmosis
POHA	preoperative holding area
POHI	physically or otherwise health impaired
POHS	presumed ocular histoplasmosis syndrome
POI	Personal Orientation Inventory
	postoperative instructions
POIK	poikilocytosis
POL	physician's office laboratory
	premature onset of labor
POLY	polychromic erythrocytes
	polymorphonuclear leukocyte
POLY-CHR	polychromatophilia

POM	pain on motion		plans of treatment
	polyoximethylene		potassium
	prescription-only		potential
	medication	POU	placenta, ovaries, and
POMC	pro-opiomelanocortin		uterus
POMP	prednisone, vincristine	POV	privately owned vehicle
	(Oncovin), methotrexate,	POW	prisoner of war
	and mercaptopurine	POX	pulse oximeter (reading)
POMR	problem-oriented medical	PP	near point of
	record		accommodation
POMS	Profile of Mood States		paradoxical pulse
PONI	postoperative narcotic		partial upper and lower
	infusion		dentures
PONV	postoperative nausea and		pedal pulse
	vomiting		peripheral pulses
POOH	postoperative open heart		pin prick
	(surgery)		pink puffer (emphysema)
POP	pain on palpation		Planned Parenthood
	persistent		plasmapheresis
	occipitoposterior		plaster of paris
	plaster of paris		poor person
	popliteal		posterior pituitary
	posterior oral pharynx		postpartum
POp	postoperative		postprandial
poplit	popliteal		presenting part
POPs	progesterone-only pills		private patient
POR	physician of record		prophylactics
	problem-oriented record		protoporphyria
PORP	partial ossicular		proximal phalanx
	replacement prosthesis		pulse pressure
PORR	postoperative recovery		push pills
	room	P-P	probability-probability
PORT	perioperative respiratory		(plots)
	therapy	PIIIP	aminoterminal type three
	portable		protocollegan
	postoperative respiratory		propeptide
	therapy	PPIX	protoporphyrin nine
POS	parosteal osteosarcoma	P&P	pins and plaster
	physician's order sheet		policy and procedure
	point-of-service	PPA	palpation, percussion, and
	positive		auscultation
poss	possible		phenylpropanolamine
post	post mortem examination		phenylpyruvic acid
	(autopsy)		postpartum amenorrhea
post op	postoperative	PP&A	palpation, percussion, and
Post Sag	posterior sagittal diameter		auscultation
D		PPAS	post-polio atrophy
post tib	posterial tibial		syndrome
POT	peak occupancy time	PPB	parts per billion

	pleuropulmonary blastoma		Present Pain Intensity
	positive pressure		proton pump inhibitor
	breathing	PPK	population pharmaco-kinetics
PPBE	postpartum breast engorgement	PPL	pars plana lensectomy
PPBS	post prandial blood sugar	PPLO	pleuro-pneumonia-like organisms
PPC	plaster of paris cast		
	progressive patient care	PPLOV	painless progressive loss of vision
PPCD	posterior polymorphous corneal dystrophy	PPM	parts per million
PPCF	plasma prothrombin conversion factor		permanent pacemaker persistent pupillary membrane
PPD	packs per day	PPMA	post-poliomyelitis muscular atrophy
	posterior polymorphous dystrophy		
	postpartum day	PPMS	psychophysiologic musculoskeletal (reaction)
	probing pocket depth		
	purified protein derivative (of tuberculin)	PPN	peripheral parenteral nutrition
P & PD	percussion & postural drainage	PPNAD	primary pigmented nodular adrenocortical disease
PPD-B	purified protein derivative, Battey		
		PPNG	penicillinase producing *Neisseria gonorrhoeae*
PPD-S	purified protein derivative, standard		
PPE	personal protective equipment	PPO	prefered provider organization
PPES	pedal pulses equal and strong	PPOB	postpartum obstetrics
		PPP	patient prepped and positioned
PPF	pellagra preventive factor		pedal pulse present peripheral pulses palpable (present)
	plasma protein fraction		
PPG	photoplethysmography		platelet-poor plasma
	postprandial glucose		postpartum psychosis
	pylorus-preserving gastrectomy		preferred practice patterns
PPGI	psychophysiologic gastrointestinal (reaction)		proportional pulse pressure (SBP minus DBP)/SBP
PPH	postpartum hemorrhage		protamine paracoagulation phenomenon
	primary pulmonary hypertension	PPPBL	peripheral pulses palpable both legs
PPHN	persistent pulmonary hypertension of the newborn	PPPG	postprandial plasma glucose
PPHx	previous psychiatric history	PPPM	per patient, per month
PPIX	protoporphyrin nine	PPQ	Postoperative Pain Questionnaire
PPI	benzylpenicilloylpolysine		
	patient package insert	PPR	patient progress record

PPr	periodontal prophylactics		Puerto Rican
PPRC	Physician Payment Review Commission		pulmonic regurgitation
			pulse rate
PPROM	prolonged premature rupture of membranes	P=R	pupils equal in size and reaction
pPROM	premature rupture of the membranes before 37 weeks gestation	P & R	pelvic and rectal
			pulse and respiration
PPS	peripheral pulmonary stenosis	PR-2	Bennett pressure ventilator
	postpartum sterilization	PRA	panel reactive antibodies (organ transplants)
	postperfusion syndrome		plasma renin activity
	postpoliomyelitis syndrome	PRAT	platelet radioactive antiglobulin test
	postpump syndrome	PRBC	packed red blood cells
	prospective payment system	PRC	packed red cells
			peer review committee
PPSS	peripheral protein sparing solution	PRCA	pure red cell aplasia
		PRD	polycystic renal disease
PPT	person, place, and time	PRE	passive resistance exercises
PPTL	postpartum tubal ligation		progressive resistive exercise
PPU	perforated peptic ulcer		
PPV	pars plana vitrectomy		proton relaxation enhancement
	patent processus vaginalum	Pred	prednisone
	positive predictive value	preg	Pregestimil® (infant formula)
	positive-pressure ventilation		
PPVT	Peabody Picture Vocabulary Test	PREMIE	premature infant
		pre-op	before surgery
PPY	packs per year (cigarettes)	prep	prepare for surgery
PQ	pronator quadratus		preposition
pQCT	peripheral quantitative computed tomography	PRERLA	pupils round, equal, react to light and accommodation
PQOCN	Psychiatric Questionnaire Obsessive-Compulsive Neurosis	prev	prevent
			previous
PR	far point of accommodation	PRFD	percutaneous radio-frequency denervation
	pack removal		
	partial remission	PRFNB	percutaneous radio-frequency facet nerve block
	patient relations		
	per rectum	PRG	phleborheogram
	premature	PRH	past relevant history
	profile		preretinal hemorrhage
	progressive resistance	PRI	Pain Rating Index
	prolonged remission		Patient Review Instrument
	prone	prim	primary
	Protestant		

PRIMIP	primipara (1st pregnancy)	PRO MYELO	promyelocytes
PR interval	part of the electrocardiographic cycle from onset of atrial depolarization on onset of ventricular depolarization	PRON	pronation
		PROS	prostate
			prosthesis
		PROT REL	protrusive relationship
PRISM	Pediatric Risk of Mortality Score	prov	provisional
		PROVIMI	proteins, vitamins, and minerals
PRK	photorefractive keratectomy	PROX	proximal
PRL	prolactin	PRP	panretinal photocoagulation
PRLA	pupils react to light and accommodation		patient recovery plan
PRM	partial rebreathing mask		penicllinase-resistant penicillin
	phosphoribomutase		pityriasis rubra pilaris
	photoreceptor membrane		platelet rich plasma
	prematurely ruptured membrane		polyribose ribitol phosphate
	primidone		poor progression of R wave in precordial leads
PRMF	preretinal macular fibrosis		
PRM-SDX	pyrimethamine; sulfadoxine		progressive rubella panencephalitis
PRN	as occasion requires	PrP	prion protein
PRO	Professional Review Organization	PRP-D	*Haemophilus influenzae,* type b diphtheria conjugate vaccine
	proline		
	pronation	PRPP	5-phosphoribosyl-1-pyrophosphate
	protein		
	prothrombin	PRP-T	polysaccharide tetanus conjugate vaccine
prob	probable		
PROCTO	procotoscopic	PRRE	pupils round regular, and equal
	proctology		
PROG	prognathism	PRRERLA	pupils round, regular, equal; react to light and accommodation
	prognosis		
	program		
	progressive	PRS	prolonged respiratory support
PROM	passive range of motion		
	premature rupture of membranes	PRSP	penicillinase-resistant synthetic penicillins
ProMACE	prednisone, methotrexate, calcium leucovorin, doxorubicin (Adriamycin), cyclophosphamide, and etoposide	PRSs	positive rolandic spikes
		PRT	protamine response test
		PRTCA	percutaneous rotational transluminal coronary angioplasty
PROMM	passive range of motion machine	PRTH-C	prothrombin time control
Promy	promyelocyte	PRV	polycythemia rubra vera

PRVEP	pattern reversal visual evoked potentials
PRW	past relevant work
	polymerized ragweed
PRX	panoramic facial x-ray
PRZ	prazepam
PRZF	pyrazofurin
PS	paradoxic sleep
	paranoid schizophrenia
	pathologic stage
	performance status
	peripheral smear
	physical status
	plastic surgery (surgeon)
	polysulfone (filter)
	posterior synechiae
	posterior synechiotomy
	pressure support
	protective services
	pulmonary stenosis
	pyloric stenosis
	serum from pregnant women
P/S	polyunsaturated to saturated fatty acids ratio
P & S	pain and suffering
	paracentesis and suction
	permanent and stationary
PS I	healthy patient with localized pathological process
PS II	a patient with mild to moderate systemic disease
PS III	a patient with severe systemic disease limiting activity but not incapacitating
PS IV	a patient with incapacitating systemic disease
PS V	moribund patient not expected to live
	(These are American Society of Anesthesiologists' physical status patient classifications. Emergency operations are designated by "E" after the classification.)
PSA	poly-substance abuse
	product selection allowed
	prostate-specific antigen
PsA	psoriatic arthritis
PSAD	prostate-specific antigen density
PSAG	*Pseudomonas aeruginosa*
PSAV	prostate-specific antigen velocity
PSBO	partial small bowel obstruction
PSC	Pediatric Symptom Checklist
	percutaneous suprapubic cystostomy
	posterior subcapsular cataract
	primary sclerosing cholangitis
	pronation spring control
	pubosacrococcygeal (diameter)
PSCC	posterior subcapsular cataract
PSC Cat	posterior subcapsular cataract
PSCH	peripheral stem cell harvest
PSCO	posterior semicircular canal
PSCP	posterior subcapsular precipitates
PSCT	peripheral stem cell transplant
PSCU	pediatric special care unit
PSD	psychosomatic disease
PSDS	palmar surface desensitization
PSE	portal systemic encephalopathy
	pseudoephedrine
PSF	posterior spinal fusion
PSG	polysomnogram
PSIG	pounds per square inch gauge
PSGN	post-streptococcal glomerulonephritis

PSH	past surgical history		progressive systemic
	post spinal headache		sclerosis
PSHx	past surgical history	PST	paroxysmal supraventricu-
PSI	Physiologic Stability		lar tachycardia
	Index		Patient Service
	pounds per square inch		Technician
	punctate subepithelial		platelet survival time
	infiltrate		postural stress test
PSIC	pediatric surgical	PSTT	placental site
	intensive care		trophoblastic tumor
PSIS	posterior superior iliac	PSV	pressure supported
	spine		ventilation
PSM	presystolic murmur	PSVT	paroxysmal supraventricu-
PSMA	personal self-maintenance		lar tachycardia
	activities	PSW	psychiatric social worker
	progressive spinal	PSY	pre-sexual youth
	muscular atrophy	PT	cisplatin
	prostate specific		parathormone
	membrane antigen		parathyroid
PSMF	protein-sparing modified		paroxysmal tachycardia
	fasting (Blackburn diet)		patient
PSMS	Physical Self Maintenance		phage type
	Scale		phenytoin
PSNP	progressive supra-nuclear		phototoxicity
	palsy		physical therapy
PSO	pelvic stabilization		pine tar
	orthosis		pint
	physician supplemental		posterior tibial
	order		preterm
	Polysporin ointment		prothrombin time
	proximal subungual	Pt	platinum
	onychomycosis	P/T	piperacillin/tazobactam
pSO₂	arterial oxygen saturation		(Zosyn®)
P/sore	pressure sore	P1/2T	pressure one-half time
PSP	pancreatic spasmolytic	P&T	paracentesis and tubing
	peptide		(of ears)
	phenolsulfonphthalein		peak and trough
	photostimulable phosphor		permanent and total
	progressive supranuclear		Pharmacy and
	palsy		Therapeutics
PSRBOW	premature spontaneous		(Committee)
	rupture of bag of	PTA	percutaneous transluminal
	waters		angioplasty
PSRT	photostress recovery test		Physical Therapy
PSS	painful shoulder syndrome		Assistant
	pediatric surgical service		plasma thromboplastin
	physiologic saline		antecedent
	solution (0.9% sodium		post-traumatic amnesia
	chloride)		pretreatment anxiety

	prior to admission		pharmacy to dose
	pure-tone average		prior to delivery
PTAB	popliteal-tibial artery bypass	PTDM	post-transplant diabetes mellitus
PTB	patellar tendon bearing	PTDP	permanent transvenous demand pacemaker
	prior to birth		
	pulmonary tuberculosis	PTE	pretibial edema
PTBA	percutaneous transluminal balloon angioplasty		proximal tibial epiphysis
			pulmonary thromboembolectomy
PTBD	percutaneous transhepatic biliary drain		
			pulmonary thromboembolism
PTBD-EF	percutaneous transhepatic biliary drainage—enteric feeding	PTED	pulmonary thromboembolic disease
PTBS	post-traumatic brain syndrome	PTF	pentoxifylline
			post-tetanic facilitation
PTB-SC-SP	patellar tendon bearing-supracondylar-suprapatellar	PTFE	polytetrafluoroethylene
		PTG	parathyroid gland
		PTGBD	percutaneous transhepatic gallbladder drainage
PTC	patient to call		
	percutaneous transhepatic cholangiography	PTH	parathyroid hormone
			post-transfusion hepatitis
	plasma thromboplastin components		prior to hospitalization
		PTHC	percutaneous transhepatic cholangiography
	post-tetanic count		
	premature tricuspid closure	PTHrP	parathyroid hormone-related protein
	prior to conception	PTJV	percutaneous transtracheal jet ventilation
	pseudotumor cerebri		
PT-C	prothrombin time control	PTK	phototherapeutic keratectomy
PTCA	percutaneous transluminal coronary angioplasty	PTL	pre-term labor
			Sodium Pentothal®
PTCDLF	pregnancy, term, complicated delivered, living female	PTLD	post-transplant lymphoproliferative disorder
PTCDLM	pregnancy, term, complicated delivered, living male	PTM	patient monitored
			posterior trabecular meshwork
PTCL	peripheral T-cell lymphoma	PTMC	percutaneous transvenous mitral commissurotomy
PTCR	percutaneous transluminal coronary recanalization		
		PTMDF	pupils, tension, media, disk, and fundus
PTCRA	percutaneous transluminal coronary rotational atherectomy	PT-NANB	posttransfusion non-A, non-B (hepatitis C)
PTD	period to discharge	PTNB	preterm newborn
	permanent and total disability	pTNM	postsurgical resection-pathologic staging of cancer
	persistent trophoblastic disease		

PTO	part-time occlusion (eye patch)	PTX	paclitaxel
			parathyroidectomy
	please turn over		pelvic traction
	proximal tubal obstruction		pentoxifylline
PTP	posterior tibial pulse		phototherapy
PTPM	post-traumatic progressive myelopathy		pneumothorax
		PTZ	pentylenetetrazol
PTPN	peripheral (vein) total parenteral nutrition		phenothiazine
		PU	pelvic-ureteric
P to P	point to point		pelviureteral
PTR	paratesticular rhabdomyosarcoma		peptic ulcer
			pregnancy urine
	patella tendon reflex	PUA	pelvic (examination) under anesthesia
	patient to return		
	prothrombin time ratio	PUB	pubic
PT-R	prothrombin time ratio	PUBS	percutaneous umbilical blood sampling
PTRA	percutaneous transluminal renal angioplasty		
		PUC	pediatric urine collector
PTS	patellar tendon suspension	PUD	partial upper denture
	Pediatric Trauma Score		peptic ulcer disease
	permanent threshold shift		percutaneous ureteral dilatation
	prior to surgery		
PTSD	post-traumatic stress disorder	PUE	pyrexia of unknown etiology
PTT	partial thromboplastin time	PUF	pure ultrafiltration
		PUFA	polyunsaturated fatty acids
	platelet transfusion therapy		
		PUFFA	polyunsaturated free fatty acids
PTT-C	partial thromboplastin time control		
		pul.	pulmonary
PTTW	patient tolerated traction well	PULP	pulpotomy
		PULSES	(physical profile) physical condition, upper limb functions, lower limb functions, sensory components, excretory functions, and support factors
PTU	pain treatment unit		
	pregnancy, term, uncomplicated		
	propylthiouracil		
PTUCA	percutaneous transluminal ultrasonic coronary angioplasty		
		Pulse A	pulse apical
		PULSE OX	pulse oximetry
PTUDLF	pregnancy, term, uncomplicated delivered, living female	Pulse R	pulse radial
		PUN	plasma urea nitrogen
		PUND	pregnancy, uterine, not delivered
PTUDLM	pregnancy, term, uncomplicated delivered, living male		
		PUNL	percutaneous ultrasonic nephrolithotripsy
PTV	posterior tibial vein		
PTWTKG	patient's weight in kilograms	PUO	pyrexia of unknown origin

PUP	percutaneous ultrasonic pyelolithotomy	PVD	patient very disturbed
			peripheral vascular disease
PU/PL	partial upper and lower dentures		posterior vitreous detachment
PUPPP	pruritic urticarial papules and plaque of pregnancy		premature ventricular depolarization
PUS	percutaneous ureteral stent	PVDA	prednisone, vincristine, daunorubicin, and asparaginase
	preoperative ultrasound		
PUVA	psoralen-ultraviolet-light (treatment)	PVE	perivenous encephalomy-elitis
PUW	pick-up walker		premature ventricular extrasystole
PV	papillomavirus		
	per vagina		prosthetic value endocarditis
	plasma volume	PVF	peripheral visual field
	polio vaccine	PVFS	postviral fatigue syndrome
	polycythemia vera		
	popliteal vein	PVGM	perifoveolar vitreoglial membrane
	portal vein		
	postvoiding	PVH	periventricular hemorrhage
	prenatal vitamins		periventricular hyperintensity
	projectile vomiting		
	pulmonary vein		pulmonary vascular hypertension
P & V	peak and valley (this is a dangerous abbreviation, use peak and trough)	PVI	peripheral vascular insufficiency
		PVK	penicillin V potassium
	pyloroplasty and vagotomy	PVL	peripheral vascular laboratory
PVA	polyvinyl alcohol		periventricular leukomalacia
	Prinzmetal's variant angina	PVM	paraverteabral muscle
PVAD	prolonged venous access devices		proteins, vitamins, and minerals
PVB	cisplatin, (Platinol) vinblastine, and bleomycin	PVMS	paravertebral muscle spasms
		PVN	peripheral venous nutrition
	paravertebral block		
	porcelain veneer bridge	PVNS	pigmented villonodular synovitis
	premature ventricular beat		
PVC	polyethylene vacuum cup	PVO	peripheral vascular occlusion
	polyvinyl chloride		
	porcelain veneer crown		pulmonary venous occlusion
	postvoiding cystogram		
	premature ventricular contraction	PVo	pulmonary valve opening
	pulmonary venous congestion	PVo$_2$	partial pressure (tension) of oxygen, vein
Pvco$_2$	partial pressure (tension) of carbon dioxide, vein		

PVOD	pulmonary vascular obstructive disease		representing atrial depolarization
PVP	cisplatin and etoposide	PWB	partial weight bearing
	penicillin V potassium		psychological well-being
	peripheral venous pressure	PWBL	partial weight bearing, left
	polyvinylpyrrolidone	PWBR	partial weight bearing, right
	postero-ventral pallidotomy	PWD	patients with diabetes
P-VP-B	cisplatin, etoposide, and bleomycin		powder
		PWI	pediatric walk-in clinic
PVR	peripheral vascular resistance		posterior wall infarct
	perspective volume rendering	PWLV	posterior wall of left ventricle
	postvoiding residual	PWM	pokeweed mitogens
	proliferative vitreoretinopathy	PWMI	posterior wall myocardial infarction
	pulmonary vascular resistance	PWO	persistent withdrawal occlusion
	pulse-volume recording	PWP	pulmonary wedge pressure
PVRI	pulmonary vascular resistance index	PWS	port-wine stain
PVS	percussion, vibration and suction	PWV	polistes wasp venom
			velocity of the pulse wave
	peripheral vascular surgery	Px	physical exam
	peritoneovenous shunt		pneumothorax
	persistent vegetative state		prognosis
			prophylaxis
	Plummer-Vinson syndrome	PXAT	paroxysmal atrial tachycardia
	pulmonic valve stenosis	PXE	pseudoxanthoma elasticum
PVT	paroxysmal ventricular tachycardia	PXF	pseudoexfoliation
	previous trouble	PXS	dental prophylaxis (cleaning)
	private	PY	pack years (see pk yrs)
PVTT	tumor thrombus in the portal vein	PYE	person-years of exposure
		PYHx	packs per year history
PW	pacing wires	PYLL	potential years of life lost
	patient waiting		
	plantar wart	PYP	pyrophosphate
	posterior wall	PYP®	technetium Tc 99m pyrophosphate kit
	pulse width		
	puncture wound	PZ	peripheral zone
P&W	pressures and waves	PZA	pyrazinamide
PWA	persons with AIDS		pyrazoloacridine
P wave	part of the electrocardiographic cycle	PZD	partial zonal dissection
		PZI	protamine zinc insulin

Q

Q	every
	quadriceps
QA	quality assurance
QAC	before every meal (this is a dangerous abbreviation)
QALE	quality-adjusted life expectancy
QALYs	quality-adjusted life years
QAM	every morning (this is a dangerous abbreviation)
QB	blood flow
QC	quad cane
	quality control
	quick catheter
QCA	quantitative coronary angiography
QCT	quantitative computed tomography
QD	dialysate flow
	every day (this is a dangerous abbreviation as it is read as four times daily)
QDAM	once daily in the morning
QDPM	once daily in the evening
QDS	United Kingdom abbreviation for four times a day
QE	quinidine effect
QED	every even day (this is a dangerous abbreviation as it will be read as four times daily-QID)
	quick and early diagnosis
QEE	quadriceps extension exercise
q4h	every four hours
qh	every hour
qhs	every night (this is a dangerous abbreviation as it is read as every hour-QHR and four times daily-QID)
QIAD	Quantitative Inventory of Alcohol Disorders
qid	four times daily
QIDM	four times daily with meals and at bedtime
QIG	quantitative immunoglobulins
QIW	four times a week (this is a dangerous abbreviation)
QJ	quadriceps jerk
QL	quality of life
QLI	Quality of Life Index
QM	every morning (this is a dangerous abbreviation as it will not be understood)
QMB	qualified Medicare beneficiary
QMI	Q wave myocardial infarction
QMRP	qualified mental retardation professional
QMT	quantitative muscle testing
q.n.	every night (this is a dangerous abbreviation as it is read as every hour)
q.n.s.	quantity not sufficient
qod	every other day (this is a dangerous abbreviation as it is read as every day or four times a day)
qoh	every other hour (this is a dangerous abbreviation as it is read as every day or four times a day)
qohs	every other night (this is a dangerous abbreviation as it is not recognized)
QOL	quality of life
QON	every other night (this is a dangerous abbreviation)
qpm	every evening (this is a dangerous abbreviation)
QPOS	Quality Point of Service

213

QP/QS	ratio of pulmonary blood to systemic blood flow	rate
QR	quiet room	reacting
QRC	qualitative radiocardiography	rectal
		rectum
QRS	part of electrocardiographic wave representing ventricular depolarization	regular
		regular insulin
		resistant
		respiration
QS	every shift	reticulocyte
	quadriceps set	retinoscopy
	quadrilateral socket	right
	sufficient quantity	roentgen
		rub
qs ad	a sufficient quantity to make	r recombinant
		ℝ̂ registered trademark
		right
QS&L	quarters, subsistence, and laundry	RA radiographic absorptiometry
Qs/Qt	intrapulmonary shunt fraction	rales
		renal artery
QSP	physiological shunt fraction	repeat action
		retinoic acid
qt	quart	rheumatoid arthritis
QTB	quadriceps tendon bearing	right arm
QTC	quantitative tip cultures	right atrium
QTL	quantitative trait locus	right auricle
Q-TWiST	quality-adjusted time without symptoms (of disease) and toxicity	room air
		rotational atherectomy
		RAA renin-angiotensin-aldosterone
QUAD	quadrant	
	quadriceps	right atrial abnormality
	quadriplegic	RAAS renin-angiotensin-aldosterone system
QU	quiet	
QUART	quadrantectomy, axillary dissection, and radiotherapy	RAB rice (rice cereal), applesauce, and banana (diet)
QW	every week (this is a dangerous abbreviation)	RABG room air blood gas
		RAC right atrial catheter
QWB	Quality of Well-Being (scale)	RACCO right anterior caudocranial oblique
QWK	once a week (this is a dangerous abbreviation)	RACT recalcified whole-blood activated clotting time
Q4wk	every four weeks	RAD ionizing radiation unit
		radical
		radiology
	R	reactive airway disease
		right axis deviation
		RADCA right anterior descending coronary artery
R	radial	RADISH rheumatoid arthritis

	diffuse idiopathic skeletal hyperostosis	RAST	radioallergosorbent test
RADS	ionizing radiation units	RAT	right anterior thigh
	rapid assay delivery systems	RA test	test for rheumatoid factor
	reactive airway disease syndrome	RATG	rabbit antithymocyte globulin
RAE	right atrial enlargement	RATx	radiation therapy
RAEB	refractory anemia, erythroblastic	R(AW)	airway resistance
RAF	rapid atrial fibrillation	RB	relieved by
RAFF	rectus abdominis free flap		retinoblastoma
RAFT	Rehabilitative Addicted Family Treatment		retrobulbar
			right breast
RAG	room air gas		right buttock
RAH	right atrial hypertrophy	R & B	right and below
RAHB	right anterior hemiblock	RBA	right basilar artery
rAHF	antihemophilic factor (recombinant)		right brachial artery
		RBB	right breast biopsy
RAID	radioimmunodetection	RBBB	right bundle branch block
RAIU	radioactive iodine uptake	RBBX	right breast biopsy examination
RALT	routine admission laboratory tests	RBC	ranitidine bismuth citrate
RAM	radioactive material		red blood cell (count)
	rapid alternating movements	RBCD	right border cardiac dullness
	rectus abdominis myocutaneous	RBCM	red blood cell mass
		RBC s/f	red blood cells spun filtration
RAN	resident's admission notes	RBCV	red blood cell volume
R₂AN	second year resident's admission notes	RBD	right border of dullness
		RBE	relative biologic effectiveness
RANTES	regulated upon activation, normal T cell expressed and secreted	RBF	renal blood flow
		RBG	random blood glucose
		RBL	Roche Biomedical Laboratory
RAO	right anterior oblique		
RAP	right atrial pressure	RBON	retrobulbar optic neuritis
RAPA	radial artery pseudoaneurysm	RBOW	rupture bag of water
		RBP	retinol-binding protein
RAQ	right anterior quadrant	RBRVS	Medicare resource-based relative-value scale
RAPD	relative afferent pupillary defect		
		RBS	random blood sugar
RAR	right arm reclining	RBT	rational behavior therapy
RARs	retinoic acid receptors	RBV	right brachial vein
RAS	recurrent aphthous stomatitis	RC	race
	renal artery stenosis		radiocarpal (joint)
	reticular activating system		Red Cross
	right arm, sitting		report called
RASE	rapid-acquisition spin echo		retrograde cystogram
			retruded contact (position)
			right coronary
			Roman Catholic

	root canal		reticulum cell sarcoma
	rotator cuff		Royal College of
R/C	reclining chair		Surgeons
R & C	reasonable and customary	RCT	randomized clinical trial
RCA	radiographic contrast		Registered Care
	agent		Technologist
	radionuclide cerebral		root canal therapy
	angiogram		Rorschach Content Test
	right carotid artery	RCV	red cell volume
	right coronary artery	RCX	ramus circumflexus
RCBF	regional cerebral blood	RD	radial deviation
	flow		Raynaud's disease
RCC	rape crisis center		reaction of degeneration
	renal cell carcinoma		reflex decay
	Roman Catholic Church		Registered Dietitian
RCCA	right common carotid		renal disease
	artery		respiratory disease
RCCT	randomized controlled		respiratory distress
	clinical trial		restricted duty
RCD	relative cardiac dullness		retinal detachment
RCE	right carotid		Reye's disease
	endarterectomy		right deltoid
RCF	Reiter complement		ruptured disk
	fixation	RDA	recommended daily
RCF®	enteral nutrition		allowance
	product		Registered Dental
RCH	residential care home		Assistant
RCHF	right-sided congestive	RDB	randomized double-blind
	heart failure		(trial)
RCIP	rape crisis intervention	RDCS	Registered Diagnostic
	program		Cardiac Sonographer
RCL	range of comfortable	RDD	renal dose dopamine
	loudness	RDE	remote data entry
RCM	radiographic contrast	RDEA	right deviation of
	media		electrical axis
	retinal capillary	RDG	right dorsogluteal
	microaneurysm	RDH	Registered Dental
	right costal margin		Hygienist
RCP	respiratory care plan	RDI	respiratory disturbance
	Royal College of		index
	Physicians	RDIH	right direct inguinal
RCPM	raven colored progressive		hernia
	matrices	RDLBBB	rate-dependent left bundle
RCPT	Registered Cardiopulmo-		branch block
	nary Technician	RDM	right deltoid muscle
RCR	replication-competent	RDMS	Registered Diagnostic
	retrovirus (assay)		Medical Sonographer
	rotator cuff repair	RDOD	retinal detachment, right
RCS	repeat cesarean section		eye

RDOS	retinal detachment, left eye	R-EEG	resting electroencephalogram
RDP	random donor platelets	REEGT	Registered Electroencephalogram Technologist
	right dorsoposterior	REF	referred
RDPE	reticular degeneration of the pigment epithelium		refused
RDS	research diagnostic criteria		renal erythropoietic factor
	respiratory distress syndrome	ref →	refer to
		REG	radioencephalogram
RDT	regular dialysis (hemodialysis) treatment	Reg block	regional block anesthesia
		regurg	regurgitation
		rehab	rehabilitation
RDTD	referral, diagnosis, treatment, and discharge	REL	relative
			religion
		RELE	resistive exercise, lower extremities
RDVT	recurrent deep vein thrombosis	REM	rapid eye movement
RDW	red (cell) distribution width		recent event memory
			remission
RE	concerning		roentgen equivalent unit
	rectal examination	REMS	rapid eye movement sleep
	reflux esophagitis	REO	respiratory and enteric orphan (viruses)
	regarding		
	regional enteritis	REP	rapid electrophoresis
	reticuloendothelial		repair
	retinol equivalents		repeat
	right ear		report
	right eye	REP CK	rapid electrophoresis creatine kinase
	rowing ergometer		
R & E	rest and exercise	repol	repolarization
	round and equal	REPS	repetitions
R↑E	right upper extremity	REPT	Registered Evoked Potential Technologist
R↓E	right lower extremity		
RE ✔	recheck	RER	renal excretion rate
READM	readmission	RES	recurrent erosion syndrome
REC	rear end collision		resection
	recommend		resident
	record		reticuloendothelial system
	recovery	RESC	resuscitation
	recreation	RESP	respirations
	recur		respiratory
RECA	right external carotid artery	REST	restoration
		RET	retention
RECT	rectum		reticulocyte
RED SUBS	reducing substances		retina
			retired
REE	resting energy expenditure		return
RE-ED	re-education		right esotropia

ret detach	retinal detachment		right frontoposterior
retic	reticulocyte	RFS	rapid frozen section
RETRO	retrograde		refeeding syndrome
RETRX	retractions		relapse-free survival
REUE	resistive exercise, upper extremities	RFT	right frontotransverse
			routine fever therapy
REV	reverse	RFTC	radio-frequency thermocoagulation
	review		
	revolutions	RFV	reason for visit
RF	radio frequency		right femoral vein
	reduction fixation	RG	right (upper outer) gluteus
	renal failure	R/G	red/green
	respiratory failure	RGM	right gluteus medius
	restricted fluids	RGO	reciprocating gait orthosis
	rheumatic fever	RH	right hemisphere
	rheumatoid factor	Rh	Rhesus factor in blood
	right foot	RH	reduced haloperidol
	risk factor		relative humidity
	radiofrequency		rest home
R&F	radiographic and fluoroscopic		retinal hemorrhage
			right hand
RFA	right femoral artery		right hyperphoria
	right forearm		room humidifier
	right frontoanterior	Rh+	Rhesus positive
RFB	retained foreign body	Rh−	Rhesus negative
	radial flow chromatography	RHA	right hepatic artery
		rHA	recombinant human albumin
	residual functional capacity		
		RHB	raise head of bed
RFE	return flow enema		right heart border
RFFIT	rapid fluorescent focus inhibition test	RH/BSO	radial hysterectomy and bilateral salpingo-oophorectomy
RFg	visual fields by Goldmann-type perimeter		
		RHC	respiration has ceased
			right heart catheterization
RFIPC	Rating Form of IBD (inflammatory bowel disease) Patient Concerns		right hemicolectomy
		RHD	radial head dislocation
			relative hepatic dullness
			rheumatic heart disease
RFL	radionuclide functional lymphoscintigraphy	rh-DNase	dornase alfa (Pulmozyme)
		RHF	right heart failure
	right frontolateral	RHG	right hand grip
RFLF	retained fetal lung fluid	r-hGH(m)	mammalian-cell–derived recombinant human growth hormone (Serostim)
RFLP	restriction fragment length polymorphism (patterns)		
RFM	rifampin	RHH	right homonymous hemianopsia
RFP	request for payment		
	request for proposal	RHINO	rhinoplasty

218

RHL	right hemisphere lesions	RIJ	right internal jugular
	right heptic lobe	RIMA	right internal mammary
rhm	roentgens per hour at one		anastamosis
	meter	RIND	reversible ischemic
RHO	right heel off		neurologic defect
Rho(D)	immune globulin to an	RIO	right inferior oblique
	Rh-negative woman		(muscle)
RhoGAM®	Rho (D) immune globulin	RIOJ	recurrent intrahepatic
RHR	resting heart rate		obstructive jaundice
RHS	right hand side	RIP	radioimmunoprecipitin
RHT	right hypertropia		test
rHuEPO	recombinant human		rapid infusion pump
	erythropoietin		respiratory inductance
RHV	right hepatic vein		plethysmograph
RHW	radiant heat warmer	RIPA	ristocetin-induced platelet
RI	refractive index		agglutination
	regular insulin	RIR	right inferior rectus
	renal insufficiency	RIS	responding to internal
	respiratory illness		stimuli
	rooming in	RISA	radioactive iodinated
RIA	radioimmunoassay		serum albumin
RIAT	radioimmune antiglobulin	RIST	radioimmunosorbent test
	test	RIT	radioimmunotherapy
RIBA	recombinant immunoblot		Rorschach Inkblot Test
	assay	RITA	right internal thoracic
RIC	right iliac crest		artery
	right internal carotid	RIVD	ruptured intervertebral
	(artery)		disk
RICA	right internal carotid	RIX	radiation-induced
	artery		xerostomia
RICE	rest, ice, compression,	RJ	radial jerk (reflex)
	and elevation	RK	radial keratotomy
RICM	right intercostal margin		right kidney
RICS	right intercostal space	RKS	renal kidney stone
RICU	respiratory intensive care	RKT	Registered Kinesiothera-
	unit		pist
RID	radial immunodiffusion	RL	right lateral
	ruptured intervertebral		right leg
	disk		right lower
RIE	rocket immunoelectro-		right lung
	phoresis		Ringer's lactate
RIF	rifampin	R → L	right to left
	right iliac fossa	RLB	right lateral bending
	right index finger		right lateral border
	rigid internal fixation	RLBCD	right lower border of
RIG	rabies immune globulin		cardiac dullness
RIGS	radioimmunoguided	RLC	residual lung capacity
	surgery	RLD	related living donor
RIH	right inguinal hernia		right lateral decubitus

219

	ruptured lumbar disk
RLDP	right lateral decubital position
RLE	right lower extremity
RLF	retrolental fibroplasia
	right lateral femoral
RLG	right lateral gaze
RLL	right liver lobe
	right lower lid
	right lower lobe
RLN	recurrent laryngeal nerve
	regional lymph node(s)
RLND	regional lymph node dissection
RLQ	right lower quadrant
RLQD	right lower quadrant defect
RLR	right lateral rectus
RLS	restless legs syndrome
	Ringer's lactate solution
	stammerer who has difficulty in enunciating R, L, and S
RLSB	right lower scapular border
	right lower sternal border
RLT	right lateral thigh
RLTCS	repeat low transverse cesarean section
RLWD	routine laboratory work done
RLX	right lower extremity
RM	radical mastectomy
	repetitions maximum
	respiratory movement
	risk manager (management)
	risk model
	room
R&M	routine and microscopic
1-RM	single repetition maximum lift
RMA	Registered Medical Assistant
	right mentoanterior
RMCA	right main coronary artery
	right middle cerebral artery
RMCAT	right middle cerebral artery thrombosis

RMCL	right midclavicular line
RMD	rapid movement disorder
RME	resting metabolic expenditure
	right mediolateral episiotomy
RMEE	right middle ear exploration
RMF	right middle finger
RMK #1	remark number 1
RML	right mediolateral
	right middle lobe
RMLE	right mediolateral episiotomy
RMO	responsible medical officer
RMP	right mentoposterior
RMR	resting metabolic rate
	right medial rectus
RMS	red-man syndrome
	Rehabilitation Medicine Service
	repetitive motion syndrome
	rhabdomyosarcoma
RMS®	rectal morphine sulfate (suppository)
RMSB	right middle sternal border
RMSE	root mean square error
RMSF	Rocky Mountain spotted fever
RMT	Registered Music Therapist
	right mentotransverse
RMV	respiratory minute volume
RN	Registered Nurse
	right nostril (nare)
Rn	radon
R/N	renew
RNA	radionuclide angiography
	ribonucleic acid
RNC	Registered Nurse, Certified
RNCD	Registered Nurse, Chemical Dependency
RNCNA	Registered Nurse Certified in Nursing Administration

RNCNAA	Registered Nurse Certified in Nursing Administration Advanced	Romb	Romberg
		ROMCP	range of motion complete and painfree
RNCS	Registered Nurse Certified Specialist	ROMI	rule out myocardial infarction
RND	radical neck dissection	ROMSA	right otitis media, suppurative, acute
RNEF	resting (radio-) nuclide ejection fraction	ROMSC	right otitis media, suppurative, chronic
RNF	regular nursing floor	ROMWNL	range of motion within normal limits
RNFL	retinal nerve fiber layer		
RNLP	Registered Nurse, license pending	ROP	retinopathy of prematurity right occiput posterior
RNP	Registered Nurse Practitioner ribonucleoprotein	ROPE	regional organ physical examination
RNS	replacement normal saline (0.9% sodium chloride)	ROR	the French acronym for measles-mumps-rubella vaccine
RNST	reactive nonstress test	R or L	right or left
RNUD	recurrent nonulcer dyspepsia	RoRx	radiation therapy
RO	reality orientation	ROS	review of systems rod outer segments
	relative odds	ROSC	restoration of spontaneous circulation
	report of		
	reverse osmosis	ROSS	review of signs and symptoms
	routine order(s)		
	Russian Orthodox	ROT	remedial occupational therapy
R/O	rule out		right occipital transverse
ROA	right occiput anterior		rotator
ROAC	repeated oral doses of activated charcoal	ROU	recurrent oral ulcer
		ROUL	rouleaux
ROAD	reversible obstructive airway disease	RP	radial pulse
ROC	receiver operating characteristic		radical prostatectomy
			radiopharmaceutical
	record of contact		Raynaud's phenomenon
	resident on call		restorative proctocolectomy
	residual organic carbon		
ROG	rogletimide		retinitis pigmentosa
ROH	rubbing alcohol		retrograde pyelogram
ROI	region of interest		root plane
ROIDS	hemorrhoids	RPA	radial photon absorptiometry
ROIH	right oblique inguinal hernia		Registered Physician's Assistant
ROJM	range of joint motion		restenosis postangioplasty
ROL	right occipitolateral		ribonuclease protection assay
ROM	range of motion		
	right otitis media		right pulmonary artery
	rupture of membranes		

RPAC	Registered Physician's Assistant Certified		Reiter protein reagin
		RPT	Registered Physical Therapist
RPC	root planing and curettage		
RPCF	Reiter protein complement fixation	RPTA	Registered Physical Therapist Assistant
RPD	removable partial denture	RPV	right portal vein
RPE	rating of perceived exertion		right pulmonary vein
		RQ	respiratory quotient
	retinal pigment epithelium	RR	recovery room
RPEP	right pre-ejection period		regular rate
	retinal pigment epithelium		regular respirations
RPF	relaxed pelvic floor		relative risk
	renal plasma flow		respiratory rate
RPFT	Registered Pulmonary Function Technologist		retinal reflex
		R/R	rales-rhonchi
RPG	retrograde percutaneous gastrostomy	R&R	rate and rhythm
			recent and remote
	retrograde pyelogram		recession and resection
RPGN	rapidly progressive glomerulonephritis		resect and recess (muscle surgery)
RPH	retroperitoneal hemorrhage		rest and recuperation
			remove and replace
RPI	resting pressure index	RRA	radioreceptor assay
	reticulocyte production index		Registered Record Administrator
RPh	Registered Pharmacist		right radial artery
RPHA	reverse passive hemagglutination		right renal artery
		RRAM	rapid rhythmic alternating movements
RPICA	right posterior internal carotid artery		
		RRC	cohort relative risk
RPICCE	round pupil intracapsular cataract extraction	RRCT, no(m)	regular rate, clear tones, no murmurs
RPL	retroperitoneal lymphadenectomy	RRD	rhegmatogenous retinal detachment
RPLC	reversed-phase liquid chromatography	RRE	round, regular, and equal (pupils)
RPLND	retroperitoneal lymph node dissection	RRED®	Rapid Rare Event Detection
RPN	renal papillary necrosis	RREF	resting radionuclide ejection fraction
	resident's progress notes		
R₂PN	second year resident's progress notes	RRI	renal resistive index
		RRM	right radial mastectomy
RPO	right posterior oblique	RRMS	relapsing-remitting multiple sclerosis
RPP	radical perineal prostatectomy	RRNA	Resident Registered Nurse Anesthetist
	rate-pressure product		
	retropubic prostatectomy	rRNA	ribosomal ribonucleic acid
RPR	rapid plasma reagin (test for syphilis)	RRND	right radical neck dissection

RROM	resistive range of motion	RSD	reflex sympathetic dystrophy
R rot	right rotation		
RRP	radical retropubic prostatectomy	RSDS	reflex-sympathetic dystrophy syndrome
RRR	recovery room routine regular rhythm and rate	RSE	right sternal edge
		RSI	repetitive strain (stress) injury
RRRN	round, regular, and react normally		
		R-SICU	respiratory-surgical intensive care unit
RRR͞M	regular rate and rhythm without murmur		
		RSLR	reverse straight leg raise
RRT	Registered Respiratory Therapist	RSM	remote study monitoring
		RSNI	round spermatid nuclear injection
RRVO	repair relaxed vaginal outlet		
		RSO	right salpingooophorec- tomy
RRVS	recovery room vital signs		
RS	Raynaud's syndrome		right superior oblique
	Reiter's syndrome	RSOP	right superior oblique palsy
	restart		
	Reye's syndrome	RSP	rapid straight pacing
	rhythm strip		right sacroposterior
	right side	RSR	regular sinus rhythm
	Ringer's solution		relative survival rate
R/S	rest stress		right superior rectus
	rupture spontaneous	RSRI	renal:systemic renin index
R & S	restraint and seclusion	RSSE	Russian spring-summer encephalitis
R/S I	resuscitation status one (full resuscitative effort)		
		RST	right sacrum transverse
		RSTs	Rodney Smith tubes
R/S II	resuscitation status two (no code, therapeutic measures only)	RSV	respiratory syncytial virus right subclavian vein
		RSVC	right superior vena cava
R/S III	resuscitation status three (no code, comfort measures only)	RSW	right-sided weakness
		RT	radiation therapy
			Radiologic Technologist
RSA	right sacrum anterior		recreational therapy
	right subclavian artery		rectal temperature
RSB	right sternal border		renal transplant
RSC	right subclavian (artery) (vein)		repetition time
			respiratory therapist
RScA	right scapuloanterior		reverse transcriptase
RSCL	Rotterdam Symptom Check List		right
			right thigh
RScP	right scapuloposterior		room temperature
RSCS	respiratory system compliance score	R/t	related to
		RTA	ready to administer
rscu-PA	recombinant, single-chain, urokinase-type plasminogen activator		renal tubular acidosis
			road traffic accident
		t-RA	tretinoin (*trans*-retinoic acid)

RTAE	right atrial enlargement	RT₃U	resin triiodothyronine
RTAH	right anterior hemiblock		uptake
RTAT	right anterior thigh	RTUS	realtime ultrasound
RTB	return to baseline	RTW	return to ward
RTC	return to clinic		return to work
	round the clock		Richard Turner Warwick
RTCA	ribavirin		(urethroplasty)
RTER	return to emergency room	RTWD	return to work
rt. ↑ ext.	right upper extremity		determination
RTF	ready-to-feed	RTx	radiation therapy
	return to flow		renal transplantation
RTFS	return to flying status	RU	residual urine
RTI	respiratory tract infection		resin uptake
	reverse transcriptase		retrograde ureterogram
	inhibitor		right upper
RTK	rhabdoid tumor of the		routine urinalysis
	kidney	RU 486	mifepristone
RTL	reactive to light	RUA	routine urine analysis
RTM	regression to the mean	RUE	right upper extremity
	routine medical care	RUG	retrograde urethrogram
RTMD	right mid-deltoid	RUL	right upper lid
rTMS	repetitive transcranial		right upper lobe
	magnetic stimulation	RUOQ	right upper outer quadrant
RTN	renal tubular necrosis	rupt.	ruptured
RTNM	retreatment staging of	RUQ	right upper quadrant
	cancer	RUQD	right upper quadrant
RTO	return to office		defect
RTOG	Radiation Therapy	RURTI	recurrent upper
	Oncology Group		respiratory tract
RTP	renal transplant patient		infection
	return to pharmacy	RUSB	right upper scapular
rtPA	alteplase (recombinant		border
	tissue-type plasminogen		right upper sternal border
	activator)	RUV	residual urine volume
RT-PCR	reverse transcription	RUX	right upper extremity
	polymerase chain	RV	rectovaginal
	reaction		residual volume
RTR	return to room		respiratory volume
RT (R)	Radiologic Technologist		retinal vasculitis
	(Registered)		return visit
RTRR	return to recovery room		right ventricle
RTS	raised toilet seat		rubella vaccine
	real time scan	RVA	rabies vaccine, adsorbed
	Resolve Through Sharing		right ventricular apex
	return to school		right vertebral artery
	return to sender	RVAD	right ventricular assist
	Revised Trauma Score		device
RTT	Respiratory Therapy	RVCD	right ventricular
	Technician		conduction deficit

RVD	relative vertebral density	RVU	relative-value units
	renal vascular disease	RVV	rubella vaccine virus
RVDP	right ventricular diastolic pressure	RVVT	Russell's viper venom time
RVE	right ventricular enlargement	RW	radiant warmer
			ragweed
RVEDP	right ventricular end-diastolic pressure		red welt
			rolling walker
RVEF	right ventricular ejection fraction	R/W	return to work
		RWM	regional wall motion
RVET	right ventricular ejection time	RWP	ragweed pollen
		RWS	ragweed sensitivity
RVF	Rift Valley fever	RXRs	retinoid X receptors
	right ventricular function	Rx	drug
	right visual field		medication
RVG	radionuclide ventriculography		pharmacy
			prescription
	right ventrogluteal		radiotherapy
RVH	renovascular hypertension		take
	right ventricular hypertrophy		therapy
			treatment
RVHT	renovascular hypertension	RXN	reaction
RVI	right ventricle infarction	RXT	radiation therapy
RVIDd	right ventricle internal dimension diastole		right exotropia
RVL	right vastus lateralis		
RVO	relaxed vaginal outlet		
	retinal vein occlusion		
	right ventricular outflow		**S**
	right ventricular overactivity		
RVOT	right ventricular outflow tract		
RVOTH	right ventricular outflow tract hypertrophy	S	sacral
RVP	right ventricular pressure		second (s)
RVR	rapid ventricular response		sensitive
	renal vascular resistance		serum
	right ventricular rhythm		single
RVS	rabies vaccine, adsorbed		sister
RVSP	right ventricular systolic pressure		son
			sponge
RVSW	right ventricular stroke work		subjective findings
			suicide
RVSWI	right ventricular stroke work index		suction
			sulfur
RVT	renal vein thrombosis		supervision
RV/TLC	residual volume to total lung capacity ratio		susceptible
		/S/	signature

s̄	without (this is a dangerous abbreviation)		short arm cast
			substance abuse counselor
S'	shoulder	SACC	short arm cylinder cast
S₁	first heart sound	SACD	subacute combined
S⁻¹...S⁻⁴	suicide risk classifications		degeneration
S₂	second heart sound	SACH	soft ankle, cushioned heel
S₃	third heart sound		solid ankle, cushion heel
	(ventricular filling	SACT	sinoatrial conduction time
	gallop)	SAD	seasonal affective disorder
S₄	fourth heart sound (atrial		Self-Assessment
	gallop)		Depression (scale)
S₁...S₅	sacral vertebra or nerves		source-axis distance
	1 through 5		subacromial decompres-
SI to SIV	symbols for the first to		sion
	fourth heart sounds		subacute dialysis
SA	sacroanterior		sugar, acetone, and
	salicylic acid		diacetic acid
	semen analysis		sugar and acetone
	Sexoholics Anonymous		determination
	sinoatrial		superior axis deviation
	sleep apnea	SADL	simulated activities of
	slow acetylator		daily living
	Spanish American	SADR	suspected adverse drug
	Staphylcococcus aureus		reaction
	subarachnoid	SADS	Schedule for Affective
	substance abuse		Disorders and
	suicide alert		Schizophrenia
	suicide attempt	SADS-C	Schedule for Affective
	surface area		Disorders And
	surgical assistant		Schizophrenia – Change
	sustained action		Version
S/A	same as	SAE	serious adverse event
	sugar and acetone		short above elbow (cast)
S&A	sugar and acetone	SAEKG	signaled average
SAA	same as above		electrocardiogram
	serum amyloid A	SAESU	Substance Abuse
	Stokes-Adams attacks		valuating Screen Unit
SAAG	serum-ascites albumin	SAF	Self-Analysis Form
	gradient	SAFHS	sonic accelerated fracture
SAB	serum albumin		healing system
	sino-atrial block		self-articulating femoral
	Spanish American Black		Spanish-American female
	spontaneous abortion	Sag D	sagittal diameter
	subarachnoid bleed	SAH	subarachnoid hemorrhage
	subarachnoid block		systemic arterial
SAC	segmental antigen		hypertension
	challenge	SAHS	sleep apnea/hypopnea
	serum aminoglycoside		(hypersomnolence)
	concentration		syndrome

SAI	Sodium Amytal® interview	SARA	sexually acquired reactive arthritis
SAL	salicylate		system for anesthetic and respiratory administration analysis
	Salmonella		
	sterility assurance level		
SAL 12	sequential analysis of 12 chemistry constituents	SARAN	senior admitting resident's admission note
SAM	methylprednisolone sodium succinate (Solu-Medrol®), aminophylline, and metaproterenol (Metaprel®)	SARC	seasonal allergic rhinoconjunctivitis
		S Arrh	sinus arrhythmia
		SART	standard acid reflux test
		SAS	saline, agent, and saline
			scalenus anticus syndrome
	selective antimicrobial modulation		see assessment sheet
			Self-rating Anxiety Scale
	self-administered medication		short arm splint
			sleep apnea syndrome
	sleep apnea monitor		Social Adjustment Scale
	Spanish-American male		Specific Activity Scale
	systolic anterior motion		subarachnoid space
SAN	side-arm nebulizer		sulfasalazine
	sinoatrial node		synthetic absorbable sutures
	slept all night		
SANC	short arm navicular cast	SASA	Sex Abuse Survivors Anonymous
sang	sanguinous		
SANS	Schedule (Scale) for the Assessment of Negative Symptoms	SASH	saline, agent, saline, and heparin
		SASP	sulfasalazine (salicylazo-sulfapyridine)
	sympathetic autonomic nervous system	SAT	methylprednisolone sodium succinate (Solu-Medrol®), aminophylline, and terbutaline
SAO	small airway obstruction		
SaO₂	arterial oxygen percent saturation		
			saturated
SAPD	self-administration of psychotropic drugs		saturation
			Saturday
SAPH	saphenous		Senior Apperception Test
SAPS	short arm plaster splint		speech awareness threshold
	Simplified Acute Physiology Score		
			subacute thyroiditis
SAPS II	Simplified Acute Physiology Score version II	SATC	substance abuse treatment clinic
SAQ	short arc quad	SATL	surgical Achilles tendon lengthening
SAR	seasonal allergic rhinitis		
	Senior Assistant Resident	SATP	substance abuse treatment program
	sexual attitudes reassessment		
		SATS	refers to oxygen saturation levels
	structural activity relationships		

SATU	substance abuse treatment unit		subacute bacterial endocarditis
SAVD	spontaneous assisted vaginal delivery	SBFT	small bowel follow through
SB	safety belt	SBG	stand-by guard
	sandbag	SBGM	self blood glucose monitoring
	scleral buckling		
	seat belt	SBH	State Board of Health
	seen by	SBI	systemic bacterial infection
	Sengstaken-Blakemore (tube)		
		SBJ	skin, bones, and joints
	sick boy	SBK	spinnbarkeit
	side bend	SBL	sponge blood loss
	side bending	SB-LM	Stanford-Binet Intelligence Test-Form LM
	sinus bradycardia		
	small bowel		
	spina bifida	SBO	small bowel obstruction
	sponge bath	SBOD	scleral buckle, right eye
	stand-by	SBOH	State Board of Health
	Stanford-Binet (test)	SBOM	soybean oil meal
	sternal border	SBOS	scleral buckle, left eye
	stillbirth	SBP	school breakfast program
	stillborn		scleral buckling procedure
	stone basketing		small bowel phytobezoars
Sb	antimony		spontaneous bacterial peritonitis
SB+	wearing seat belt		
SB−	not wearing seat belt		systolic blood pressure
SBA	serum bactericidal activity	SBQC	small based quad cane
	standby angioplasty	SBR	sluggish blood return
	standby assistant (assistance)		strict bed rest
		SBS	shaken baby syndrome
	Summary Basis of Approval		short bowel syndrome
			side-by-side
SBAC	small bowel adenocarcinoma		small bowel series
		SBT	serum bactericidal titers
SBB	stereotactic breast biopsy	SBTB	sinus breakthrough beat
SBBO	small-bowel bacterial overgrowth	SBTT	small bowel transit time
		SBV	single binocular vision
SBC	sensory binocular cooperation	SBX	symphysis, buttocks, and xiphoid
	single base cane	SC	schizophrenia
	standard bicarbonate		self-care
	strict bed confinement		serum creatinine
SBD	straight bag drainage		service connected
SBE	saturated base excess		sick call
	self-breast examination		sickle-cell
	short below elbow (cast)		Snellen's chart
	shortness of breath on exertion		spinal cord
			sport cord

	sternoclavicular
	subclavian
	subclavian catheter
	subcutaneous
	succinylcholine
	sulfur colloid
$\bar{s}c$	without correction (without glasses)
S&C	sclerae and conjunctivae
SCA	sickle cell anemia
	subclavian artery
	subcutaneous abdominal (block)
	superior cerebellar artery
SCa	serum calcium
SCAD	short chain acyl-coenzyme A dehydrogenase
SCAN	suspected child abuse and neglect
SCAP	stem cell apheresis
SCAT	sheep cell agglutination titer
	sickle cell anemia test
SCB	strictly confined to bed
SCBC	small cell bronchogenic carcinoma
SCBE	single-contrast barium enema
SCBF	spinal cord blood flow
SCC	sickle cell crisis
SCC	short course chemotherapy (for tuberculosis)
	small cell carcinoma
	squamous cell carcinoma
SCCA	semi-closed circle absorber
	squamous cell carcinoma antigen
SCCa	squamous cell carcinoma
SCCE	squamous cell carcinoma of the esophagus
SCCHN	squamous cell carcinoma of the head and neck
SCCI	subcutaneous continuous infusion
SCD	sequential compression device
	service connected disability
	sickle cell disease
	spinal cord disease
	subacute combined degeneration
	sudden cardiac death
ScDA	scapulodextra anterior
SCDM	soybean-casein digest medium
ScDP	scapulodextra posterior
SCE	sister chromatid exchange
	soft cooked egg
	specialized columnar epithelium
SCEMIA	self-contained enzymatic membrane immunoassay
SCEP	somatosensory cortical evoked potential
SCF	special care formula
	stem cell factor
SCFA	short-chain fatty acid
SCFE	slipped capital femoral epiphysis
SCG	seismocardiography
	serum Chemogram
	sodium cromoglycate
SCh	succinylcholine chloride
SCHISTO	schistocytes
SCHIZ	schizocytes
	schizophrenia
SCHLP	supracricord hemilaryngopharyngec-tomy
SCHNC	squamous cell head and neck cancer
SCI	spinal cord injury
	subcoma insulin
SCID	severe combined immunodeficiency disorders (disease)
	structured clinical interview for DSM-III-R
SCII	Strong-Campbell Interest Inventory
SCIP	Screening and Crisis Intervention Program

SCIPP	sacrococcygeal to inferior pubic point	SCr	serum creatinine
SCIU	spinal cord injury unit	sCR	soluble complement receptor
SCIV	subclavian intravenous	SC/RP	scaling and root planing
SCI-WORA	spinal cord injury without radiographic abnormalities	SC-RNV	subcutaneous radionuclide venography
SCL	skin conductance level symptom checklist	SCS	spinal cord stimulation splatter control shield suspected catheter sepsis
SCL-90	Symptoms Checklist—90 items	SCSAX	subcostal short axis
ScLA	scapulolaeva anterior	SCSIT	Southern California Sensory Integration Tests
SCLAX	subcostal long axis		
SCLC	small-cell lung cancer		
SCLD	sickle cell lung disease	SCT	Sertoli cell tumor sex chromatin test sickel cell trait sugar coated tablet
SCLE	subcutaneous lupus erythematosis		
ScLP	scapulolaeva posterior		
SCLs	synthetic combinatorial libraries soft contact lenses	SCTX	static cervical traction
		SCU	self-care unit special care unit
SCM	scalene muscle sensation, circulation, and motion spondylitic caudal myelopathy sternocleidomastoid supraclavicular muscle	SCUCP	small cell undifferentiated carcinoma of the prostate
		SCUF	slow continuous ultrafiltration
		SCUT	schizophrenia, chronic undifferentiated type
SCMD	senile choroidal macular degeneration	SCV	subclavian vein subcutaneous vaginal (block)
SCMV	serogroup C meningococcal vaccine	SD	scleroderma senile dementia severe deficit sleep deprived septal defect severely disabled shoulder disarticulation single dose skin dose somatic dysfunction spasmodic dysphonia spontaneous delivery stable disease standard deviation standard diet step-down sterile dressing straight drainage
SCN	special care nursery suprachiasmatic nucleus		
SCOB	Schedule-Controlled Operant Behavior		
SCOP	scopolamine		
SCOPE	arthroscopy		
SCP	sodium cellulose phosphate standardized care plan		
S-CPK	serum creatine phosphokinase		
SCR	special care room (seclusion room) spondylitic caudal radioculopathy stem cell rescue		

	streptozocin and doxorubicin		standard deviation of the mean
	sudden death	S/D/M	systolic, diastolic, mean
	surgical drain	SD/N	signal-difference-to-noise ratio
S & D	seen and discussed		
	stomach and duodenum	SDP	sacrodextra posterior
S/D	sharp/dull		single donor platelets
	systolic-diastolic ratio		stomach, duodenum, and pancreas
SDA	sacrodextra anterior		
	same day admission	SDR	selective dorsal rhizotomy
	serotonin/dopamine antagonist	SDS	same day surgery
			Self-Rating Depression Scale
	Seventh-Day Adventist		
	steroid-dependent asthmatic		sodium dodecyl sulfate
			somatropin deficiency syndrome
SDAT	senile dementia of Alzheimer's type		
			Speech Discrimination Score
SDB	Sabouraud dextrose broth		
	self-destructive behavior		standard deviation score
	sleep disordered breathing		sudden death syndrome
SDBP	seated diastolic blood pressure	SDSO	same day surgery overnight
	standing diastolic blood pressure	SDS-PAGE	sodium dodecyl sulfate – polyacrylamide gel electrophoresis
	supine diastolic blood pressure	SDT	sacrodextra transversa
SDC	serum digoxin concentration		speech detection threshold
		SDU	step-down unit
	serum drug concentration	SE	saline enema (0.9% sodium chloride)
	Sleep Disorders Center		
	sodium deoxycholate		self-examination
SD&C	suction, dilation, and curettage		side effect
			soft exudates
SDD	selective digestive (tract) decontamination		spin echo
			staff escort
	sterile dry dressing		standard error
SDDT	selective decontamination of the digestive tract		Starr-Edwards (valve, pacemaker)
SDES	symptomatic diffuse esophageal spasm	Se	selenium
		S/E	suicidal and eloper
SDH	subdural hematoma	SEA	sheep erythrocyte agglutination (test)
SDI	Sandimmune (cyclosporine)		
			Southeast Asia
SDII	sudden death in infancy		synaptic electronic activation
SDL	serum digoxin level		
	serum drug level	SEAR	Southease Asia refugee
	speech discrimination loss	SEC	second
			secondary
SDM	soft drusen maculopathy		secretary

231

	steric exclusion chromatography	SER-IV	supination external rotation, type 4 fracture
SECG	scalp electrocardiogram	SERO-	serosanguineous
SECL	seclusion	SANG	
SECPR	standard external cardiopulmonary resuscitation	SERs	somatosensory evoked responses
SED	sedimentation	SES	socioeconomic status
	skin erythema dose		standard electrolyte solution
	socially and emotionally disturbed	SET	social environmental therapy
	spondyloepiphyseal dysplasia		systolic ejection time
SED-NET	severely emotional disturbed - network	SEWHO	shoulder-elbow-wrist-hand orthosis
sed rt	sedimentation rate	SF	salt free
SEER	Surveillance, Epidemiology, and End Results (program)		saturated fat
			scarlet fever
			seizure frequency
			seminal fluid
SEG	segment		soft feces
	sonoencephalogram		sound field
segs	segmented neutrophils		spinal fluid
SEH	spinal epidural hematomas		sugar free
			symptom-free
	subependymal hemorrhage		synovial fluid
SEI	subepithelial (comeal) infiltrate	S&F	soft and flat
		SF-6	sulfahexafluoride
SELFVD	sterile elective low forceps vaginal delivery	SF 36	Short Form 36
		SFA	saturated fatty acids
			superficial femoral artery
SEM	scanning electron microscopy	SFB	single frequency bioimpedance
	semen	SFC	spinal fluid count
	slow eye movement		subarachnoid fluid collection
	standard error of mean		
	systolic ejection murmur	SFD	scaphoid fossa depression
SEMI	subendocardial myocardial infarction		small for dates
		SFEMG	single-fiber electromyography
SENS	sensitivity		
	sensorium	SFH	schizophrenia family history
SEP	separate		
	serum electrophoresis	SFP	simulated fluorescence process
	somatosensory evoked potential		simultaneous foveal perception
	systolic ejection period		spinal fluid pressure
SEQ	sequela		
SER	scanning equalization radiography	SFPT	standard fixation preference test
	signal enhancement ratio	SFS	split function studies

SFTR	sagittal, frontal, transverse, rotation	SH2	sarc homology region 2
		SHA	super heated aerosol
SFUP	surgical follow-up	SHAL	standard hyperalimentation
SFV	superficial femoral vein		
SFW	shell fragment wound	SHAS	supravalvular hypertrophic aortic stenosis
SG	salivary gland		
	scrotography		
	serum glucose	S Hb	sickle hemoglobin screen
	side glide	SHBG	sex hormone-binding globulin
	skin graft		
	specific gravity	SHEENT	skin, head, eyes, ears, nose, and throat
	Swan-Ganz (catheter)		
SGA	small for gestational age	SHGT	somatic-cell human gene therapy
	subjective global assessment (dietary history and physical examination)		
		SHI	standard heparin infusion
		Shig	*Shigella*
	substantial gainful activity (employment)	SHL	sudden hearing loss
			supraglottic horizontal laryngectomy
SGC	Swan-Ganz catheter		
SGD	straight gravity drainage	SHO	Senior House Officer
SGE	significant glandular enlargement	SHR	scapulohumeral rhythm
		SHS	student health service
s̄ gl	without correction (without glasses)	SHx	social history
		SI	International System of Units
SGM	serum glucose monitoring		sacroiliac
SGOT	serum glutamic oxalo-acetic transaminase (same as AST)		sagittal index
			sector iridectomy
			self-inflicted
SGPT	serum glutamic pyruvic transaminase (same as ALT)		sensory integration
			seriously ill
			sexual intercourse
SGS	second-generation sulfonylurea		small intestine
			strict isolation
	subglottic stenosis		stress incontinence
SGTCS	secondarily generalized tonic-clonic seizures		stroke index
			suicidal ideation
SH	serum hepatitis	Si	silicon
	sexual harassment	S & I	suction and irrigation
	short	SIA	small intestinal atresia
	shoulder	SIADH	syndrome of inappropriate antidiuretic hormone secretion
	shower		
	social history		
	sulfhydryl (group)	SIAT	supervised intermittent ambulatory treatment
	surgical history		
S&H	speech and hearing	SIB	self-injurious behavior
	suicidal and homicidal	SIBC	serum iron-binding capacity
S/H	suicidal/homicidal ideation		
		sibs	siblings

233

SIC	self-intermittent catherization	SIS	sister
			Surgical Infection Stratification (system)
	squamous intraepithelial cells	SISI	Short Increment Sensitivity Index
SICD	sudden infant crib death		
SICT	selective intracoronary thrombolysis	SISS	severe invasion streptococcal syndrome
SICU	surgical intensive care unit	SIT	silicon-intensified target
			Slossen Intelligence Test
SIDA	French and Spanish abbreviation for AIDS		sperm immobilization test
			surgical intensive therapy
SIDD	syndrome of isolated diastolic dysfunction	SIT BAL	sitting balance
		SIT TOL	sitting tolerance
SIDERO	siderocyte	SIV	simian immunodeficiency virus
SIDFF	superimposed dorsiflexion of foot		
		SIVP	slow intravenous push
SIDS	sudden infant death syndrome	SIW	self-inflicted wound
		SJCRH	St. Jude Children's Research Hospital
SIEP	serum immunoelectro-phoresis		
		S-JRA	systemic juvenile rheumatoid arthritis
SIG	let it be marked (appears on prescription before directions for patient)	SJS	Stevens-Johnson syndrome
			Swyer-James syndrome
	sigmoidoscopy	SK	seborrheic keratosis
Signal 99	patient in cardiac or respiratory distress		senile keratosis
			SmithKline®
SIJ	sacroiliac joint		solar keratosis
SIL	seriously ill list		streptokinase
	sister-in-law	S & K	single and keeping (baby)
SILFVD	sterile indicated low forceps vaginal delivery	SKAO	supracondylar knee-ankle orthosis
SILV	simultaneous independent lung ventilation		
		SKB	SmithKline Beecham
SIM	selective ion monitoring	SKC	single knee to chest
	Similac®	SK-SD	streptokinase streptodornase
SIMCU	surgical intermediate care unit		
		SL	scapholunate
Sim c̄ Fe	Similac with iron®		sensation level
SIMV	synchronized intermittent mandatory ventilation		sentinel lymphadenectomy
			serious list
SIN	salpingitis isthmica nodose		shortleg
			slight
SIP	Sickness Impact Profile		sublingual
	stroke in progression	S/L	slit lamp (examination)
SIQ	sick in quarters	SLA	sacrolaeva anterior
SIR	standardized incidence rate (ratio)		sex and love addictions
			slide latex agglutination
SIRS	systemic inflammatory response syndrome		The Satisfaction with Life Areas

SLAA	Sex and Love Addicts Anonymous	SLPMS	short-leg posterior-molded splint
SLAC	scapholunate advanced collapse	SLR	straight leg raising
		SLRT	straight leg raising test
SLAP	serum leucine amino-peptidase	SLS	second-look sonography
			short leg splint
SLB	short leg brace		single limb support
SLC	short leg cast	SLT	scanning laser tomography
SLCC	short leg cylinder cast		swing light test
SLCG	sulfolithocholyglycine		
SLCT	Sertoli-Leydig cell tumor	SLT	sacrolaeva transversa
SLE	slit lamp examination	SLTEC	Shiga-like toxin-producing *Escherichia coli*
	St. Louis encephalitis		
	systemic lupus erythematosus		
		sl. tr.	slight trace
SLEX	slit lamp examination (biomicroscopy)	SLUD	salivation, lacrimation, urination, and defecation
SLFVD	sterile low forceps vaginal delivery		
		SLV	since last visit
SLGXT	symptom limited graded exercise test	SLWB	severely low birth weight
		SLWC	short leg walking cast
SLK	superior limbic keratoconjunctivitis	SM	sadomasochism
			skim milk
SLL	second look laparotomy		small
	small lymphocytic lymphoma		sports medicine
			Stairmaster®
SLMFVD	sterile low mid-forceps vaginal delivery		streptomycin
			systolic motion
SLMMS	slightly more marked since		systolic murmur
		SMA	sequential multiple analyzer
SLMP	since last menstrual period		simultaneous multichannel auto-analyzer
SLN	sentinel lymph node(s)		spinal muscular atrophy
	superior laryngeal nerve		superior mesenteric artery
SLNTG	sublingual nitroglycerin		supplementary motor area
SLNWBC	short leg nonweight-bearing cast	SMA-6	sequential multipler analyzer for sodium, potassium, CO_2, chloride, glucose, and BUN
SLNWC	short leg non-walking cast		
SLO	scanning laser ophthalmoscope		
	second look operation	SMA-7	sodium, potassium, CO_2, chloride, glucose, BUN, and creatinine
	Smith-Lemi-Opitz (syndrome)		
	streptolysin O		
SLOA	short leave of absence	SMA-12	glucose, BUN, uric acid, calcium, phosphorus, total protein, albumin, cholesterol, total bilirubin, alkaline
SLP	speech language pathology		
SLPI	secretory leukocyte protease inhibitor		

	phosphatase, SGOT, and LDH	SMILE	safety, monitoring, intervention, length of stay and evaluation
SMA-18	SMA-12 + SMA−6		sustained maximal inspiratory lung exercises
SMA-23	includes the entire SMA-12 plus sodium, potassium, CO$_2$, chloride, direct bilirubin, triglyceride, SGPT, indirect bilirubin, R fraction, and BUN/creatinine ratio	SMIT	standard mycological identification techniques
		SMN	second malignant neoplasia
SMAO	superior mesenteric artery occlusion	SMO	Senior Medical Officer
			slip made out
SMAR	self-medication administration record	SMON	subacute myelo-opticoneuropathy
		SMP	self-management program
SMAS	superficial musculoapo-neurotic system	SMPN	sensorimotor polyneuropathy
	superior mesenteric artery syndrome	SMR	senior medical resident
			skeletal muscle relaxant
SMAST	Short Michigan Alcoholism Screening Test		standardized mortality ratio
			submucosal resection
SMB	simulated moving bed	SMRR	submucous resection and rhinoplasty
SMBG	self-monitoring blood glucose	SMS	scalded mouth syndrome
SMC	special mouth care		senior medical student
SMCA	sorbitol MacConkey agar		somatostatin
SMCD	senile macular chorio-retinal degeneration		stiff-man syndrome
SMD	senile macular degeneration	SMSA	standard metropolitan statistical area
SMDA	Safe Medical Defice Act	SMV	submentovertical
SME	significant medical event		superior mesenteric vein
SMF	streptozocin, mitomycin, and fluorouracil	SMVT	sustained monomorphic ventricular tachycardia
SMFVD	sterile mid-forceps vaginal delivery	SMX-TMP	sulfamethoxazole and tri-methoprim (SMZ-TMP)
SMG	submandibular gland	SN	sciatic notch
SMH	state mental hospital		staff nurse
SMI	sensory motor integration (group)		student nurse
			suprasternal notch
	severely mentally impaired		superior nasal
	small volume infusion	Sn	tin
	suggested minimum increment	S/N	signal to noise ratio
	sustained maximal inspiration	SNA	specimen not available
			Student Nursing Assistant
		SNa	serum sodium
		SNAP	scheduled nursing activities program

236

	Score for Neonatal Acute Physiology
	sensory nerve action potential
SNAP-PE	Score for Neonatal Acute Physiology-Perinatal Extension
SNAT	suspected non-accidental trauma
SNB	scalene node biopsy
SNC	skilled nursing care
SNCV	sensory nerve conduction velocity
SND	single needle device
	sinus node dysfunction
SNDA	Supplemental New Drug Application
SNE	subacute necrotizing encephalomyelopathy
SNEP	student nurse extern program
SNF	skilled nursing facility
SnF$_2$	stannous fluoride
SNF/MR	skilled nursing facility for the mentally retarded
SNGFR	single nephron glomerular filtration rate
SNHL	sensorineural hearing loss
SNIP	strict no information in paper
SNM	student nurse midwife
SnMp	tin-mesoporphyrin
SNOOP	Systematic Nursing Observation of Psychopathology
SNP	simple neonatal procedure
	sodium nitroprusside
SNR	signal-to-noise ratio
SNRT	sinus node recovery time
SNS	sterile normal saline (0.9% sodium chloride)
	sympathetic nervous system
SNT	sinuses, nose, and throat
	suppan nail technique
SNV	Sin Nombre virus
	skilled nursing visit
	spleen necrosis virus
SO	second opinion
	sex offender
	shoulder orthosis
	significant other
	special observation
	sphincter of Oddi
	standing orders
	suboccipital
	superior oblique
	supraoptic
	supraorbital
	sutures out
	sympathetic ophthalmia
S-O	salpingo-oophorectomy
S&O	salpingo-oophorectomy
SO$_3$	sulfite
SO$_4$	sulfate
SOA	serum opsonic activity
	spinal opioid analgesia
	supraorbital artery
	swelling of ankles
SOAA	signed out against advice
SOAM	sutures out in the morning
SOAMA	signed out against medical advice
SOAP	subjective, objective, assessment, and plans
SOAPIE	subjective, objective, assessment, plan, implementation, (intervention), and evaluation
SOB	see order book
	shortness of breath (this abbreviation has caused problems)
	side of bed
SOBE	short of breath on exertion
SOBOE	short of breath on exertion
SOC	see old chart
	socialization
	standard of care
	state of consciousness
S & OC	signed and on chart (e.g. permit)
SOD	sinovenous occlusive disease
	superoxide dismutase

	surgical officer of the day		spouse
SODAS	spheriodal oral drug absorption system		stand and pivot
			stand pivot
SOG	suggestive of good		status post
SOH	sexually oriented hallucinations		systolic pressure
		sp	species
SoHx	social history	S/P	status post
SOI	slipped on ice	SP 1	suicide precautions number 1
	surgical orthotopic implantation (implant)	SP 2	suicide precautions number 2
	syrup of ipecac	SPA	albumin human (formerly known as salt-poor albumin)
SOL	solution		
	space occupying lesion		serum prothrombin activity
SOL I	special observations level one (there are also SOL II and SOL III)		single photon absorptiometry
SOM	secretory otitis media		Speech Pathology and Audiology
	serous otitis media		stimulation produced analgesia
	somatization		
SOMI	sterno-occipital mandibular immobilizer		student physician's assistant
Sono	sonogram		subperiosteal abscess
SONP	solid organs not palpable		suprapubic aspiration
SOOL	spontaneous onset of labor	SPAC	satisfactory postanesthesia course
SOP	standard operating procedure	SPAG	small particle aerosol generator
SOPM	sutures out in afternoon (or evening)	SPAMM	spatial modulation of magnetization
SOR	sign own release	SPBI	serum protein bound iodine
SOS	if there is need	SPBT	suprapubic bladder tap
	may be repeated once if urgently required (Latin: si opus sit)	SPC	statistical process control
			suprapubic catheter
	self-obtained smear	SPCT	simultaneous prism and cover test
	suicidal observation status		
SOSOB	sit on side of bed	SPD	subcorneal pustular dermatosis
SOT	solid organ transplant		
	something other than		Supply, Processing, and Distribution (department)
	stream of thought		
	superficial ocular trauma		suprapubic drainage
SP	sacrum to pubis	SPE	serum protein electrophoresis
	sequential pulse		
	serum protein		superficial punctate erosions
	shoulder press		
	spastic dysphonia		
	speech		
	Speech Pathologist		
	spinal		

SPEB	streptococcal pyrogenic exotoxins B	SpO₂	oxygen saturation by pulse oximeter
SPEC	specimen	spont	spontaneous
	streptococcal pyrogenic exotoxins C	SPP	Sexuality Preference Profile
Spec Ed	special education		species (specus)
SPECT	single photon emission computed tomography		super packed platelets
			suprapubic prostatectomy
SPEEP	spontaneous positive end-expiratory pressure	SPR	surface plasmon resonance
SPEP	serum protein electrophoresis	SPRAS	Sheehan Patient Rated Anxiety Scale
SPET	single-photon emission tomography	SP-RIA	solid-phase radioimmunoassay
SPF	split products of fibrin	SPROM	spontaneous premature rupture of membrane
	sun protective factor		
sp fl	spinal fluid	SPS	shoulder pain and stiffness
SPG	scrotopenogram		simple partial seizure
	sphenopalatine ganglion		sodium polyethanol sulfonate
SpG	specific gravity		
SPH	severely and profoundly handicapped		sodium polystyrene sulfonate
	sighs per hour		status post surgery
	spherocytes		systemic progressive sclerosis
SPHERO	spherocytes		
SPI	speech processor interface	SPT	skin prick test
	surgical peripheral iridectomy	SP TAP	spinal tap
		SPTs	second primary tumors
SPIA	solid phase immunoabsorbent assay	SP TUBE	suprapubic tube
SPIF	spontaneous peak inspiratory force	SPTX	static pelvic traction
		SPU	short procedure unit
S-PIN	Steinmann pin	SPVR	systemic peripheral vascular resistance
SPL	sound pressure level		
SPL®	Staphylococcal Phage Lysate	SQ	status quo
			subcutaneous (this is a dangerous abbreviation)
SPLATTT	split anterior tibial tendon transfer	Sq CCa	squamous cell carcinoma
SPK	superficial punctate keratitis	SQE	subcutaneous emphysema
		SQM	square meter(s)
SPM	scanning probe microscopy	SR	screen
SPMA	spinal progressive muscle atrophy		sedimentation rate
			see report
SPMSQ	Short Portable Mental Status Questionnaire		senior resident
			service record
SPN	solitary pulmonary nodule		side rails
	student practical nurse		sinus rhythm
SPO	status postoperative		slow release
			smooth-rough

	social recreation	SRP	septorhinoplasty
	stretch reflex		stapes replacement
	superior rectus		prosthesis
	sustained release	SRR	surgical recovery room
	suture removal	SRS	somatostatin receptor
	system review		scintigraphy
S/R	strong/regular (pulse)	s̄RS	without redness or
S&R	seclusion and restraint		swelling
SRA	steroid-resistant asthma	SRS-A	slow-reacting substance of
SRAN	surgical resident		anaphylaxis
	admission note	SRSV	small round structured
SRBC	sheep red blood cells		viruses
	sickle red blood cells	SRT	sedimentation rate test
SRBOW	spontaneous rupture of		sleep-related tumescence
	bag of waters		speech reception threshold
SRD	service-related disability		surfactant replacement
	sodium-restricted diet		therapy
SRE	skeletal related event		sustained release
SRF	somatotropin releasing		theophylline
	factor	SRU	side rails up
	subretinal fluid	SRUS	solitary rectal ulcer
SRF-A	slow releasing factor of		syndrome
	anaphylaxis	SR ↑ X2	both siderails up
SRGVHD	steroid-resistant graft-	SS	half
	versus-host disease		sacrosciatic
SRH	signs of recent		saline (sodium chloride
	hemorrhage		0.9%) soak
SRI	serotonin re-uptake		saline solution (0.9%
	inhibitor		sodium chloride)
SRICU	surgical respiratory		saliva sample
	intensive care unit		salt sensitivity (sensitive)
SRIF	somatotropin-		salt substitute
	release inhibiting factor		serotonin syndrome
	(somatostatin)		serum sickness
SRMD	stress-related mucosal		sickle cell
	damage		Sjögren's syndrome
SR/NE	sinus rhythm, no ectopy		sliding scale
SRNV	subretinal neovasculariza-		slip sent
	tion		Social Security
SRNVM	subretinal neovascular		social service
	membrane		somatostatin
SRO	sagittal ramus osteotomy		steady state
	single room occupancy		step stool
	sustained-release oral		subaortic stenosis
SROCPI	Self-Rating Obsessive-		susceptible
	Compulsive Personality		suprasciatic (notch)
	Inventory		symmetrical strength
SROM	spontaneous rupture of	SS#	Social Security number
	membrane	S & S	shower and shampoo

	signs and symptoms	SSF	subscapular skinfold
	sling and swathe	SSG	sodium stibogluconate
	soft and smooth (prostate)		sublabial salivary gland
	support and stimulation	SSI	sliding scale insulin
	swish and spit		sub-shock insulin
	swish and swallow		superior sector iridectomy
SSA	sagittal split advancement		Supplemental Security
	salicylsalicylic acid		Income
	(salsalate)	SSKI	saturated solution of
	Sjögren's syndrome		potassium iodide
	antigen A	SSL	subtotal supraglottic
	Social Security		laryngectomy
	Administration	SSM	short stay medical
	sulfasalicylic acid (test)		skin surface microscopy
SSC	sign symptom complex		superficial spreading
	silver sulfadiazine and		melanoma
	chlorhexidine	SSN	severely subnormal
	Similac® and special care		Social Security number
	Special Services for	SSO	short stay observation
	Children		(unit)
	stainless steel crown		Spanish speaking only
SSc	systemic sclerosis	SSOP	Second Surgical Opinion
SSCA	single shoulder contrast		Program
	arthrography	SSP	short stay procedure (unit)
SSCP	single strand	SSPE	subacute sclerosing
	conformational		panencephalitis
	polymorphism	SSPL	saturation sound pressure
	substernal chest pain		level
SSCr	stainless steel crown	SSPU	surgical short procedure
SSCU	surgical special care unit		unit
SSCVD	sterile spontaneous	SSR	substernal retractions
	controlled vaginal		sympathetic skin response
	delivery	SSRFC	surrounding subretinal
SSD	serosanguineous drainage		fluid cuff
	sickle cell disease	SSRI	selective serotonin
	silver sulfadiazine		reuptake inhibitor
	Social Security disability	SSS	layer upon layer
	source to skin distance		scalded skin syndrome
SSDI	Social Security disability		Scandinavian Stroke Scale
	income		Sepsis Severity Score
SSE	saline solution enema		short stay service (unit)
	(0.9% sodium chloride)		sick sinus syndrome
	skin self-examination		skin and skin structures
	soapsuds enema		sterile saline soak
	systemic side effects	SSSB	sagittal split setback
SSEH	spontaneous spinal	SSSIs	skin and skin structure
	epidural hematoma		infections
SSEPs	somatosensory evoked	SSSS	staphylococcal scalded
	potentials		skin syndrome

SST	sagittal sinus thrombosis	STAXI	State-Trait Anger Expression Inventory
SSU	short stay unit		
SSX	sulfisoxazole acetyl	STB	stillborn
S/SX	signs/symptoms	STBAL	standing balance
ST	esotropic	ST BY	stand by
	sacrum transverse	STC	serum theophylline concentration
	Schiotz's tonometry		
	shock therapy		soft tissue calcification
	sinus tachycardia		special treatment center
	skin test		stimulate to cry
	slight trace		stroke treatment center
	smokeless tobacco		subtotal colectomy
	sore throat		sugar tongue cast
	speech therapist	ST CLK	station clerk
	speech therapy	STD	sexually transmitted disease(s)
	sphincter tone		
	split thickness		skin test dose
	spondee threshold		skin to tumor distance
	station (obstetrics)		sodium tetradecyl sulfate
	stomach	STD TF	standard tube feeding
	straight	STEAM	stimulated-echo acquisition mode
	stress testing		
	stretcher	STEM	scanning transmission electron microscopic
	subtotal		
	Surgical Technologist	Stereo	steropsis
	survival time	STET	single photon emission tomography
	synapse time		
S & T	sulfamethoxazole and trimethoprim (SMZ-TMP or SMX-TMP)		submaximal treadmill exercise test
		STETH	stethoscope
STA	second trimester abortion	STF	special tube feeding
	superficial temporal artery		standard tube feeding
		STG	stillborn
stab.	polymorphonuclear leukocytes (white blood cells, in nonmature form)		short-term goals
			split-thickness graft
			superior temporal gyri
		STH	soft tissue hemorrhage
			somatotrophic hormone
STAI	State-Trait Anxiety Inventory		subtotal hysterectomy
			supplemental thyroid hormone
STAI-I	State-Trait-Anxiety Index—I		
		STHB	said to have been
STA-MCA	superficial temporary artery-middle cerebral artery (bypass)	STI	soft tissue injury
			sum total impression
		STILLB	stillborn
STAPES	stapedectomy	STIR	short TI (tau) inversion recovery
staph	Staphylococcus aureus		
stat	immediately	STIs	systolic time intervals
STATINS	HMG-CoA reductase inhibitors	STJ	scapulothoracic joint
			subtalar joint

242

STK	streptokinase		serial thrombin time
STL	sent to laboratory		skin temperature test
	serum theophylline level		soft tissue tumor
STLE	St. Louis encephalitis	STT#1	Schirmer tear test one
STLOM	swelling, tenderness, and limitation of motion	STT#2	Schirmer tear test two
		STTb	basal Schirmer tear test
STM	short-term memory	STTOL	standing tolerance
	streptomycin	STU	shock trauma unit
STMT	Seat Movement		surgical trauma unit
STNM	surgical evaluative staging of cancer	STV	short-term variability
		STV+	short-term variability-present
STNR	symmetrical tonic neck reflex	STV 0	short-term variability-absent
S to	sensitive to	STV inter	short-term variability-intermittent
STOP	sensitive, timely, and organized programs (battered spouses)		
		STX	stricture
		STZ	streptozocin
STORCH	syphilis, toxoplasmosis, other agents, rubella, cytomegalovirus, and herpes (maternal infections)	S&U	supine and upright
		SU	sensory urgency
			Somogyi units
			stroke unit
			supine
STP	short-term plans	S/U	shoulder/umbilicus
	sodium thiopental	SUA	serum uric acid
STPD	standard temperature and pressure—dry		single umbilical artery
STPI	State-Trait Personality Inventory	SUB	Skene's urethra and Bartholin's glands
STR	sister	Subcu	subcutaneous
	small tandem repeat	SUBCUT	subcutaneous
	stretcher	Subepi M Inj	subepicardial myocardial injury
Strab	strabismus		
strep	streptococcus	SUBL	sublingual
	streptomycin	SUB-MAND	submandibular
Str Post MI	strictly posterior myocardial infarction	sub q	subcutaneous (this is a dangerous abbreviation since the q is mistaken for every, when a number follows)
STS	serologic test for syphilis short-term survivors sodium tetradecyl sulfate sodium thiosulfate soft tissue sarcoma soft tissue swelling Surgical Technology Student	
		SUD	sudden unexpected death
		SuDBP	supine diastolic blood pressure
		SUDS	Subjective Unit of Distress (Disturbance) (Discomfort) Scale
STSG	split thickness skin graft		
STSS	streptococcal-induced toxic shock syndrome		sudden unexplained death syndrome
STT	scaphoid, trapezium trapezoid		

SUI	stress urinary incontinence suicide	SVC-RPA	superior vena cava and right pulmonary artery (shunt)
SUID	sudden unexplained infant death	SVCS	superior vena cava syndrome
SULF-PRIM	sulfamethoxazole and trimethoprim	SVD	single vessel disease spontaneous vaginal delivery
SUN	serum urea nitrogen		
SUNDS	sudden unexplained nocturnal death syndrome	SVE	sterile vaginal examination
			Streptococcus viridans endocarditis
SUO	syncope of unknown origin	SV&E	suicidal, violent, and eloper
SUP	stress ulcer prophylaxis		
	superior	SVG	saphenous vein graft
	supination	SVI	seminal vesicle invasion
	supinator		stroke volume index
	symptomatic uterine prolapse	S VISC	serum viscosity
		SVL	severe visual loss
supp	suppository	SVN	small volume nebulizer
SUR	suramin	SVO$_2$	mixed venous oxygen saturation
	surgery		
	surgical	SVP	spontaneous venous pulse
Surgi	Surgigator	SVPB	supraventricular premature beat
SUUD	sudden unexpected, unexplained death		
		SVPC	supraventricular premature contraction
SUX	succinylcholine		
	suction	SVR	supraventricular rhythm
SUZI	subzonal insertion		systemic vascular resistance
SV	seminal vesical		
	severe	SVRI	systemic vascular resistance index
	sigmoid volvulus		
	single ventricle	SVT	supraventricular tachycardia
	single vessel		
	snake venom	SVVD	spontaneous vertex vaginal delivery
	stock volume		
	subclavian vein	SW	sandwich
Sv	sievert (radiation unit)		sea water
SV40	simian virus 40		seriously wounded
SVA	small volume admixture		short wave
SVB	saphenous vein bypass		Social Worker
SVBG	saphenous vein bypass graft		stab wound
			sterile water
SVC	slow vital capacity	S&W	soap and water
	subclavian vein compression	S/W	somewhat
		SWA	Social Work Associate
	superior vena cava	SWD	short wave diathermy
SVCO	superior vena cava obstruction	SWFI	sterile water for injection
		SWG	standard wire gauge

244

SWI	sterile water for injection			is a dangerous
	surgical wound infection			abbreviation)
S&WI	skin and wound isolation			temperature
SWO	superficial white			tender
	onychomycosis			tension
SWOG	Southwest Oncology			testicles
	Group			thoracic
SWOT	strengths, weaknesses,			thymine
	opportunities, threats			trace
	(analysis)	t		teaspoon (5 mL) (this is a
SWP	small whirlpool			dangerous abbreviation)
SWR	surface wrinkling	T+		increase intraocular
	retinopathy			tension
	surgical waiting room	T-		decreased intraocular
SWS	sheltered workshop			tension
	slow wave sleep	T°		temperature
	social work service	$T_{1/2}$		half-life
	student ward secretary	T_1		tricuspid first sound
	Sturge-Weber syndrome	T_2		tricuspid second sound
SWT	stab wound of the throat	T-2		dactinomycin,
SWU	septic work-up			doxorubicin,
Sx	signs			vincristine, and
	surgery			cyclophosphamide
	symptom	T_3		triiodothyronine
SXA	single-energy x-ray			(liothyronine)
	absorptiometry	T3		Tylenol® with codeine 30
SXR	skull x-ray			mg (this is a dangerous
SYN	synovial			abbreviation)
SYN Fl	synovial fluid	T_4		levothyroxine
SYPH	syphilis			thyroxine
SYR	syrup	$T_{3/4}$ind		triiodothyronine to
SYS BP	systolic blood pressure			thyroxine index
SZ	schizophrenic	T-7		free thyroxine factor
	seizure	T-10		methotrexate, calcium
	suction			leucovorin rescue,
SZN	streptozocin			doxorubicin, cisplatin,
				bleomycin,
				cyclophosphamide, and
				dactinomycin
		$T_1...T_{12}$		thoracic nerve 1 through 12
				thoracic vertebra

T

				1 through 12
		TA		Takayasu's arteritis
				temperature axillary
				temporal arteritis
				therapeutic abortion
				tracheal aspirate
T	inverted T wave			traffic accident
	tablespoon (15 mL) (this			tricuspid atresia

245

	truncus arteriosus	TAHL	thick ascending limb of Henle's loop
Ta	tonometry applanation		
T&A	tonsillectomy and adenoidectomy	T Air	air puff tonometry
		TAL	tendon Achilles lengthening
	tonsils and adenoids		total arm length
T(A)	axillary temperature	T ALCON	Alcon® tonometry
TA-55	stapling device	TAML	therapy-related acute
TAA	Therapeutic Activities Aide		myelogenous leukemia
	thoracic aortic aneurysm	TAM	tamoxifen
	total ankle arthroplasty		teenage mother
	transverse aortic arch		total active motion
	triamcinolone acetonide		tumor-associated macrophages
	tumor associated antigen (antibodies)	TAN	Treatment Authorization Number
TAAA	thoracoabdominal aortic aneursym		tropical ataxic neuropathy
		TANI	total axial (lymph) node irradiation
TAB	tablet		
	therapeutic abortion	TAO	thromboangitis obliterans
	triple antibiotic (bacitracin, neomycin, and polymyxin—this is a dangerous abbreviation)		troleandomycin
		TAP	tonometry by applanation
			transabdominal preperitoneal (laparoscopic hernia repair)
TAC	tetracaine, Adrenalin® and cocaine		
		TAPP	transabdominal preperitoneal polypropylene (mesh-plasty)
	tibial artery catheter		
	total abdominal colectomy		
	total allergen content		
	triamcinolone cream	T APPL	applanation tonometry
TAD	transverse abdominal diameter	TAPVC	total anomalous pulmonary venous connection
TADAC	therapeutic abortion, dilation, aspiration, and curettage		
		TAPVD	total anomalous pulmonary venous drainage
TAE	transcatheter arterial embolization		
		TAPVR	total anomalous pulmonary venous return
TAF	tissue angiogenesis factor		
TAG	tumor-associated glycoprotein		
		TAR	thrombocytopenia with absent radius
TA-GVHD	transfusion-associated graft-versus-host disease		
			total ankle replacement
			treatment authorization request
TAH	total abdominal hysterectomy		
		TARA	total articular replacement arthroplasty
	total artificial heart		
TAHBSO	total abdominal hysterectomy, bilateral salpingo-oophorectomy	TART	tumorectomy plus radiotherapy

TAS	therapeutic activities specialist	T bili	total bilirubin
	turning against self	TBK	total body potassium
	typical absence seizures	tbl	tablespoon (15 mL)
TAT	tell a tale	TBLB	transbronchial lung biopsy
	tetanus antitoxin	TBLC	term birth, living child
	'til all taken	TBLF	term birth, living female
	thematic apperception test	TBLI	term birth, living infant
	thrombin-antithrombin III complex	TBLM	term birth, living male
	transactivator of transcription	TBM	tracheobronchomalacia
	turnaround time		tubule basement membrane
TAUC	time-averaged urea concentration		tuberculous meningitis
TAX	cefotaxime	TBN	total body nitrogen
TB	Tapes for the Blind	TBNA	transbronchial needle aspiration
	terrible burning		treated but not admitted
	thought broadcasting	TBNa	total body sodium
	toothbrush	TBOCS	Tale-Brown Obsessive-Compulsive Scale
	total base	TBP	thyroxine-binding protein
	total bilirubin		total-body photographs
	total body		total body protein
	tuberculosis		tuberculous peritonitis
TBA	to be absorbed	TBPA	thyroxine-binding prealbumin
	to be added		
	to be administered	TBR	total bed rest
	to be admitted	TBS	tablespoon (15ml)(this is a dangerous abbreviation)
	to be announced		
	to be arranged		
	total body (surface) area		total serum bilirubin
T-bar	device used in respiratory therapy	TBSA	total body surface area
			total burn surface area
TBAGA	term birth appropriate for gestational age	tbsp	tablespoon (15 mL)
		TBT	tolbutamide test
TBB	transbronchial biopsy		tracheal bronchial toilet
TBC	to be cancelled		transbronchoscopic balloon tipped
	total blood cholesterol	TBV	total blood volume
	total body clearance		transluminal balloon valvuloplasty
	tuberculosis		
TBD	to be determined	TBW	total body water
TBE	tick-born encephalitis	TBZ	thiabendazole
T-berg	Trendelenburg (position)	TC	team conference
TBF	total body fat		terminal cancer
TBG	thyroxine-binding globulin		thioguanine and cytarabine
TBI	toothbrushing instruction		thoracic circumference
	total body irradiation		throat culture
	traumatic brain injury		tissue culture

	tolonium chloride	^{99m}Tc	technetium Tc 99m
	total cholesterol	DTPA	pentetate
	to (the) chest	TCE	tetrachloroethylene
	tracheal collar	T cell	small lymphocyte
	trauma center	^{99m}TcGHA	technetium Tc 99m
	true conjugate		gluceptate
	tubocurarine	TCH	turn, cough,
Tc	technetium		hyperventilate
T/C	telephone call	TCHRs	traditional Chinese herbal
	ticarcillin-clavulanic acid		remedies
	(Timentin)	TCI	to come in
	to consider	TCID	tissue culture infective
3TC	lamivudine (Epivir)		dose
TC7	Interceed®	TCIE	transient cerebral
T&C	turn and cough		ischemic episode
	type and crossmatch	TCL	tibial collateral ligament
T&C#3	Tylenol® with 30 mg	TCM	tissue culture media
	codeine		traditional Chinese
TCA	thioguanine and		medicine
	cytarabine		transcutaneous (oxygen)
	trichloroacetic acid		monitor
	tricuspid atresia	^{99m}Tc-	technetium Tc 99m
	tricyclic antidepressant	MAA	albumin microaggre-
	tumor chemosensitivity		gated
	assay	TCMH	tumor-direct cell-mediated
	tumor clonogenic assays		hypersensitivity
TCABG	triple coronary artery	TCMS	transcranial cortical
	bypass graft		magnetic stimulation
TCAD	tricyclic antidepressant	TCMZ	trichloromethiazide
TCAR	tiazofurin	TCN	tetracycline
TCB	to call back		triciribine phosphate
	tumor cell burden		(tricyclic nucleoside)
TCBS agar	thiosulfate-citrate-bile	TCNS	transcutaneous nerve
	salt-sucrose agar		stimulator
TCC	transitional cell carcinoma	TCNU	tauromustine
TCD	transcerebellar diameter	TcO$_4^-$	pertechnetate
	transcranial Doppler	TCOM	transcutaneous oxygen
	(ultrasonography)		monitor
	transverse cardiac	TCP	transcutaneous pacing
	diameter		tranylcypromine
TCCB	transitional cell carcinoma		tumor control probability
	of bladder	TcPCO$_2$	transcutaneous carbon
TC/CL	ticarcillin-clavulanate		dioxide
	(Timentin)	TcPO$_2$	transcutaneous oxygen
TCD	transcystic duct	^{99m}TcPYP	technetium Tc 99m
TCDB	turn, cough, and deep		pyrophosphate
	breath	TCR	T-cell receptor
TCDD	tetrachlorodibenzo-p-	TCRE	transcervical resection of
	dioxin		the endometrium

[99m]TcSC	technetium Tc 99m sulfur colloid	TDT	tentative discharge tomorrow
TCT	thyrocalcitonin		Trieger Dot Test
	tincture		tumor doubling time
TCU	transitional care unit	TdT	terminal deoxynucleotidyl transferase
TCVA	thromboembolic cerebral vascular accident	TDWB	touch down weight bearing
TD	Takayasu's disease	TDx®	fluorescence polarization immunoassay
	tardive dyskinesia	TE	echo time
	temporary disability		tennis elbow
	test dose		terminal extension
	tetanus-diphtheria toxoid (pediatric use)		tooth extraction
	tidal volume		toxoplasmic encephalitis
	tone decay		trace elements
	total disability		tracheoesophageal
	transverse diameter		transesophageal echocardiography
	travelers' diarrhea	T&E	testing and evaluation
	treatment discontinued		training and evaluation
Td	tetanus-diphtheria toxoid (adult type)		trial and error
TDAC	tumor-derived activated cell (cultures)	TEA	thromboendarterectomy
TDD	telephone device for the deaf	TEBG	testosterone-estradiol binding globulin
	thoracic duct drainage	TeBG	testeosterone binding globulin
TDE	total daily energy (requirement)	TEC	total eosinophil count
TDF	testis determining factor		toxic Escherichia coli
	tumor dose fractionation		transient erythroblastopenia of childhood
TDI	tolerable daily intake		transluminal extraction-endarterectomy catheter
	toluene diisocyanate		triethyl citrate
TDK	tardive diskinesia	T&EC	trauma and emergency center
TDL	thoracic duct lymph	TED	thyroid eye disease
TDM	therapeutic drug monitoring	TEDS®	anti-embolism stockings
TDMAC	tridodecylmethyl ammonium chloride	TEE	total energy expended
TDN	totally digestible nutrients		transnasal endoscopic ethmoidectomy
	transdermal nitroglycerin		transesophageal echocardiography
TDNTG	transdermal nitroglycerin	TEF	tracheoesophageal fistula
TDNWB	touchdown non-weight-bearing	TEG	thromboelastogram (thromboelastography)
TdP	torsades de pointes	TEI	total episode of illness
TDPWB	touchdown partial weight-bearing		
TdR	thymidine		
TDS	three times a day (United Kingdom)		

	transesophageal imaging		to follow
TEL	telemetry		tube feeding
	telephone	TFA	topical fluoride application
tele	telemetry		trans fatty acids
TEM	transmission electron microscopy		trifluoroacetic acid
TEMP	temperature	TFB	trifascicular block
	temporal	TFBC	The Family Birthing Center
	temporary		
TEN	tension (intraocular pressure)	TFC	time to following commands
	toxic epidermal necrolysis	TFCC	transjugular fibrocartilage complex
TEN®	Total Enteral Nutrition	TFF	tangential flow filtration
TENS	transcutaneous electrical nerve stimulation	TF-Fe	transferrin-bound iron
		TFL	tensor fasciae latae
TEP	total extraperitoneal (laparoscopic hernia repair)	TFM	transverse friction massage
		TFR	total fertility rate
	tracheoesophageal puncture	TFT	trifluridine (trifluorothy-midine)
	tubal ectopic pregnancy	TFTs	thyroid function tests
TER	terlipressin	TG	triglycerides
	total elbow replacement	6-TG	thioguanine
	total energy requirement	TGA	transient global amnesia
	transurethral electroresection		transposition of the great arteries
TERB	terbutaline	TGE	transmissible gastroenteritis
TERC	Test of Early Reading Comprehension	TGFA	triglyceride fatty acid
TERM	full-term	TGF	transforming growth factor
	terminal		
tert.	tertiary	TGF-$_\beta$	transforming growth factor-beta
TES	thoracic endometriosis syndrome	TGGE	temperature-gradient gel electrophoresis
	treatment emergent symptoms	TGR	tenderness, guarding, and rigidity
TESI	thoracic epidural steroid injection	TGS	tincture of green soap
		TGs	triglycerides
TESS	Treatment Emergent Symptom Scale	TGT	thromboplastin generation test
TET	transcranial electrostimu-lation therapy	TGV	thoracic gas volume
			transposition of great vessels
	treadmill exercise test		
TEU	token economy unit	TGXT	thallium-graded exercise test
TEV	talipes equinovarus (deformity)		
		TH	thrill
TF	tactile fremitus		thyroid hormone
	tail flick (reflex)		
	tetralogy of Fallot		

	total hysterectomy	TICS	diverticulosis
T&H	type and hold	TICU	thoracic intensive care unit
THA	tacrine (tetrahydroacridine) Cognex		transplant intensive care unit
	total hip arthroplasty		trauma intensive care unit
	transient hemispheric attack	TID	three times a day
THAL	thalassemia	TIDM	three times daily with meals
THBI	thyroid hormone binding index	TIE	transient ischemic episode
THBR	thyroid hormone-binding ratio	TIG	tetanus immune globulin
THAM®	tromethamine	TIH	tumor-inducing hypercalcemia
THC	tetrahydrocannabinol (dronabinol)	TIL	tumor-infiltrating lymphocytes
	thigh circumference	%tile	percentile
	transhepatic cholangiogram	TIMP	tissue inhibitor of metalloproteinase
TH-CULT	throat culture	TIN	three times a night (this is a dangerous abbreviation)
tHcy	total homocysteine		
THE	transhepatic embolization		tubulointerstitial nephritis
Ther Ex	therapeutic exercise	tinct	tincture
THF	thymic humoral factor	TIND	Treatment Investigational New Drug (application)
THI	transient hypogammaglobulinemia of infancy	TINEM	there is no evidence of malignancy
THKAFO	trunk-hip-knee-ankle-foot orthosis	TIP	toxic interstitial pneumonitis
THP	take home packs	TIPS	transjugular intrahepatic portosystemic shunt (stent)
	total hip prosthesis		
	transhepatic portography		
	trihexyphenidyl (Artane)	TIPSS	transjugular intrahepatic portosystemic shunt (stent)
THR	target heart rate		
	total hip replacement		
	training heart rate	TIS	tumor *in situ*
THTV	therapeutic home trial visit	TISS	Therapeutic Intervention Scoring System
THV	therapeutic home visit	TIT	*Treponema (pallidum)* immobilization test
TI	terminal ileus		
	thought insertion		triiodothyronine (liothyronine)
	transischial		
	transverse diameter of inlet	TIUP	term intrauterine pregnancy
	tricuspid insufficiency	TIVA	total intravenous anethesia
TIA	transient ischemic attack		
TIB	tibia	TIVC	thoracic inferior vena cava
TIBC	total iron-binding capacity		
TIC	paclitaxel (Taxol), ifosamide, and cisplain	+tive	positive
	trypsin-inhibitor capacity	TIW	three times a week (this is

	a dangerous abbreviation)	TLR	tonic labyrinthine reflex
TJ	tendon jerk	TLS	tumor lysis syndrome
	triceps jerk	TLSO	thoracic lumbar sacral orthosis
TJA	total joint arthroplasty	TLSSO	thoracolumbosacral spinal orthosis
TJN	tongue jaw neck (dissection)	TLT	tonsillectomy
	twin jet nebulizer	TLV	total lung volume
TJR	total joint replacement	TM	temperature by mouth
TK	thymidine kinase		Thayer-Martin (culture)
	toxicokinetics		trabecular meshwork
TKA	total knee arthroplasty		trademark
	tyrosine kinase activity		transcendental meditation
TKD	tokodynamometer		treadmill
TKE	terminal knee extension		tropical medicine
TKIC	true knot in cord		tumor
TKNO	to keep needle open		tympanic membrane
TKP	thermokeratoplasty	T & M	type and crossmatch
	total knee prosthesis	TMA	thrombotic microangiopathy
TKO	to keep open		transcription mediated amplification
TKR	total knee replacement		transmetatarsal amputation
TKVO	to keep vein open		
TL	team leader	T/MA	tracheostomy mask
	transverse line	TMAS	Taylor Manifest Anxiety Scale
	trial leave		
	tubal ligation	T_{max}	temperature maximum
T/L	terminal latency	t_{max}	time of occurrence for maximum (peak) drug concentration
Tl	thallium		
TLA	translumbar arteriogram (aortogram)		
TLAC	triple lumen arrow catheter	TMB	tetramethylberizidine
			transient monocular blindness
TL BLT	tubal ligation, bilateral		trimethoxybenzoates
TLC	tender loving care	TMC	transmural colitis
	thin layer chromatography		triamcinolone
	T-lymphocyte choriocarcinoma	TMCA	trimethylcolchicinic acid
	total lung capacity	TMCN	triamcinolone
	total lymphocyte count	TMD	temporomandibular dysfunction (disorder)
	triple lumen catheter		treating physician
TLD	thermoluminescent dosimeter	TME	thermolysin-like metalloendopeptidase
TLE	temporal lobe epilepsy		total mesorectal excision
TLI	total lymphoid irradiation		
	translaryngeal intubation	TMET	tread mill exercise test
TLK	thermal laser keratoplasty	TMI	threatened myocardial infarction
TLNB	term living newborn		
TLP	transitional living program		transmandibular implant

	transmural infarct		transrectal needle biopsy (of the prostate)
TMJ	temporomandibular joint		Tru-Cut® needle biopsy
TMJD	temporomandibular joint dysfunction	TNBP	transurethral needle biopsy of prostate
TMJS	temporomandibular joint syndrome	TND	term, normal delivery
TML	tongue midline treadmill	TNDM	transient neonatal diabetes mellitus
TMM	torn medial meniscus total muscle mass	TNF	tumor necrosis factor
Tmm	McKay-Marg tension	TNF-bp	tumor necrosis factor binding protein
TMNG	toxic multinodular goiter	TNG	nitroglycerin
		TNI	total nodal irradiation
TMP	thallium myocardial perfusion transmembrane pressure trimethoprim	TNM	primary tumor, regional lymph nodes, and distant metastasis (used with subscripts for the staging of cancer)
TMP/SMZ	trimethoprim and sulfamethoxazole (correct name is sulfamethoxazole and trimethoprin; SMZ-TMP)	TNS	transcutaneous nerve stimulation (stimulator) Tullie-Niebörg syndrome
		TNT	triamcinolone and nystatin
		TNTC	too numerous to count
TMR	trainable mentally retarded transmyocardial revascularization	TO	old tuberculin telephone order time off tincture of opium (warning: this is NOT paregoric) total obstruction transfer out
TMST	treadmill stress test		
TMT	tarsometatarsal teratoma with malignant transformation treadmill test tympanic membrane thermometer		
		T(O)	oral temperature
		T/O	time out
		T&O	tubes and ovaries
TMTC	too many to count	TOA	time of arrival tubo-ovarian abscess
TMTX	trimetrexate		
TM-WKTM	tender mass with known tissue malignancy	TOAA	to affected areas
		TOB	tobacco tobramycin
TMX	tamoxifen		
TMZ	temazepam temozolomide	TOC	total organic carbon
		TOCE	transcatheter oily chemoembolization
TN	normal intraocular tension team nursing temperature normal	TOCO	tocodynamometer
		TOD	intraocular pressure of the right eye time of death time of departure tubal occlusion device
T&N	tension and nervousness tingling and numbness		
TNA	total nutrient admixture		
TNB	term newborn transnasal butorphanol	TOF	tetralogy of Fallot

	time of flight		treating physician
	total of four		trigger point
	train-of-four	T:P	trough-to-peak ratio
TOGV	transposition of the great vessels	T & P	temperature and pulse turn and position
TOH	throughout hospitalization	TPA	alteplase, recombinant
TOL	tolerate trial of labor		(tissue plasminogen activator)
TOLA	temporary leave of absence		third-party administrator tissue polypeptide antigen
TOLD	Test of Language Development		total parenteral alimentation
TOM	tomorrow transcutaneous oxygen monitor	TPAL	term infant(s), premature infant(s), abortion(s), living children
Tomo	tomography	TPC	total patient care
TON	tonight	TPD	tropical pancreatic
TOP	termination of pregnancy		diabetes
	Topografov (virus) topotecan	TPE	therapeutic plasma exchange
TOPO	topotecan		total placental estrogens
TOPO 1	topoisermerase		total protective
TOPV	trivalent oral polio		environment
	vaccine	TPF	trained participating father
TOR	toremifene	TPH	thromboembolic
TORC	Test of Reading Comprehension		pulmonary hypertension trained participating
TORCH	toxoplasmosis, other (syphillis, hepatitis, zoster), rubella,cytome-	TPHA	husband *Treponema pallidum* hemagglutination
	galovirus, and herpes	T PHOS	triple phosphate crystals
	simplex (maternal infections)	TPI	*Treponema pallidum* immobilization
TORP	total ossicular replacement prosthesis	TPL T plasty	thromboplastin tympanoplasty
TOS	intraocular pressure of the	TPM	temporary pacemaker
	left eye	TPN	total parenteral nutrition
	thoracic outlet syndrome	TPO	thyroid peroxidase
TOT BILI	total bilirubin		thrombopoietin
TOV	trial of void		trial prescription order
TOWL	Test of Written Language	TPP	thiamine pyrophosphate
TP	temperature and pressure	TP & P	time, place, and person
	temporoparietal	TPPN	total peripheral parenteral
	therapeutic pass		nutrition
	thrombophlebitis	TPPV	trans pars plana
	Todd's paralysis		vitrectomy
	toilet paper	TPR	temperature
	total protein		temperature, pulse, and
	"T" piece		respiration

	total peripheral resistance		total radical-trapping
TPRI	total peripheral resistance index		antioxidant parameter
			thrombospondin-related
T PROT	total protein		anonymous protein
TPT	time to peak tension		trapezium
	transpyloric tube		trapezius muscle
	treadmill performance test	TRAS	transplant renal artery
TPU	tropical phagedenic ulcer		stenosis
T-putty	Theraputty	TRB	return to baseline
TPVR	total peripheral vascular	TRBC	total red blood cells
	resistance	TRC	tanned red cells
TQM	total quality management	TRD	tongue-retaining
TR	therapeutic recreation		device
	time to repeat		traction retinal
	tincture		detachment
	to return		treatment-resistant
	trace		depression
	transfusion reaction	TRDN	transient respiratory
	transplant recipients		distress of the newborn
	treatment	Tren	Trendelenburg
	tremor	TRH	protirelin (thyrotropin-
	tricuspid regurgitation		releasing hormone)
	tumor registry		(Relefact TRH®;
T(R)	rectal temperature		Thypinone®)
T & R	tenderness and rebound	TRI	trimester
	treated and released	T₃RIA	triiodothyronine level by
TRA	therapeutic recreation		radioimmunoassay
	associate	TRIC	trachoma inclusion
	to run at		conjunctivitis
TRAb	thyrotropin-receptor	TRICH	*Trichomonas*
	antibody	TRIG	triglycerides
TRACH	tracheal	TRISS	Trauma Related Injury
	tracheostomy		Severity Score
TRAFO	tone-reducing ankle/foot	TR-LSC	time-resolved liquid
	orthosis		scintillation counting
TRAM	transverse rectus	TRM-SMX	trimethoprim-
	abdominis		sulfamethoxazole
	myocutaneous (flap)		(correct name is
	transverse rectus		sulfamethoxazole and
	abdominum muscle		trimethoprin; SMZ-
TRAMP	transversus and rectus		TMP; SMX-TMP)
	abdominis musculo-	tRNA	transfer ribonucleic acid
	peritoneal (flap)	TRNBP	transrectal needle biopsy
Trans D	transverse diameter		prostate
TRANS	transfusion reaction	TRND	Trendelenburg
Rx		TRNG	tetracycline-resistant
TRAP	tartrate-resistant		*Neisseria gonorrhoeae*
	(leukocyte) acid	TRO	to return to office
	phophatase	TROM	total range of motion

TRP	tubular reabsorption of phosphate	TSB	total serum bilirubin trypticase soy broth
TRPT	transplant	TSBB	transtracheal selective bronchial brushing
TRS	Therapeutic Recreation Specialist the real symptom	TSC	technetium sulfur colloid theophylline serum concentration
TRT	thermoradiotherapy thoracic radiation therapy treatment-related toxicity		total symptom complex
TR/TE	time to repetition and time to echo in spin (echo sequence of magnetic resonance imaging)	TSD	target to skin distance Tay-Sachs disease
		TSDP	tapered steroid dosing package
T_3RU	triiodothyronine resin uptake	TSE	targeted systemic exposure transmissible spongiform encephalopathy
TRUS	transrectal ultrasonography	T set	tracheotomy set
TRUSP	transrectal ultrasonography of the prostate	TSE	testicular self-examination total skin examination
TRZ	triazolam	TSF	tricep skin fold
TS	Tay-Sachs (disease) temperature sensitive	TSGs	tumor suppressor genes
	test solution thoracic spine	TSH	thyroid-stimulating hormone (thyrotropin)
	toe signs Tourette's syndrome	TSH-RH	thyrotropin-releasing hormone
	transsexual	T-SKULL	trauma skull
	Trauma Score	tsp	teaspoon (5 mL)
	tricuspid stenosis triple strength	TSP	thrombospondin total serum protein tropical spastic paraparesis
	Turner's syndrome		
T/S	trimethoprim/ sulfamethoxazole (correct name is sulfamethoxazole and trimethoprin)	TSPA	thiotepa
		T-SPINE	thoracic spine
		TSR	total shoulder replacement
		TSS	total serum solids toxic shock syndrome
T&S	type and screen	TSST	toxic shock syndrome toxin
Ts	Schiotz tension T suppressor cell	TST	titmus stereocuity test trans-scrotal testosterone
TSAb	thyroid stimulating antibodies		treadmill stress test tuberculin skin test(s)
TSA	toluenesulfonic acid total shoulder arthroplasty	TSTA	tumor-specific transplantation antigens
	type-specific antibody	T&T	tobramycin and ticarcillin
TSAR®	tape surrounded Appli-rulers		touch and tone
TSAS	Total Severity Assessment Score	TT	Test Tape® tetanus toxoid thrombin time

	thrombolytic therapy		time to pregnancy
	thymol turbidity		time to tumor progression
	tilt table		time-to-progression
	tonometry	TTR	transthyretin
	total thyroidectomy		triceps tendon reflex
	transit time	TTS	tarsal tunnel syndrome
	transtracheal		temporary threshold shift
	tuberculin tested		through the skin
	twitch tension		transdermal therapeutic
	tympanic temperature		system
T/T	trace of ___ /trace of ___		transfusion therapy
T&T	tympantomy and tube		service
	(insertion)	TTT	tilt table test
TT4	total thyroxine		tolbutamide tolerance test
TTA	total toe arthroplasty		total tourniquet time
TTAT	toe touch as tolerated		turn-to-turn transfusion
TTC	transtracheal catheter	TTUTD	tetanus toxoid up-to-date
TTD	tarsal tunnel	TTVP	temporary transvenous
	decompression		pacemaker
	temporary total disability	TTWB	touch toe weight bearing
	transverse thoracic	TTx	thrombolytic therapy
	diameter	TU	Todd units
TTDM	thallim threadmill		transrectal ultrasound
TTE	transthoracic		transurethral
	echocardiography		tuberculin units
TTF	time to treatment failure	1-TU	1 tuberculin unit
TTI	Teflon tube insertion	5-TU	5 tuberculin units
	transfer to intermediate	250-TU	250 tuberculin units
TTII	thyrotropin-binding	TUE	transurethral extraction
	inhibitory	TUF	total ultrafiltration
	immunoglobulins	TUIBN	transurethral incision of
TTJV	transtracheal jet		bladder neck
	ventilation	TUIP	transurethral incision of
TTM	total tumor mass		the prostate
TTN	transient tachypnea of the	TULIP®	transurethral
	newborn		ultrasound-guided
TTNA	transthoracic needle		laser-induced
	aspiration		prostatectomy (system)
TTNB	transient tachypnea of the	TUMT	transurethral microwave
	newborn		therapy
TTO	time trade-off	TUN	total urinary nitrogen
	to take out	TUNA	transurethral needle
	transfer to open		ablation
	transtracheal oxygen	TUPR	transurethral prostatic
TTOD	tetanus toxoid outdated		resection
TTOT	transtracheal oxygen	TUR	transurethral resection
	therapy	T₃UR	triiodothyronine uptake
TTP	thrombotic thrombocy-		ratio
	topenic purpura	TURB	turbidity

TURBN	transurethral resection bladder neck		TWA	time-weighted average
			TWAR	*Chlamydia psittaci*
TURBT	transurethral resection bladder tumor		T wave	part of the electrocardiographic cycle, representing a portion of ventricular repolarization
TURP	transurethral resection of prostate			
TURV	transurethral resection valves		TWD	total white and differential count
TURVN	transurethral resection of vesical neck		TWE	tapwater enema
			TWETC	tapwater enema 'til clear
TUU	transureteroureterostomy		TWG	total weight gain
TUV	transurethral valve		TWH	transitional wall hyperplasia
TV	television			
	temporary visit		TWHW ok	toe walking and heel walking all right
	tidal volume			
	transvenous		TWI	T-wave inversion
	trial visit		TWR	total wrist replacement
	Trichomonas vaginalis		T1WT	T1 weighted image
	tricuspid value		TWWD	tap water wet dressing
T/V	touch-verbal		Tx	therapy
TVC	triple voiding cystogram			traction
	true vocal cord			transcription
TVc	tricuspid valve closure			transfuse
TVD	triple vessel disease			transplant
TVDALV	triple vessel disease with an abnormal left ventricle			transplantation
				treatment
				tympanostomy
TVF	tactile vocal fremitus		T & X	type and crossmatch
TVH	total vaginal hysterectomy		TXA_2	thromboxane A_2
TVN	tonic vibration response		TXB_2	thromboxane B_2
TVP	tensor veli palatini (muscle)		TXE	Timoptic-XE®
			TXL	paclitaxel (Taxol) (this is a dangerous abbreviation as it can be read as TXT)
	transvenous pacemaker			
	transvesicle prostatectomy			
TVR	tricuspid valve replacement		TXM	type and crossmatch
			TXS	type and screen
TVS	transvaginal sonography		TXT	docetaxel (Taxotere) (this is a dangerous abbreviation as it can be read as TXL)
TVSC	transvaginal sector scan			
TVU	total volume of urine			
TVUS	transvaginal ultrasound			
TW	tapwater		TYCO #3	Tylenol® with 30 mg of codeine (#1=7.5 mg, #2=15 mg and #4=60 mg of codeine present)
	test weight			
	thought withdrawal			
	T-wave			
TW2	Tanner-Whitehouse mark 2 (bone-age assessment)		Tyl	Tylenol®
				tyloma (callus)
5TW	five times a week (this is a dangerous abbreviation)		TYMP	tympanogram

TZ	temozolomide
	transition zone
TZD	thiazolidinedione

U

U	Ultralente Insulin®
	units (this is the most dangerous abbreviation —spell out "unit")
	unknown
	upper
	urine
Ⓤ	Kosher
U/1	1 finger breadth below umbilicus
1/U	1 finger over umbilicus
U/	at umbilicus
U100	100 units per milliliters
UA	umbilical artery
	unauthorized absence
	uncertain about
	unstable angina
	upper airway
	upper arm
	uric acid
	urinalysis
UAC	umbilical artery catheter
	under active
	upper airway congestion
UA/C	uric acid to creatinine (ratio)
UAD	upper airway disease
UAE	urinary albumin excretion
UAL	umbilical artery line
	up *ad lib*
UA&M	urinalysis and microscopy
UAO	upper airway obstruction
UAPF	upon arrival patient found
UAS	upstream activating sequence

UASA	upper airway sleep apnea
UAT	up as tolerated
UAVC	univentricular atrioventricular connection
UBC	University of British Columbia (brace)
UBD	universal blood donor
UBF	unknown black female
	uterine blood flow
UBI	ultraviolet blood irradiation
UBM	unknown black male
UBO	unidentified bright object
UBW	usual body weight
UC	ulcerative colitis
	umbilical cord
	unchanged
	unconscious
	Unit clerk
	United Church of Christ
	urea clearance
	urinary catheter
	urine culture
	usual care
	uterine contraction
U&C	urethral and cervical
	usual and customary
UCB	umbilical cord blood
UCD	urine collection device
	usual childhood diseases
UCE	urea cycle enzymopathy
UCG	urinary chorionic gonadotropins
UCHD	usual childhood diseases
UCHI	usual childhood illnesses
UCHS	uncontrolled hemorrhagic shock
UCI	urethral catheter in
	usual childhood illnesses
UCL	uncomfortable loudness level
UCLP	unilateral cleft lip and palate
UCO	urethral catheter out
UCP	urethral closure pressure
UCR	unconditioned response
	usual, customary, and reasonable

UCRE	urine creatinine	UG	until gone
UCRP	universal coagulation reference plasma		urinary glucose urogenital
UCS	unconscious	UGA	under general anesthesia
UC&S	urine culture and sensitivity		urogenital atrophy
UCX	urine culture	UGCR	ultrasound-guided compression repair
UD	as directed	UGDP	University Group Diabetes Project
	ulnar deviation urethral dilatation	UGH	uveitis, glaucoma, and hyphema (syndrome)
	urethral discharge urodynamics	UGI	upper gastrointestinal series
	uterine distension	UGIH	upper gastrointestinal (tract) hemorrhage
UDC	uninhibited detrusor (muscle) capacity	UGIS	upper gastrointestinal series
	usual diseases of childhood	UGIT	upper gastrointestinal tract
UDCA	ursodeoxycholic acid	UGI	upper gastrointestinal
UDN	updraft nebulizer	w/SBFT	(series) with small
UDO	undetermined origin		bowel follow through
UDP	unassisted diastolic pressure	UGK	urine, glucose, and ketones
UDPGT	uridinediphospho-glucuronyl transferase	UGP	urinary gonadotropin peptide
UDS	unconditioned stimulus	UH	umbilical hernia
UDT	undescended testicle(s)		unfavorable history University Hospital
UE	under elbow undetermined etiology	UHBI	upper hemibody irradiation
	upper extremity	UHDDS	Uniform Hospital Discharge Data Set
UES	undifferentiated embryonal sarcoma	UHP	University Health Plan
	upper esophageal sphincter	UI	urinary incontinence
UESP	upper esophageal sphincter pressure	UIB	Unemployment Insurance Benefits
UF	ultrafiltration until finished	UIBC	unbound iron binding capacity
UFC	urine-free cortisol		unsaturated iron binding capacity
UFF	unusual facial features	UID	once daily (this is a dangerous abbreviation, spell out "once daily")
UFFI	urea formaldehyde foam insulation		
UFH	unfractionated heparin		
UFN	until further notice		
UFO	unflagged order unidentified foreign object	UIEP	urine (urinary) immunoelectrophoresis
UFOV	useful field of view	UIP	usual interstitial pneumonitis
UFR	ultrafiltration rate		
UFT	uracil and futrafur	UIQ	upper inner quadrant
UFV	ultrafiltration volume	UJ	universal joint (syndrome)

UK	United Kingdom		undetermined origin
	unknown		ureteral orifice
	urine potassium		urinary output
	urokinase	UOP	urinary output
UK IC	urokinase intracoronary	UOQ	upper outer quadrant
UKO	unknown origin	Uosm	urinary osmolality
UL	Unit Leader	✔ up	check up
	upper left	UP	unipolar
	upper lid		ureteropelvic
	upper limb	U/P	urine to plasma
	upper lobe		(creatinine)
U/L	upper and lower	UPC	unknown primary
U & L	upper and lower		carcinoma
ULLE	upper lid, left eye	UPDRS	Unified Parkinson's
ULN	upper limits of normal		Disease Rating Scale
ULPA	ultra-low particulate air	UPEP	urine protein
ULQ	upper left quadrant		electrophoresis
ULRE	upper lid, right eye	UPG	uroporphyrinogen
ULSB	upper left sternal border	UPIN	unique physician
ULYTES	electrolytes, urine		identification number
UM	unmarried	UPJ	ureteropelvic junction
Umb A Line	umbilical artery line	UPLIF	unilateral posterior lumbar
			interbody fusion
Umb V Line	umbilical venous line	UPO	metastatic carcinoma of
			unknown primary
umb ven	umbilical vein		origin
UMCD	uremic medullary cystic	UPOR	usual place of residence
	disease	UPP	urethral pressure profile
UMN	upper motor neuron	UPPP	uvulopalatopharyngo-
	(disease)		plasty
UN	undernourished	U/P ratio	urine to plasma ratio
	urinary nitrogen	UPSC	uterine papillary serous
UNA	urinary nitrogen		carcinoma
	appearance	UPT	uptake
UNa	urine sodium		urine pregnancy test
unacc	unaccompanied	UR	unrelated
UNC	uncrossed		upper respiratory
UNDEL	undelivered		upper right
UNG	ointment		urinary retention
UNK	unknown		utilization review
UNL	upper normal levels	UR AC	uric acid
UNOS	United Network for	URD	undifferentiated
	Organ Sharing		respiratory disease
UN/P	unpatched eye	URG	urgent
UN/P OD	unpatched right eye	URI	upper respiratory infection
UN/P OS	unpatched left eye	URIC A	uric acid
UNS	unsatisfactory	url	unrelated
UNSAT	unsatisfactory	UR&M	urinalysis, routine and
UO	under observation		microscopic

URO	urology		up to date
UROL	Urologist	*ut dict*	as directed
	urology	UTF	usual throat flora
UROB	urobilinogen	UTI	urinary tract infection
URQ	upper right quadrant	UTL	unable to locate
URS	ureterorenoscopy	UTM	urinary-tract
URSB	upper right sternal border		malformations
URT	uterine resting tone	UTMDACC	University of Texas M.D.
URTI	upper respiratory tract		Anderson Cancer
	infection		Center
US	ultrasonography	UTO	unable to obtain
	unit secretary		upper tibial osteotomy
USA	unit services assistant	UTS	ulnar tunnel syndrome
	United States Army		ultrasound
	unstable angina	UUD	uncontrolled unsterile
USAF	United States Air Force		delivery
USAN	United States Adopted	UUN	urinary urea nitrogen
	Names	UV	ultraviolet
USAP	unstable angina pectoris		ureterovesical
USB	upper sternal border		urine volume
U-SCOPE	ureteroscopy	UVA	ultraviolet A light
USCVD	unsterile controlled		ureterovesical angle
	vaginal delivery	UVB	ultraviolet B light
USDA	United States Department	UVC	umbilical vein catheter
	of Agriculture	UVH	univentricular heart
USG	ultrasonography	UVJ	ureterovesical junction
USH	United Services for	UVL	ultraviolet light
	Handicapped		umbilical venous line
	usual state of health	UVR	ultraviolet radiation
USI	urinary stress	UVT	unsustained ventricular
	incontinence		tachycardia
USM	ultrasonic mist	U/WB	unit of whole blood
USMC	United States Marine	UW	unilateral weakness
	Corps	UWF	unknown white female
USN	ultrasonic nebulizer	UWM	unknown white male
	United States Navy		unwed mother
USOGH	usual state of good health		
USOH	usual state of health		
USP	unassisted systolic		
	pressure		
	United States		
	Pharmacopeia		**V**
USPHS	United States Public		
	Health Service		
USUCVD	unsterile uncontrolled		
	vaginal delivery		
USVMD	urine specimen volume	V	five
	measuring device		gas volume
UTD	unable to determine		minute volume

	vaccinated	VAD	vascular (venous) access device
	vagina		
	vein		ventricular assist device
	ventricular		Veterans Administration Domiciliary
	verb		
	verbal		vincristine, doxorubicin (Adriamycin), and dexamethasone
	vertebral		
	very		
	viral	VaD	vascular dementia
	vitamin	VADCS	ventricular atrial distal coronary sinus
	vomiting		
$\dot{V}$	ventilation (L/min)	VADRIAC	vincristine, doxorubicin (Adriamycin), and cyclophosphamide
+V	positive vertical divergence		
V1	fifth cranial nerve, ophthalmic division		
		VAERS	Vaccine Adverse Events Reporting System
V2	fifth cranial nerve, maxillary division	VAG	vagina
V3	fifth cranial nerve, mandibular division	VAG HYST	vaginal hysterectomy
V_1 to V_6	precordial chest leads	VAH	Veterans Administration Hospital
VA	vacuum aspiration		
	valproic acid	VAHBE	ventricular atrial His bundle electrocardiogram
	Veterans Administration		
	visual acuity	VAHRA	ventricular atrial height right atrium
V_A	alveolar gas volume		
V&A	vagotomy and antrectomy	VAIN	vaginal intraepithelial neoplasia
VAB	vinblastine, dactinomycin (actinomycin D), bleomycin		
		VALE	visual acuity, left eye
VAC	ventriculo-arterial connections	VAMC	Veterans Affairs Medical Center
	vincristine, dactinomycin (actinomycin D), and cyclophosphamide	VAMP®	venous arterial management protection system
		VAMS	Visual Analogue Mood Scale
	vincristine, doxorubicin (Adriamycin), and cyclophosphamide	VANCO/P	vancomycin-peak
		VANCO/T	vancomycin-trough
VA cc	distance visual acuity with correction	VAOD	visual acuity, right eye
		VAOS	visual acuity, left eye
VA ccl	near visual acuity with correction	VA OS LP with P	visual acuity, left eye, left perception with projection
VAC EXT	vacuum extractor		
VACO	Veterans Administration Central Office	VAP	ventilator-associated pneumonia
			venous access port
VACTERL	vertebral, anal, cardiac, tracheal, esophageal, renal, and limb anomalies		vincristine, asparaginase, and prednisone
		VAPCS	ventricular atrial proximal coronary sinus

VAPP	vaccine-associated paralytic poliomyelitis	VBD	vinblastine, bleomycin, and cisplatin
VAR	variant	VBG	venous blood gas
VARE	visual acuity, right eye		vertical banded gastroplasty
VAS	vasectomy	VBGP	vertical banded gastroplasty
	vascular		
	Visual Analogue Scale (Score)	VBI	vertebrobasilar insufficiency
VASC	Visual-Auditory Screen Test for Children	VBL	vinblastine
VA sc	distance visual acuity without correction	VBP	vinblastine, bleomycin, and cisplatin
VA scl	near visual acuity without correction	VBS	vertebral-basilar system
		VC	color vision
VASPI	Visual Analogue Self Assessment Scales For Pain Intensity		etoposide and carboplatin
			pulmonary capillary blood volume
VAS RAD	vascular radiology		vena cava
VAT	video-assist thoracoscopy		verbal cues
VATER	vertebral, anal, tracheal, esophageal, and renal anomalies		vincristine
			vital capacity
			vocal cords
VATH	vinblastine, doxorubicin (Adriamycin), thiotepa, and fluoxymesterone (Halotestin)	V&C	vertical and centric (a bite)
		VCA	vasoconstrictor assay
		VCAM	vascular cell adhesion molecule
VATS	video assisted thoracic surgery	VCAP	vincristine, cyclophospha-mide, doxorubicin (Adriamycin), and prednisone
VB	Van Buren (catheter)		
	venous blood		
	vinblastine		
	vinblastine and bleomycin	Vcc	vision with correction
VB_1	first voided bladder specimen	VCCA	velocity common carotid artery
VB_2	second midstream bladder specimen	VCD	vocal cord dysfunction
		VCG	vectorcardiography
VB_3	voided bladder specimen after expression of prostatic secretions		voiding cystogram
		VCO	ventilator CPAP oxyhood
		VCR	video cassette recorder
VBAC	vaginal birth after cesarean		vincristine sulfate
		VCT	venous clotting time
VBAI	vertebrobasilar artery insufficiency	VCTS	vitreal corneal touch syndrome
VBAP	vincristine, carmustine, doxorubicin (Adriamycin), and prednisone	VCU	voiding cystourethrogram
		VCUG	vesicoureterogram
			voiding cystourethrogram
VBC	vinblastine, bleomycin, and cisplatin	VD	venereal disease
			viral diarrhea
			voided

	volume of distribution	V/E	violence and eloper
V_D	deadspace volume	VEA	ventricular ectopic activity
V_d	volume of distribution		viscoelastic agent
V&D	vomiting and diarrhea	VEB	ventricular ectopic beat
VDA	venous digital angiogram	VEC	vecuronium
	visual discriminatory acuity		velocity-encoded cine
VDAC	vaginal delivery after cesarean	VECG	vector electrocardiogram
VDD	atrial synchronous ventricular inhibited pacing	VED	vacuum erection device vacuum extraction delivery ventricular ectopic depolarization
VDDR I	vitamin D dependency rickets type I	VEE	Venezuelan equine encephalitis
VDDR II	vitamin D dependency rickets type II	VEF	visually evoked field
VDG	venereal disease–gon- orrhea	VEG VEGF	vegetation (bacterial) vascular endothelial growth factor
Vdg	voiding	VENT	ventilation
VDH	valvular disease of the heart		ventilator ventral ventricular
VDJ	variable diversity joining		
VDL	vasodepressor lipid visual detection level	VEP	visual evoked potential
VDO	varus derotational osteotomy	VER	ventricular escape rhythm visual evoked responses
VD or M	venous distention or masses	VES VET	ventricular extrasystoles veteran
VDP	vinblastine, dacarbazine, and cisplatin (Platinol)	VF	Veterinarian veterinary left leg (electrode)
VDRF	ventilator dependent respiratory failure		ventricular fibrillation visual field
VDRL	Venereal Disease Research Laboratory (test for syphilis)	VFC	vocal fremitus Vaccines for Children (program)
VDRR	vitamin D-resistant rickets	VFD	visual fields
VDS	vasodepressor syncope venereal disease—syphilis vindesine	VFFC	visual fields full to confrontation
VDT	video display terminal	VFI	visual fields intact Visual Functioning index
VD/VT	dead space to tidal volume ratio	V. Fib	ventricular fibrillation
VE	vaginal examination	VFP	vitreous fluorophotometry
	vertex	VFPN	Volu-feed premie nipple
	Vietnam era	VFRN	Volu-feed regular nipple
	visual examination	VFT	venous filling time
	vitamin E vocational evaluation		ventricular fibrillation threshold
V_E	minute volume (expired)	VG	vein graft

	ventricular gallop		vasoactive intracorporeal
	ventrogluteal		pharmacotherapy
	very good		very important patient
V&G	vagotomy and		vinblastine, ifosfamide,
	gastroenterotomy		and cisplatin (Platinol)
VGAD	vein of Galen aneurysmal		voluntary interruption of
	dilatation		pregnancy
VGAM	vein of Galen aneurysmal	VIPomas	vasoactive intestinal
	malformation		peptide-secreting
VGH	very good health		tumors
VH	vaginal hysterectomy	VIQ	Verbal Intelligence
	Veterans Hospital		Quotient (part of
	viral hepatitis		Wechsler tests)
	vitreous hemorrhage	VIS	Visual Impairment
	von Herrick (grading		Service
	system)	VISC	vitreous infusion suction
VH I	very narrow anterior		cutter
	chamber angles	VISI	volar intercalated
VH II	moderately narrow		segmental instability
	anterior chamber angles	VIT	venom immunotherapy
VH III	moderately wide open		vital
	anterior chamber angles		vitamin
VH IV	wide open anterior	VIT CAP	vital capacity
	chamber angles	VIU	visual internal
VHD	valvular heart disease		urethrotomy
VHL	von Hippel-Lindau	*VIZ*	namely
	disease (complex)	V-J	ventriculo-jugular (shunt)
VI	six	VKC	vernal keratoconjunctivitis
	volume index	VKDB	vitamin K deficiency
via	by way of		bleeding
vib	vibration	VKH	Vogt-Koyanagi-Harada's
VIBS	Victim's Information		disease
	Bureau Service	VL	left arm (electrode)
VICA	velocity internal carotid		vial
	artery	VLA	very-late antigen
VICP	Vaccine Injury	V-LAP	video laser ablation of
	Compensation Program		prostate
VID	videodensitometry	VLBW	very low birth weight
VIG	vaccinia immune globulin		(less than 1500 g)
VIH	Spanish and French	VLCD	very low calorie diet
	abbreviation for human	VLCFA	very long chain fatty
	immunodeficiency virus		acids
VIN	vulvar intraepithelial	VLDL	very low density
	neoplasm		lipoprotein
VIP	etopside (VePesid),	VLE	vision left eye
	ifosfamide, and	VLH	ventrolateral nucleus of
	cisplatin (Platinol)		the hypothalamus
	vasoactive intestinal	VLM	visceral larva migrans
	peptide	VLP	virus-like particle

VLR	vastus lateralis release		variegate porphyria
VM	ventilated mask		venipuncture
	ventimask		venous pressure
	Venturi mask		ventriculo-peritoneal
	vestibular membrane		visual perception
VM 26	teniposide	V & P	vagotomy and
VMA	vanillylmandelic acid		pyloroplasty
VMCP	vincristine, melphalan,		ventilation and perfusion
	cyclophosphamide, and	VP-16	etoposide
	prednisone	VPA	valproic acid
VMD	vertical maxillary		ventricular premature
	deficiency		activation
VME	vertical maxillary excess	V-Pad	sanitary napkin
VMH	ventromedial	VPB	ventricular premature beat
	hypothalamus	VPC	ventricular premature
VMO	vastus medalis oblique		contractions
VMR	vasomotor rhinitis	VPD	ventricular premature
VMS	vanilla milkshake		depolarization
VN	visiting nurse	VPDF	vegetable protein diet plus
VNA	Visiting Nurses'		fiber
	Association	VPDs	ventricular premature
VNB	vinorelbine		depolarizations
VNC	vesicle neck contracture	VPI	velopharyngeal
VNTR	variable number of		incompetence
	tandem repeat(s)		velopharyngeal
VO	verbal order		insufficiency
VO$_2$	oxygen consumption	VPL	ventro-posterolateral
VOCAB	vocabulary	VPLS	ventilation-perfusion lung
VOCOR	void on-call to operating		scan
	room	VPM	venous pressure module
VOCTOR	void on-call to operating	VPR	volume pressure response
	room	VPS	valvular pulmonic
VOD	veno-occlusive disease		stenosis
	vision right eye	VPT	vascularized patellar
VOE	vascular occlusive episode		tendon
VO$_2$I	oxygen consumption index	VQ	ventilation perfusion
VOL	volume	VR	right arm (electrode)
	voluntary		valve replacement
VOM	vomited		venous resistance
VOO	continuous ventricular		ventricular rhythm
	asynchronous pacing		verbal reprimand
VOR	vestibular ocular reflex		vocational rehabilitation
VOS	vision left eye	VRA	visual reinforcement
VOSS	visual observation		audiometry
	shivering score		visual response
VOT	Visual Organization Test		audiometry
VOU	vision both eyes	VRB	vinorelbine (Navelbine)
VP	etoposide (VePesid) and	VRC	vocational rehabilitation
	cisplatin (Platinol)		counselor

VRE	vancomycin-resistant enterococci	v. tach.	ventricular tachycardia
	vision right eye	VTE	venous thromboembolism
VRI	viral respiratory infection	VTEC	verotoxin-producing *Escherichia coli*
VRL	ventral root, lumbar		
VRP	vocational rehabilitation program	VT-NS	ventricular tachycardia non-sustained
VRSA	vancomycin-resistant *Staphylococcus aureus*	VTOP	voluntary termination of pregnancy
VRT	variance of resident time	VTP	voluntary termination of pregnancy
	ventral root, thoracic	VT-S	ventricular tachycardia sustained
	vertical radiation topography	VT/VF	ventricular tachycardia/fibrillation
	Visual Retention Test		
	vocational rehabilitation therapy	VTX	vertex
		V/U	verbalize understanding
VRTA	Vocational Rehabilitation Therapy Assistant	VUJ	vesico ureteral junction
		VUR	vesicoureteric reflux
VRU	ventilator rehabilitation unit	VV	varicose veins
		V-V	ventriculovenous (shunt)
VS	vagal stimulation	V&V	vulva and vagina
	versus *(vs)*	V/V	volume to volume ratio
	very sensitive	VVC	vulvovaginal candidiasis
	visit	VVD	vaginal vertex delivery
	visited	VVETP	Vietnam Veterans Evaluation and Treatment Program
	vital signs (temperature, pulse, and respiration)		
VSADP	vocational skills assessment and development program	VVFR	vesicovaginal fistula repair
		V/VI	grade 5 on a 6 grade basis
VSBE	very short below elbow (cast)	VVI	ventricular demand pacing
VSD	ventricular septal defect	VVOR	visual-vestibulo-ocular-reflex
VSI	visual motor integration		
VSMC	vascular smooth muscle cell	VVR	ventricular response rate
		VVT	ventricular synchronous pacing
VSN	vital signs normal		
VSO	vertical subcondylar oblique	VW	vessel wall
		VWD	ventral wall defect
VSOK	vital signs normal		von Willebrand disease
VSR	venous stasis retinopathy	vWF	von Willebrand factor
VSS	vital signs stable	VWM	ventricular wall motion
V_{ss}	apparent volume of distribution	V_x	vitrectomy
		V-XT	V-pattern exotropia
VSSAF	vital signs stable, afebrile	VY	surgical replacement flap
VSV	vesicular stomatitis virus	VZ	varicella zoster
VT	validation therapy	VZIG	varicella zoster immune globulin
	ventricular tachycardia		
V_t	tidal volume	VZV	varicella zoster virus

W

W	wash
	wearing glasses
	week
	weight
	well
	white
	widowed
	wife
	with
	work
W-1	insignificant (allergies)
W-3	minimal (allergies)
W-5	moderate (allergies)
W-7	moderate-severe (allergies)
W-9	severe (allergies)
WA	when awake
	while awake
	wide awake
	with assistance
W or A	weakness or atrophy
WAF	weakness, atrophy, and fasciculation
	white adult female
WAGR	Wilms' tumor, aniridia, genitourinary malformations, and mental retardation (syndrome)
WAIS	Wechsler Adult Intelligence Scale
WAIS-R	Wechsler Adult Intelligence Scale-Revised
WAM	white adult male
WAP	wandering atrial pacemaker
WARI	wheezing associated respiratory infection
WAS	whiplash-associated disorders
	Wiskott-Aldrich syndrome
WASO	wakefulness after sleep onset
WASS	Wasserman test
WAT	word association test
WB	waist belt
	weight bearing
	well baby
	Western blot
	whole blood
WBACT	whole blood activated clotting time
WBAT	weight bearing as tolerated
WBC	weight bearing with crutches
	well baby clinic
	white blood cell (count)
WBCT	whole blood clotting time
WBD	weeks by dates (for gestational age)
WBE	weeks by examination (for gestational age)
WBH	whole-body hyperthermia
W Bld	whole blood
WBN	wellborn nursery
WBOS	wide base of support
WBPTT	whole blood partial thromboplastin time
WBQC	wide base quad cane
WBR	whole body radiation
WBRT	whole brain radiotherapy
WBS	weeks by size (for gestational age)
	whole body scan
WBTF	Waring Blender tube feeding
WBTT	weight bearing to tolerance
WBUS	weeks by ultrasound
WBV	whole blood volume
WC	ward clerk
	ward confinement
	warm compress
	wet compresses
	wheelchair
	when called
	white count
	whooping cough
	will call
	worker's compensation
WCA	work capacity assessment

WCC	well child care	WEUP	willful exposure to unwanted pregnancy
	white cell count	WF	wet film
WCE	white coat effect		white female
WCH	white coat hypertension	W/F	weakness and fatigue
WC/LC	warm compresses and lid scrubs	WFE	Williams flexion exercises
WCM	whole cow's milk	W FEEDS	with feedings
WCS	work capacity specialist	WFH	white-faced hornet
WD	ward	WFI	water for injection
	well developed	WFL	within full limits
	well differentiated		within functional limits
	wet dressing	WF-O	will follow in office
	Wilson's disease	WFR	wheel-and-flare reaction
	word	WG	Wegener's granulomatosis
	working distance	WH	walking heel (cast)
	wound		well healed
W/D	warm and dry		well hydrated
	withdrawal	WHA	warmed humidified air
W → D	wet to dry	WHNR	well healed, no residuals
W4D	Worth four-dot (test for fusion)	WHNS	well healed, no sequelae
WDCC	well-developed collateral circulation		well healed, nonsymptomatic
WDF	white divorced female		well healed, no sequelae
WDHA	watery diarrhea, hypokalemia, and achlorhydria	WHO	World Health Organization
			wrist-hand orthosis
WDHH	watery diarrhea, hypokalemia, and hypochlorhydria	WHOART	World Health Organization Adverse Reaction Terms (Terminology)
WDLL	well-differentiated lymphocytic lymphoma	WHPB	whirlpool bath
WDM	white divorced male	WHR	ratio of waist to hip circumference
WDS	word discrimination score	WHV	woodchuck hepatitis virus
WDWN-BM	well-developed, well-nourished black male	WHVP	wedged hepatic venous pressure
		WHZ	wheezes
WDWN-WF	well-developed, well-nourished white female	WI	ventricular demand pacing
			walk-in
WE	weekend	W/I	within
W/E	weekend	W+I	work and interest
WEE	Western equine encephalitis	WIA	wounded in action
		WIC	Women, Infants, and Children (program)
WEP	weekend pass	WID	widow
WESR	Westergren erythrocyte sedimentation rate		widower
		WIED	walk-in emergency department
	Wintrobe erythrocyte sedimentation rate	WIS	Ward Incapacity Scale

WISC	Wechsler Intelligence Scale for Children	W/O	water in oil
			without
WISC-R	Wechsler Intelligence Scale for Children-Revised	WOB	work of breathing
		WOP	without pain
		WP	whirlpool
WK	week	WPBT	whirlpool, body temperature
	work		
WKI	Wakefield Inventory	WPCs	washed packed cells
WKS	Wernicke-Korsakoff Syndrome	WPFM	Wright peak flow meter
		WPOA	wearing patch on arrival
WL	waiting list	WPP	Wechsler Preschool Primary Scale of Intelligence
	wave length		
	weight loss		
WLE	wide local excision	WPPSI	Wechsler Preschool Primary Scale of Intelligence
WLM	working level months		
WLS	wet lung syndrome		
WLT	waterload test	WPPSI-R	WPPSI revised
WM	wall motion	WPW	Wolff-Parkinson-White (syndrome)
	warm, moist		
	wet mount	WR	Wassermann reaction
	white male		wrist
	whole milk	WRA	with-the-rule astigmatism
WMA	wall motion abnormality	WRAT	Wide Range Achievement Test
WMD	warm moist dressings (sterile)	WRAT-R	The Wide Range Achievement Test, Revised
WMF	white married female		
WMI	wall motion index	WRBC	washed red blood cells
WML	white matter lesions (cerebral)	WRC	washed red (blood) cells
		WRIOT	Wide Range Interest-Opinion Test (for career planning)
WMM	white married male		
WMP	warm moist packs (unsterile)	WS	ward secretary
			watt seconds
	weight management program		Williams syndrome
WMS	Wechsler Memory Scale		work simplification
WMX	whirlpool, massage, and exercise		work simulation
			work status
WN	well nourished	W&S	wound and skin
WND	wound	WSepF	white separated female
WNF	well-nourished female	WSepM	white separated male
WNL	within normal limits	WSF	white single female
WNM	well-nourished male	WSM	white single male
WNLS	weighted nonlinear least squares	WSP	wearable speech processor
		WT	walking tank
WNt50	Wagner-Nelson time 50 hours		weight (wt)
			Wilms' tumor
WO	weeks old		wisdom teeth
	wide open	0WT	zero work tolerance
	written order		

W-T-D	wet to dry		XC	excretory cystogram
WTP	willingness to pay		XD	times daily
WTS	whole tomography slice		X&D	examination and diagnosis
W/U	workup		X2d	times two days
WV	whispered voice		XDP	xeroderma pigmentosum
W/V	weight-to-volume ratio		Xe	xenon
WW	Weight Watchers		^{133}Xe	xenon, isotope of mass 133
	wheeled walker		XeCT	xenon-enhanced computed tomography
WWI	World War One			
WWII	World War Two		X-ed	crossed
W/W	weight-to-weight ratio		XES	x-ray energy spectrometer
W → W	wet to wet		XFER	transfer
WWAC	walk with aid of cane		XGP	xanthogranulomatous pyelonephritis
WW Brd	whole wheat bread			
WWidF	white widowed female		XI	eleven
WWidM	white widowed male		XII	twelve
WWW	World Wide Web		XIP	x-ray in plaster
WYOU	women years of usage		XKO	not knocked out
			XL	extended release (once a day oral solid dosage form)
				extra large
				forty

X

			XLA	X-linked infantile agammaglobulinemia
			X-leg	cross leg
X	break		XLFDP	cross-linked fibrin degradation products
	cross			
	crossmatch		XLH	X-linked hypophos-phatemia
	except			
	exophoria for distance		XLJR	X-linked juvenile retinoschisis
	extra			
	female sex chromosome		XLMR	X-linked mental retardation
	start of anesthesia			
	ten		XM	crossmatch
	times		X-mat.	crossmatch
	xylocaine		XMM	xeromammography
X′	exophoria at 33 cm		XNA	xenoreactive natural antibodies
X^2	chi-square			
X+#	xyphoid plus number of fingerbreadths		XOM	extraocular movements
			XOP	x-ray out of plaster
$\bar{x}$	mean		XP	xeroderma pigmentosum
X3	orientation as to time, place and person		XR	x-ray
			XRT	radiation therapy
			XS	excessive
XBT	xylose breath test		X-SCID	X-linked severe combined immunodeficiency disease

XS-LIM	exceeds limits of procedure		Obsessive-Compulsive Scale
XT	exotropia	Yel	yellow
	extract	YF	yellow fever
	extracted	YFH	yellow-faced hornet
X(T')	intermittent exotropia at 33 cm	YFI	yellow fever immunization
X(T)	intermittent exotropia	YJV	yellow jacket venom
XU	excretory urogram	YLC	youngest living child
XULN	times upper limit of normal	YMC	young male Caucasian
		Y/N	yes/no
XV	fifteen	YO	years old
3X/WK	three times a week	YOB	year of birth
XX	normal female sex chromosome type	YOD	year of death
	twenty	YORA	younger-onset rheumatoid arthritis
XX/XY	sex karyotypes	YPC	YAG (yttrium aluminum garnet) posterior capsulotomy
XXX	thirty		
XY	normal male sex chromosome type		
XYL	Xylocaine®	YPLL	years of potential life lost before age 65
	xylose	yr	year
XYLO	Xylocaine®	YSC	yolk sac carcinoma
		YTD	year to date
		YTDY	yesterday

Y

Z

Y	male sex chromosome		
	year	Z	impedance
	yellow	ZDV	zidovudine
YAC	yeast artificial chromosome	Z-E	Zollinger-Ellison (syndrome)
YACs	yeast artificial chromosomes	ZEEP	zero end-expiratory pressure
YACP	young adult chronic patient	ZES	Zollinger-Ellison syndrome
YAG	yttrium aluminum garnet (laser)	Z-ESR	zeta erythrocyte sedimentation rate
YAS	youth action section (police)	ZIFT	zygote intrafallopian (tube) transfer
Yb	ytterbium	ZIG	zoster serum immune globulin
YBOCS	Yale-Brown		

ZIP	zoster immune plasma	z-Plasty	surgical relaxation of contracture
ZMC	zygomatic		
	zygomatic maxillary compound (complex)	ZPO	zinc peroxide
		ZPP	zinc protoporphyrin
Zn	zinc	ZPT	zinc pyrithione
ZnO	zinc oxide	ZSB	zero stools since birth
ZnOE	zinc oxide and eugenol	ZSR	zeta sedimentation rate
ZNS	zonisamide		
ZPC	zero point of charge		
	zopiclone		

Chapter 4

Symbols and Numbers

↑	above alive elevated greater than high improved increase rising up	⇓	flexor plantar response (Babinski) testes descended
		⇑	extensor extensor response (positive Babinsky) testes undescended
↑g	increasing	‖	parallel parallel bars
↓	dead decrease depressed down falling lowered normal plantar reflex restricted	√	check flexion
		#	fracture number pound weight
		∴	therefore
↓g	decreasing	∵	because
→	causes to greater than progressing results in showed to the right transfer to	Δ scan	delta scan (computed tomography scan)
		+	plus positive present
		−	absent minus negative
←	less than resulted from to the left	/	slash mark signifying per, and, or with (this is a dangerous
↔	same as stable to and from unchanging		symbol as it is mistaken for a one)

Symbol	Meaning	Symbol	Meaning
±	either positive or negative	⊖	bone conduction threshold
	no definite cause		reversible
	plus or minus	?	questionable
	very slight trace		not tested
⌐	right lower quadrant	Ø	no
	right upper quadrant		none
			without
⌐	left upper quadrant	@	at
	left lower quadrant		
>	greater than	1/2 and 1/2	half Dakin's solution and half glycerin
	left ear-bone conduction threshold	1°	first degree
≥	greater than or equal to		primary
		1:1	one-to-one individual session with staff)
<	caused by	2°	second degree
	less than		secondary
	right ear-bone conduction threshold	2×2	gauze dressing folded 2"×2"
≤	less than or equal to	3°	tertiary
≮	not less than		third degree
≯	not more than	3×	three times
∧	above	4×4	gauze dressing folded 4"×4"
	diastolic blood pressure		
	increased	5+2	cytarabine and daunorubicin
∨	below		
	systolic blood pressure	24°	twenty-four hours (24 hr is safer as the ° is seen as a zero)
≠	not equal to		
≅	approximately equal to	777	Ortho Novum 777® (a triphasic oral contraceptive)
=	equal		
	equal to		
≈	approximately		
≡	identical		
		1,000	one thousand (1^3)
×	left ear-air conduction threshold	10,000	ten thousand (1^4)
	ten	100,000	one hundred thousand (1^5)
]	left ear-masked bone conduction threshold	1,000,000	one million (1^6)
		10,000,000	ten million (1^7)
△	right ear-masked air conduction threshold	100,000,000	one hundred million (1^8)
	change	1,000,000,000	one billion (1^9)
[	right ear-masked	i	one (Roman numerals

are dangerous expressions and should not be used)

ii	two	β B	beta
iii	three	Γ γ	gamma
iiii	four	Δ δ	anion gap
iv	four (this is a dangerous abbreviation as it is read as intravenous, use 4)		change
			delta
			delta gap
			prism diopter
			temperature
			trimester
v	five	E ε	epsilon
vi	six	Z ζ	zeta
vii	seven	H η	eta
viii	eight	Θ θ	negative
ix	nine		theta
x	ten	I ι	iota
xi	eleven	K κ	kappa
xii	twelve	Λ λ	lambda
XL	forty	M μ	micro
	extended release dosage form		mu
		N ν	nu
♂	male	Ξ ξ	xi
♀	female	O o	omicron
■	deceased male	Π π	pi
●	deceased female		
□	living male	P ρ	rho
	left ear-masked air conduction threshold	Σ σ	sigma
			sum of
			summary
○	living female		
	respiration	T τ	tau
	right ear-bone conduction threshold	Y υ	upsilon
◇	sex unknown	Φ φ	phenyl
(□)	adopted living male		phi
*	birth		thyroid
†	dead	X χ	chi
	death	Ψ ψ	psi
			psychiatric
♀	standing	Ω ω	omega
O—<	recumbent position	'	feet
			minutes (as in 30')
Q	sitting position	"	inches
			seconds
♥	heart	⊙	start of an operation
A α	alpha	⊗	end of anesthesia

Numbers and letters for teeth

Two adult numbering systems and a deciduous system are shown. The adult systems are shown as numbers, whereas deciduous teeth are lettered. The system commonly used in the U.S. is 1 to 32 (shown in bold face type).

1 (18)	upper right 3rd molar
2 (17) (A)	upper right 2nd molar
3 (16) (B)	upper right 1st molar
4 (15)	upper right 2nd bicuspid
5 (14)	upper right 1st bicuspid
6 (13) (C)	upper right canine (eyetooth)
7 (12) (D)	upper right lateral incisor
8 (11) (E)	upper right central incisor
9 (21) (F)	upper left central incisor
10 (22) (G)	upper left lateral incisor
11 (23) (H)	upper left canine
12 (24)	upper left 1st bicuspid
13 (25)	upper left 2nd bicuspid
14 (26) (I)	upper left 1st molar
15 (27) (J)	upper left 2nd molar
16 (28)	upper left 3rd molar
17 (38)	lower left 3rd molar
18 (37) (K)	lower left 2nd molar
19 (36) (L)	lower left 1st molar
20 (35)	lower left 2nd bicuspid
21 (34)	lower left 1st bicuspid
22 (33) (M)	lower left canine
23 (32) (N)	lower left lateral incisor
24 (31) (O)	lower left central incisor
25 (41) (P)	lower right central incisor
26 (42) (Q)	lower right lateral incisor
27 (43) (R)	lower right canine
28 (44)	lower right 1st bicuspid
29 (45)	lower right 2nd bicuspid
30 (46) (S)	lower right 1st molar
31 (47) (T)	lower right 2nd molar
32 (48)	lower right 3rd molar

UPPER   UPPER

	Right															Left
1	**2**	**3**	**4**	**5**	**6**	**7**	**8**	**9**	**10**	**11**	**12**	**13**	**14**	**15**	**16**
18	17	16	15	14	13	12	11	21	22	23	24	25	26	27	28
A	B				C	D	E	F	G	H				I	J
T	S				R	Q	P	O	N	M				L	K
48	47	46	45	44	43	42	41	31	32	33	34	35	36	37	38
32	**31**	**30**	**29**	**28**	**27**	**26**	**25**	**24**	**23**	**22**	**21**	**20**	**19**	**18**	**17**

LOWER   LOWER

Shorthand for laboratory test values

See text for meaning of the abbreviations shown

Complete Blood Count

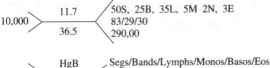

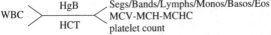

Electrolytes

142	99	sodium	chloride
4.7	25	potassium	bicarbonate

SMA 6 (Astra 7)

$$\begin{array}{c|c}142 & 99 \\ \hline 4.7 & 25\end{array}\Big\langle\begin{array}{c}12 \\ 1.0 \\ 125\end{array}\qquad\begin{array}{c|c}\text{sodium} & \text{chloride} \\ \hline \text{potassium} & \text{bicarbonate}\end{array}\Big\langle\begin{array}{l}\text{BUN} \\ \text{(creatinine)} \\ \text{glucose}\end{array}$$

Blood Gases

7.4/80/48/98/25   pH/PO_2/PCO_2/% O_2 saturation/bicarbonate

Obstetrical shorthand

$$\frac{2\ cm | 80\%}{-2\ Vtx}$$ 2 cm = dilation of cervix

80% = degree of cer-   Vtx = vertex; presen-
    vix effacement   tation of fetus,
                                            (breech = Br)

−2 = station; distance
     above (−) or
     below (+) the
     spine of the ischium measured in cm

Reflexes[1]

Reflexes are usually graded on a 0 to 4+ scale

4+   may indicate disease
       often associated with clonus
       very brisk, hyperactive (or $++++$)
3+   brisker than average
       possibly but not necessarily indicative of disease
          (or $+++$)
2+   average
       normal (or $++$)
1+   low normal
       somewhat diminished (or $+$)
0   may indicate neuropathy
       no response

Muscle strength[1]

0—No muscular contraction detected
1—A barely detectable flicker or trace of contraction
2—Active movement of the body part with gravity eliminated
3—Active movement against gravity
4—Active movement against gravity and some resistance
5—Active movement against full resistance without evident
    fatigue. This is normal muscle strength

Pulse[1]

 0   completely absent
+1   markedly impaired (or 1+, or +)
+2   modererately impaired (or 2+, or ++)
+3   slightly impaired (or 3+, or +++)
+4   normal (or 4+, or ++++)

Gradation of intensity of heart murmurs[1]

1/6 or I/VI	may not be heard in all positions
	very faint, heard only after the listener has "tuned in"
2/6 or II/VI	quiet, but heard immediately upon placing the stethoscope on the chest
3/6 or III/VI	moderately loud
4/6 or IV/VI	loud
5/6 or V/VI	very loud, may be heard with a stethoscope partly off the chest (thrills are associated)
6/6 or VI/VI	may be heard with the stethoscope entirely off the chest (thrills are associated)

Tonsil Size

0   no tonsils
1   less than normal
2   normal
3   greater than normal
4   touching

Apothecary symbols (Should never be used)

The symbols presented below are for informational use. The apothecary system should *not* be used. Only the metric system should be used. The methods of expressing the symbols, the meanings, and the equivalence are not the classic ones, nor are they accurate, but reflect the usual intended meanings when used by some older physicians in writing prescription directions.

℥ or ℥ ⁱ	dram, teaspoonful, (5 mL)	℥ or ℥ ⁱ	ounce, (30 mL)
		gr	grain (approximately 60 mg)
℥ ⁱⁱ	two drams, 2 teaspoonfuls, (10 mL)	♏	minim (approximately 0.06 mL)
℥ₛₛ	half ounce, tablespoonful, (15 mL)	gtt	drop

References

1. Bates B. A guide to physical examinations and history taking, 6th ed. Philadelphia: J.B. Lippincott; 1995.

Please forward additional meanings for these abbreviations, additional abbreviations and their meanings, or corrections to the author so that the list can be updated. Thank you. Dr. Neil M. Davis, 1143 Wright Drive, Huntingdon Valley, PA 19006-2721. FAX (215) 938 1937. E-mail med@neilmdavis.com

Additions

_____

_____

_____

_____

_____

_____

_____

_____

_____

_____

_____

_____

_____

Chapter 5

Pharmaceutical Generic Name and Trademark Cross-reference Index

Listed below is a cross-referenced index of generic and trademark drug names. Generic names begin with a lower case letter while trademarks begin with a capital letter. This partial list consists of frequently prescribed and new drugs.

The meanings of abbreviated and coded drug names can be found in chapter 2 (Lettered Abbreviations and Acronyms).

Complete indices of United States drug names can be found in current editions of Drug Facts and Comparisons[1], the American Drug Index[2], and Physicians GenRx[3]. A complete list of world-wide names may be found in Martindales.[4] These and other references should be used to determine the equivalence of products, strength designations, and dosage forms. Although several products may be listed under one generic name they may differ in strength or concentration available as is the case with estradiol transdermal (Climara, Estraderm, and Vivelle).

Some products are marketed without a trademark, as in the case of thioguanine. In such cases only the generic names are listed. When a product is often prescribed and/or labeled generically, the generic name is shown in italics.

The following abbreviations are used in this listing:

EC	enteric coated
HCl	hydrochloride
inj	injection
ophth	ophthalmic
soln	solution
SR	sustained release tablets or capsules (and other forms of extended release)

Abbokinase	urokinase
abciximab	ReoPro
Abelcet	amphotericin B lipid complex
acarbose	Precose
Accupril	quinapril HCl
Accutane	isotretinoin
acebutolol HCl	Sectral
Acel-Imune	diphtheria & tetanus toxoids & acellular pertussis vaccine
acetaminophen	Tylenol
acetazolamide	Diamox
acetohexamide	Dymelor
acetohydroxamic acid	Lithostat
acetylcholine ophth	Miochol E
acetylcysteine	Mucomyst
Achromycin	tetracycline HCl
Acthar	corticotropin
Acthrel	corticorellin ovine triflutate
Actifed	triprolidine HCl; pseudo-ephedrine HCl
Actigall	ursodiol
Activase	alteplase, recombinant
Acular	ketorolac tromethamine ophth
acyclovir	Zovirax
Adalat	nifedipine
Adalat CC	nifedipine SR
adapalene	Differin
Adapin	doxepin HCl
Adderall	amphetamine; dextroamphet-amine mixed salts
Adenocard	adenosine
adenosine	Adenocard
Adrenalin	epinephrine
Adriamycin	doxorubicin HCl
Advil	ibuprofen
AeroBid	flunisolide
Afrin nasal spray	oxymetazoline HCl
Agrelin	anagrelide
Akineton	biperiden
albendazole	Albenza
Albenza	albendazole
albumin human	Albuminar
	Albutein
	Buminate
	Plasbumin
Albuminar	albumin human
Albutein	albumin human
albuterol	Proventil
	Ventolin
Aldactazide	spironolactone; hydrochlorothia-zide
Aldactone	spironolactone
aldesleukin	Proleukin
Aldomet	methyldopa
Aldoril	methyldopa; hydrochloro-thiazide
alendronate sodium	Fosamax
Alfenta	alfentanil HCl
alfentanil HCl	Alfenta
Allegra	fexofenadine HCl
Alkeran	melphalan
allopurinol	Zyloprim
Alomide	lodoxamide tromethamine ophth soln
alprazolam	Xanax
alprostadil	Caverject
	Prostin VR
Altace	ramipril

alteplase, recombinant	Activase	amoxicillin; clavulanic acid	Augmentin
altretamine	Hexalen		
aluminum acetate	Domeboro	Amoxil	amoxicillin
		amphetamine resins	Biphetamine
aluminum carbonate	Basaljel	amphetamine; dextroamphet-	Adderall
aluminum hydroxide	Amphojel	amine mixed salts	
aluminum hydroxide; magnesium hydroxide	Maalox	Amphojel	aluminum hydroxide
		amphotericin B	Fungizone
		amphotericin B lipid complex	Abelcet
Alupent	metaproterenol sulfate		
amantadine HCl	Symmetrel	ampicillin	Omnipen Polycillin Principen
Amaryl	glimepiride		
Ambien	zolpidem tartrate		
amcinonide	Cyclocort	ampicillin sodium	Omnipen-N Polycillin-N Totacillin-N
Amicar	aminocaproic acid		
amifostine	Ethyol		Unasyn
amikacin sulfate	Amikin	ampicillin sodium; sulbactam sodium	
Amikin	amikacin sulfate		
amiloride HCl	Midamor Moduretic		
amino acid inj	Aminosyn Travasol TrophAmine	amrinone lactate	Inocor
		amsacrine	Amsidyl
		Amsidyl	amsacrine
aminocaproic acid	Amicar	Amvisc	sodium hyaluronate
aminogluteth- imide	Cytadren	Amytal	amobarbital sodium
aminophylline	aminophylline		
Aminosyn	amino acid inj	Anadrol-50	oxymetholone
amiodarone HCl	Cordarone	Anafranil	clomipramine HCl
amitriptyline HCl	Elavil Endep	anagrelide	Agrelin
amlodipine besylate	Norvasc	Anaprox	naproxen sodium
amlodipine besylate; benazepril HCl	Lotrel	anastrozole	Arimidex
		Anbesol	benzocaine
		Ancef	cefazolin sodium
amobarbital sodium	Amytal	Ancobon	flucytosine
		Androderm	testosterone transdermal system
amoxapine	Asendin		
amoxicillin	Amoxil Trimox	Anectine	succinylcholine chloride

Anexsia	hydrocodone bitartrate; acetamino-phen		immune globulin
		Ativan	lorazepam
		atovaquone	Mepron
Ansaid	flurbiprofen	atracurium besylate	Tracrium
Antabuse	disulfiram		
Antilirium	physostigmine salicylate	Atromid-S	clofibrate
		atropine sulfate tablets	Sal-Tropine
antipyrine otic	Auralgan		
Antivert	meclizine	Atrovent	ipratropium bromide
Anturane	sulfinpyrazone		
Aplisol	tuberculin skin test	Augmentin	amoxicillin; clavulanic acid
Apresazide	hydralazine HCl; hydrochloro-thiazide	Auralgan	antipyrine otic
		auranofin	Ridaura
		aurothioglucose	Solganal
Apresoline	hydralazine HCl	Aventyl	nortriptyline HCl
aprotinin	Trasylol	Avitene	collagen hemostat
AquaMEPHY-TON	phytonadione		
		Avonex	interferon beta-la
Aquasol A	vitamin A	Axid	nizatidine
Aralen	chloroquine phosphate	Azactam	aztreonam
		azatadine maleate	Optimine
Aramine	metaraminol bitartrate		
		azathioprine	Imuran
arcitumomab	CEA-Scan	azelaic acid cream	Azelex
Arduan	pipecuronium bromide		
		Azelex	azelaic acid cream
Aredia	pamidronate disodium		
		azithromycin	Zithromax
Arfonad	trimethaphan camsylate	Azmacort	triamcinolone acetonide aerosol
arginine HCl	R-Gene		
Arimidex	anastrozole	aztreonam	Azactam
Aristocort	triamcinolone acetonide	Azulfidine	sulfasalazine
Arlidin	nylidrin HCl		
Artane	trihexyphenidyl HCl		
Asendin	amoxapine		
asparaginase	Elspar		
aspirin buffered	Bufferin		
aspirin EC	Ecotrin	**B**	
astemizole	Hismanal		
Atarax	hydroxyzine HCl		
atenolol	Tenormin		
atenolol; chlorthalidone	Tenoretic		
Atgam	lymphocyte	Baciguent	bacitracin ointment

bacitracin ointment	Baciguent	betamethasone dipropionate	Diprosone
baclofen	Lioresal	betamethasone; clotrimazole cream	Lotrisone
Bactrim	sulfamethoxa-zole-trimeth-oprim		
		Betapace	sotalol
Bactroban	mupirocin nasal ointment	Betaseron	interferon beta-1b
		betaxolol	Kerlone
BAL in Oil	dimercaprol	betaxolol HCl ophth suspension	Betoptic S
Basaljel	aluminum carbonate		
BCG intravesical	TheraCys TICE BCG	betaxolol HCl ophth soln	Betoptic
beclomethasone dipropionate	Beclovent Beconase AQ Nasal Vancenase Vancenase AQ Nasal Vanceril	bethanechol chloride	Urecholine
		Betoptic	betaxolol HCl ophth soln
		Betoptic S	betaxolol HCl ophth suspension
Beclovent	beclomethasone dipropionate	Biaxin	clarithromycin
		bicalutamide	Casodex
Beconase AQ Nasal	beclomethasone dipropionate	Bicillin C-R	penicillin G benzathine; penicillin G procaine
belladonna alkaloids; phenobarbital	Donnatal		
		Bicillin L-A	penicillin G benzathine
Bellergal-S	phenobarbital; ergotamine; belladonna	Bicitra	sodium citrate; citric acid
Benadryl	diphenhydramine HCl	BiCNU	carmustine
		biperiden	Akineton
benazepril HCl	Lotensin	Biphetamine	amphetamine resins
Benemid	probenecid		
Bentyl	dicyclomine HCl	bisacodyl	Dulcolax
benzocaine	Anbesol	bisoprolol fumarate; hydrochlorothi-azide	Ziac
benzocaine; tetracaine HCl	Cetacaine		
benztropine mesylate	Cogentin	bitolterol mesylate	Tornalate
bepridil	Vascor	Blenoxane	bleomycin sulfate
beractant	Survanta		
Berroca	vitamin B complex; folic acid; vitamin C	bleomycin sulfate	Blenoxane
		Blocadren	timolol maleate
		B & O Supprettes	opium; belladonna suppositories
Betadine	povidone iodine		
Betagan	levobunolol HCl		
betamethasone	Celestone		

287

Botox	botulinum toxin type A
botulinum toxin type A	Botox
Brethaire	terbutaline sulfate aerosol
Brethine	terbutaline sulfate tablets and inj
bretylium tosylate	Bretylol
Bretylol	bretylium tosylate
Brevibloc	esmolol HCl
Brevital Sodium	methohexital sodium
Bricanyl	terbutaline sulfate tablets and inj
bromocriptine mesylate	Parlodel
brompheniramine maleate	Dimetane
brompheniramine maleate; phenylpropanolamime	Dimetapp Extentabs
Bronkometer	isoetharine HCl aerosol
Bronkosol	isoetharine HCl soln
Bucladin-S	buclizine HCl
buclizine HCl	Bucladin-S
budesonide nasal inhaler	Rhinocort
Bufferin	aspirin buffered
bumetanide	Bumex
Bumex	bumetanide
Buminate	albumin human
Buphenyl	phenylbutyrate sodium
bupivacaine HCl	Marcaine HCl
bupropion HCl	Wellbutrin
BuSpar	buspirone HCl
buspirone HCl	BuSpar
busulfan	Myleran
butabarbital sodium	Butisol
butalbital;	Fioricet

acetaminophen; caffeine	
butalbital; aspirin; caffeine	Fiorinal
Butazolidin	phenylbutazone
Butisol	butabarbital sodium
butorphanol tartrate inj	Stadol
butorphanol tartrate nasal spray	Stadol NS

C

Cafergot	ergotamine tartrate; caffeine
Calan SR	verapamil HCl SR
Calciferol	ergocalciferol
Calcimar	calcitonin
calcitonin	Calcimar
calcitonin-salmon	Miacalcin
calcium carbonate	Os-Cal 500 Tums
camphorated tincture of opium	paregoric
Camptosar	irinotecan HCl
Capastat Sulfate	capreomycin sulfate
Capitrol	chloroxine
Capoten	captopril
capreomycin sulfate	Capastat Sulfate
captopril	Capoten
Carafate	sucralfate
carbachol	Isopto Carbachol
carbamazepine	Tegretol
carbamide peroxide otic	Debrox

carbenicillin	Geocillin	ceftazidime	Ceptaz
Carbocaine	mepivacaine HCl		Fortaz
			Tazicef
carboplatin	Paraplatin		Tazidime
Cardene	nicardipine HCl	ceftibuten	Cedax
		Ceftin	cefuroxime axetil
Cardizem	diltiazem HCl	ceftizoxime sodium	Cefizox
Cardizem CD	diltiazem HCl SR		
		ceftriaxone sodium	Rocephin
Cardura	doxazosin mesylate	cefuroxime axetil	Ceftin
carisoprodol	Soma	cefuroxime sodium	Kefurox
carmustine	BiCNU		Zinacef
Carnitor	levocarnitine	Cefzil	cefprozil
carvedilol	Coreg	Celestone	betamethasone
Casodex	bicalutamide	CellCept	mycophenolate mofetil
Cataflam	diclofenac potassium		
		Centrum	vitamins; minerals
Catapres	clonidine HCl		
Caverject	alprostadil	cephalexin	Keflex
CEA-SCAN	arcitumomab	cephalexin HCl	Keftab
Ceclor	cefaclor		
Cedax	ceftibuten	cephalothin sodium	Keflin
CeeNu	lomustine		
cefaclor	Ceclor	cephapirin sodium	Cefadyl
cefadroxil	Duricef		
Cefadyl	cephapirin sodium	cephradine	Velosef
		Cephulac	lactulose
cefamandole nafate	Mandol	Ceptaz	ceftazidime
		Cerebyx	fosphenytoin sodium
cefazolin sodium	Ancef		
	Kefzol	Cerubidine	daunorubicin HCl
cefepime HCl	Maxipime		
cefixime	Suprax	Cervidil	dinoprostone vaginal insert
Cefizox	ceftizoxime sodium		
		Cetacaine	benzocaine; tetracaine HCl
Cefobid	cefoperazone sodium		
		cetirizine HCl	Zyrtec
cefonicid sodium	Monocid	Chlor-Trimeton	chlorpheniramine maleate
cefoperazone sodium	Cefobid		
Cefotan	cefotetan	chloral hydrate	chloral hydrate
cefotaxime sodium	Claforan	chlorambucil	Leukeran
		chloramphenicol	Chloromycetin
cefotetan	Cefotan	chloramphenicol ophth	Chloroptic ophth
cefoxitin sodium	Mefoxin		
cefpodoxime proxetil	Vantin	chlordiazepoxide HCl	Librium
cefprozil	Cefzil		

chlordiazepoxide HCl; amitriptyline HCl	Limbitrol
chlorhexidine gluconate	Hibiclens
chlorhexidine gluconate mouth rinse	Peridex
Chloromycetin	chloramphenicol
chloroprocaine HCl	Nesacaine
Chloroptic ophth	chloramphenicol ophth
chloroquine phosphate	Aralen
chlorothiazide	Diuril
chlorotrianisene	TACE
chloroxine	Capitrol
chlorpheniramine maleate	Chlor-Trimeton
chlorpheniramine maleate SR	Teldrin
chlorpromazine	Thorazine
chlorpropamide	Diabinese
chlorprothixene	Taractan
chlorthalidone	Hygroton
chlorthalidone; reserpine	Regroton
chlorzoxazone 250 mg	Paraflex
chlorzoxazone 500 mg	Parafon Forte DSC
Choledyl	oxtriphylline
cholestyramine	Questran
choline magnesium trisalicylate	Trilisate
Chronulac	lactulose
Chymodiactin	chymopapain
chymopapain	Chymodiactin
Cibalith-S	lithium citrate
cidofovir	Vistide
Ciloxan	ciprofloxacin ophth soln
cimetidine HCl	Tagamet

Cipro	ciprofloxacin HCl
ciprofloxacin HCl	Cipro
ciprofloxacin ophth soln	Ciloxan
cisapride	Propulsid
cisatracurium besylate	Nimbex
cisplatin	Platinol AQ
cladribine	Leustatin
Claforan	cefotaxime sodium
clarithromycin	Biaxin
Claritin	loratadine
Claritin D	loratadine; pseudoephed-rine sulfate
clemastine fumarate	Tavist
Cleocin	clindamycin HCl
clidinium bromide	Quarzan
clidinium; chlordiaze-poxide	Librax
Climara	estradiol transdermal
clindamycin HCl	Cleocin
Clinoril	sulindac
clioquinol	Vioform
clofibrate	Atromid-S
Clomid	clomiphene citrate
clomiphene citrate	Clomid
clomipramine HCl	Anafranil
clonazepam	Klonopin
clonidine HCl	Catapres
clorazepate dipotassium	Tranxene
Clorpactin WCS-90	oxychlorosene sodium
clotrimazole	Gyne-Lotrimin Lotrimin Mycelex

cloxacillin sodium	Tegopen
clozapine	Clozaril
Clozaril	clozapine
co-trimoxazole	Bactrim
	Cotrim
	Septra
	sulfamethoxazole; trimethoprim
coal tar product	Zetar
Cogentin	benztropine mesylate
Cognex	tacrine HCl
Colace	docusate sodium
ColBENEMID	probenecid; colchicine
colchicine	colchicine
Colestid	colestipol HCl
colestipol HCl	Colestid
colistimethate sodium	Coly-Mycin M
colistin sulfate	Coly-Mycin S
collagen hemostat	Avitene
collagenase	Santyl
Collyrium	tetrahydrozoline HCl ophth
Coly-Mycin M	colistimethate sodium
Coly-Mycin S	colistin sulfate
Compazine	prochlorperazine
Cordarone	amiodarone HCl
Coreg	carvedilol
Corgard	nadolol
Cortef	hydrocortisone
corticorellin ovine triflutate	Acthrel
corticotropin	Acthar
cortisone acetate	Cortone Acetate
Cortone Acetate	cortisone acetate
Cortrosyn	cosyntropin
Corvert	ibutilide fumarate
Cosmegen	dactinomycin
cosyntropin	Cortrosyn
Cotazym	pancrelipase
Cotazym-S	pancrelipase EC
Cotrim	sulfamethoxazole-trimethoprim
Coumadin	warfarin sodium
Covera HS	verapamil HCl SR bedtime formulation
Cozaar	losartan potassium
Crixivan	indinavir
cromolyn sodium	Gastrocrom
	Intal
	Nasalcrom
	Opticrom
crotamiton	Eurax
Crystodigin	digitoxin
Cuprimine	penicillamine
cyclobenzaprine HCl	Flexeril
Cyclocort	amcinonide
Cyclogyl	cyclopentolate HCl
cyclopentolate HCl	Cyclogyl
cyclophosphamide	Cytoxan
	Neosar
cycloserine	Seromycin
cyclosporine	Sandimmune
cyclosporine microemulsion capsules and oral soln	Neoral
Cycrin	medroxyprogesterone acetate
Cylert	pemoline
cyproheptadine HCl	Periactin
Cystospaz-M	hyoscyamine sulfate SR
Cytadren	aminoglutethimide
cytarabine	Cytosar-U
Cytomel	liothyronine sodium
Cytosar-U	cytarabine
Cytotec	misoprostol
Cytovene	ganciclovir
Cytoxan	cyclophosphamide

dacarbazine	DTIC-Dome
dactinomycin	Cosmegen
Dalmane	flurazepam HCl
dalteparin sodium	Fragmin
danazol	Danocrine
Danocrine	danazol
Dantrium	dantrolene sodium
dantrolene sodium	Dantrium
dapsone	dapsone
Daranide	dichlorphenamide
Daraprim	pyrimethamine
Darvocet-N 100	propoxyphene napsylate; acetaminophen
Darvon	propoxyphene HCl
Darvon Compound 65	propoxyphene HCl; aspirin; caffeine
daunorubicin citrate liposomal	DaunoXome
daunorubicin HCl	Cerubidine
DaunoXome	daunorubicin citrate liposomal
Daypro	oxaprozin
DDAVP	desmopressin acetate
Debrox	carbamide peroxide otic
Decadron	dexamethasone
Deca-Durabolin	nandrolone decanoate
Declomycin	demeclocycline HCl
deferoxamine mesylate	Desferal
Delestrogen	estradiol valerate
Deltasone	prednisone
Demadex	torsemide
demecarium bromide	Humorsol
demeclocycline HCl	Declomycin
Demerol	meperidine HCl
Demser	metyrosine
Demulen	ethynodiol diacetate; ethinyl estradiol
Depakene	valproic acid
Depakote	divalproex sodium
Depo-Medrol	methylprednisolone acetate SR
Depo-Provera	medroxyprogesterone acetate SR
Depo-Testosterone	testosterone cypionate SR
Desferal	deferoxamine mesylate
desflurane	Suprane
desipramine HCl	Norpramin
desmopressin acetate	DDAVP
Desogen	desogestrel; ethinyl estradiol
desogestrel; ethinyl estradiol	Desogen Ortho-Cept
desonide	Tridesilon
desoximetasone	Topicort
Desoxyn	methamphetamine HCl
Desyrel	trazodone HCl
dexamethasone	Decadron Hexadrol
dexchlorpheniramine maleate SR	Polaramine Repetabs
dexfenfluramine HCl	Redux
Dexferrum	iron dextran inj

dexrazoxane	Zinecard	Dilantin	phenytoin
D.H.E. 45	dihydroergot-amine mesylate	Dilaudid	hydromorphone HCl
DiaBeta	glyburide	diltiazem HCl	Cardizem
Diabinese	chlorpropamide	diltiazem HCl SR	Cardizem CD
Diamox	acetazolamide		Dilacor XR
Diapid	lypressin		Tiazac
diazepam	Valium	dimenhydrinate	Dramamine
diazepam emulsified inj	Dizac	dimercaprol	BAL in Oil
		Dimetane	brompheniramine maleate
diazoxide	Hyperstat	dinoprostone gel	Prepidil
Dibenzyline	phenoxybenz-amine HCl	dinoprostone vaginal insert	Cervidil
dibucaine	Nupercainal	dinoprostone vaginal suppositories	Prostin E2
dichlorphena-mide	Daranide		
diclofenac potassium	Cataflam	Dipentum	olsalazine sodium
diclofenac sodium	Voltaren	diphenhydramine HCl	Benadryl
diclofenac sodium SR	Voltaren-XR	diphenoxylate HCl; atropine sulfate	Lomotil
dicloxacillin sodium	Dynapen		
dicyclomine HCl	Bentyl	diphtheria & tetanus toxoids & acellular pertussis vaccine	Acel-Imune Tripedia
didanosine	Videx		
Didronel	etidronate disodium		
diethylpropion HCl	Tenuate		
diethylstilbestrol diphosphate	Stilphostrol	dipivefrin	Propine
Differin	adapalene	Diprivan	propofol
diflorasone diacetate	Florone	Diprosone	betamethasone dipropionate
Diflucan	fluconazole	dipyridamole	Persantine
diflunisal	Dolobid	dirithromycin	Dynabac
Digibind	digoxin immune fab	Disalcid	salsalate
		disopyramide phosphate	Norpace
digitoxin	Crystodigin		
digoxin	Lanoxin	disulfiram	Antabuse
digoxin capsules	Lanoxicaps	Ditropan	oxybutynin chloride
digoxin immune fab	Digibind		
		Diulo	metolazone
dihydroergota-mine mesylate	D.H.E. 45	Diuril	chlorothiazide
		divalproex sodium	Depakote
Dilacor XR	diltiazem HCl SR	Dizac	diazepam emulsified inj

dobutamine HCl	Dobutrex
Dobutrex	dobutamine HCl
docetaxel	Taxotere
docusate calcium	Surfak
docusate calcium; phenolphthalein	Doxidan
docusate sodium	Colace
docusate sodium; casanthranol	Peri-Colace
Dolobid	diflunisal
Dolophine	methadone HCl
Domeboro	aluminum acetate
Donnatal	belladonna alkaloids; phenobarbital
dopamine HCl	Intropin
Dopram	doxapram HCl
dorzolamide HCl	Trusopt
doxacurium chloride	Nuromax
doxapram HCl	Dopram
doxazosin mesylate	Cardura
doxepin HCl	Adapin Sinequan
Doxidan	docusate calcium; phenolphtha-lein
Doxil	doxorubicin, liposomal
doxorubicin HCl	Adriamycin Rubex
doxorubicin, liposomal	Doxil
doxycycline hyclate	Vibramycin
Dramamine	dimenhydrinate
Drisdol	ergocalciferol
Dristan Long Lasting	oxymetazoline HCl
Drixoral Syrup	pseudoephedrine HCl; bromphiramine maleate
dronabinol	Marinol

droperidol	Inapsine
DTIC-Dome	dacarbazine
Dulcolax	bisacodyl
Durabolin	nandrolone phenpropionate
Duragesic	fentanyl transdermal
Duramorph	morphine sulfate inj
Duranest	etidocaine HCl
Duricef	cefadroxil
Dyazide	triamterene 37.5 mg; hydro-chlorothiazide 25 mg
Dymelor	acetohexamide
Dynabac	dirithromycin
DynaCirc	isradipine
Dynapen	dicloxacillin sodium
dyphylline	Lufyllin
Dyrenium	triamterene

E

echothiophate iodide	Phospholine Iodide
Ecotrin	aspirin EC
Edecrin	ethacrynic acid
edetate disodium	Endrate
edrophonium chloride	Tensilon
E.E.S. 400	erythromycin ethylsuccinate
Effexor	venlafaxine HCl
Elavil	amitriptyline HCl
Eldepryl	selegiline HCl
Eldisine	vindesine sulfate
Elixophyllin	theophylline
Elocon	mometasone furoate

Elspar	asparaginase
Emcyt	estramustine phosphate sodium
EMLA Cream	lidocaine; prilocaine cream
E-Mycin	erythromycin
enalapril maleate	Vasotec
enalapril maleate; hydrochlorothiazide	Vaseretic
encainide HCl	Enkaid
Endep	amitriptyline HCl
Endrate	edetate disodium
Enduron	methyclothiazide
enflurane	Ethrane
Engerix-B	hepatitis B vaccine
Enkaid	encainide HCl
enoxaparin sodium	Lovenox
Entex LA	phenylpropanolamine HCl; guaifenesin SR
epinephrine	Adrenalin
epinephrine racemic	Vaponefrin
Epivir	lamivudine
epoetin alfa	Epogen Procrit
Epogen	epoetin alfa
epoprostenol sodium	Flolan
Equanil	meprobamate
Ergamisol	levamisole HCl
ergocalciferol	Calciferol Drisdol
ergoloid mesylates	Hydergine
ergonovine maleate	Ergotrate
Ergostat	ergotamine tartrate
ergotamine tartrate; caffeine	Cafergot
ergotamine tartrate	Ergostat
Ergotrate	ergonovine maleate
Ery-Tab	erythromycin EC
Erythrocin Stearate	erythromycin stearate
erythromycin	E-Mycin
erythromycin base coated particles	PCE Dispertab
erythromycin EC	Ery-Tab
erythromycin estolate	Ilosone
erythromycin ethylsuccinate	E.E.S. 400
erythromycin ethylsuccinate; sulfisoxazole	Pediazole
erythromycin stearate	Erythrocin Stearate
Eserine Sulfate	physostigmine ophth ointment
Esidrix	hydrochlorothiazide
Esimil	guanethidine monosulfate; hydrochlorothiazide
Eskalith	lithium carbonate
esmolol HCl	Brevibloc
Estinyl	ethinyl estradiol
Estrace	estradiol
Estraderm	estradiol transdermal
estradiol	Estrace
estradiol transdermal	Climara Estraderm Vivelle
estradiol vaginal ring	Estring
estradiol valerate	Delestrogen

estramustine phosphate sodium	Emcyt	etodolac	Lodine
		Etopophos	etoposide phosphate
Estratest	estrogens, esterified; methyltestosterone	etoposide	VePesid
		etoposide phosphate	Etopophos
		Etrafon	perphenazine; amitriptyline HCl
Estratest H.S.	estrogens, esterified; methyltestosterone, half strength		
		Eulexin	flutamide
		Eurax	crotamiton
		Euthroid	liotrix
Estring	estradiol vaginal ring	Eutonyl	pargyline HCl
		Ex-Lax	phenolphthalein
estrogens, conjugated	Premarin		
estrogens, conjugated; medroxyprogesterone acetate	Premphase Prempro		

F

estrogens, esterified; methyltestosterone	Estratest		
estrogens, esterified methyltestosterone, half strength	Estratest H.S.	famciclovir	Famvir
		famotidine	Pepcid
		Famvir	famciclovir
		Fareston	toremifene citrate
estropipate	Ogen	Fastin	phentermine HCl
ethacrynic acid	Edecrin	fat emulsion	Intralipid
ethambutol HCl	Myambutol		Liposyn II and III
ethchlorvynol	Placidyl		
ethinyl estradiol	Estinyl	felbamate	Felbatol
ethionamide	Trecator-SC	Felbatol	felbamate
Ethmozine	moricizine	Feldene	piroxicam
ethopropazine HCl	Parsidol	felodipine	Plendil
		fenfluramine HCl	Pondimin
ethosuximide	Zarontin		
Ethrane	enflurane	fenoprofen calcium	Nalfon
ethyl chloride	ethyl chloride		
ethynodiol diacetate; ethinyl estradiol	Demulen	fentanyl citrate	Sublimaze
		fentanyl citrate; droperidol	Innovar
Ethyol	amifostine	fentanyl transdermal	Duragesic
etidocaine HCl	Duranest		
etidronate disodium	Didronel	Feosol	ferrous sulfate
		Fer-In-Sol	ferrous sulfate
		Fergon	ferrous gluconate
		ferrous gluconate	Fergon

ferrous sulfate	Feosol	fluorescein	Fluorescite
	Fer-In-Sol	sodium soln	
ferrous sulfate	SlowFe	fluorescein	Fluor-I-Strip
SR		sodium strips	
fexofenadine	Allegra	Fluorescite	fluorescein
HCl			sodium soln
filgrastim	Neupogen	fluorometholone	FML
finasteride	Proscar	Fluothane	halothane
Fioricet	butalbital;	fluoxetine HCl	Prozac
	acetamino-	fluoxymesterone	Halotestin
	phen; caffeine	fluphenazine HCl	Permitil
Fiorinal	butalbital;		Prolixin
	aspirin;	flurazepam HCl	Dalmane
	caffeine	flurbiprofen	Ansaid
Flagyl	metronidazole	flutamide	Eulexin
flavoxate HCl	Urispas	fluticasone	Flonase
Flaxedil	gallamine	propionate	Flovent
	triethiodide	fluvastatin	Lescol
flecainide acetate	Tambocor	sodium	
Flexeril	cyclobenzaprine	fluvoxamine	Luvox
	HCl	maleate	
Flolan	epoprostenol	FML	fluorometholone
	sodium	Folex	methotrexate
Flonase	fluticasone	*folic acid*	Folvite
	propionate	Folvite	folic acid
Florinef	fludrocortisone	Forane	isoflurane
	acetate	Fortaz	ceftazidime
Florone	diflorasone	Fosamax	alendronate
	diacetate		sodium
Floropryl	isoflurophate	foscarnet	Foscavir
Flovent	fluticasone	Foscavir	foscarnet
	propionate	fosinopril	Monopril
Floxin	ofloxacin	sodium	
floxuridine	FUDR	fosphenytoin	Cerebyx
fluconazole	Diflucan	sodium	
flucytosine	Ancobon	Fragmin	dalteparin sodium
Fludara	fludarabine	FUDR	floxuridine
	phosphate	Fulvicin P/G	griseofulvin
fludarabine	Fludara	Fungizone	amphotericin B
phosphate		Furacin	nitrofurazone
fludrocortisone	Florinef	*furosemide*	Lasix
acetate			
Flumadine	rimantadine		
flunisolide	Aero Bid		
fluocinolone	Synalar		
acetonide			
fluocinonide	Lidex	**G**	
Fluor-I-Strip	fluorescein		
	sodium strips	gabapentin	Neurontin

gallamine triethiodide	Flaxedil	dextromethor-phan	
gallium nitrate	Ganite	guanabenz acetate	Wytensin
Gamimune N	immune globulin intravenous	guanadrel sulfate	Hylorel
Gammar-P IV	immune globulin intravenous	guanethidine monosulfate	Ismelin
ganciclovir	Cytovene	guanethidine monosulfate; hydrochlorothi-azide	Esimil
ganciclovir ophthalmic implant	Vitrasert		
Ganite	gallium nitrate	guanfacine HCl	Tenex
Gantanol	sulfamethoxazole	Gyne-Lotrimin	clotrimazole
Garamycin	gentamicin sulfate		
Gastrocrom	cromolyn sodium		
gemcitabine HCl	Gemzar		
gemfibrozil	Lopid		**H**
Gemzar	gemcitabine HCl		
gentamicin sulfate	Garamycin		
Geocillin	carbenicillin		
glimepiride	Amaryl		
glipizide	Glucotrol	Habitrol	nicotine transdermal system
glipizide SR	Glucotrol XL		
glucagon	glucagon	haemophilus b vaccine	Hib-Immune
Glucophage	metformin HCl		HibTITER
Glucotrol	glipizide		PedvaxHIB
Glucotrol XL	glipizide SR		ProHIBiT
glyburide	DiaBeta	halcinonide	Halog
	Micronase	Halcion	triazolam
glyburide micronized	Glynase	Haldol	haloperidol
glycopyrrolate	Robinul	Halog	halcinonide
Glynase	glyburide micronized	haloperidol	Haldol
		haloprogin	Halotex
gold sodium thiomalate	Myochrysine	Halotestin	fluoxymesterone
		Halotex	haloprogin
goserelin acetate	Zoladex	halothane	Fluothane
granisetron HCl	Kytril	Havrix	hepatitis A vaccine, inactivated
Grifulvin V	griseofulvin		
griseofulvin	Fulvicin P/G		
	Grifulvin V		
guaifenesin	Organidin NR	H-BIG	hepatitis B immune globulin
	Robitussin		
guaifenesin; codeine phosphate	Robitussin A-C	Healon	sodium hyaluronate
	Tussi-Organidin NR	*heparin sodium*	Liquaemin Sodium
guaifenesin;	Robitussin-DM		

hepatitis A vaccine, inactivated	Havrix Vaqta		extended, (human)
		hyaluronidase	Wydase
hepatitis B immune globulin	H-BIG	Hycamtin	topotecan HCl
		Hydergine	ergoloid mesylates
hepatitis B vaccine	Engerix-B Recombivax HB	hydralazine HCl	Apresoline
		hydralazine HCl; hydrochlorothi-azide	Apresazide
Herplex	idoxuridine		
Hespan	hetastarch	hydralazine; hydrochlorothi-azide; reserpine	Ser-Ap-Es
hetastarch	Hespan		
Hexadrol	dexamethasone		
Hexalen	altretamine	Hydrea	hydroxyurea
Hib-Immune	haemophilus b vaccine	*hydrochlorothi-azide*	Esidrix HydroDIURIL Oretic
Hibiclens	chlorhexidine gluconate		
HibTITER	haemophilus b vaccine	hydrocodone bitartrate; acetaminophen	Anexsia Lorcet Lortab Vicodin
Hiprex	methenamine hippurate		
Hismanal	astemizole	hydrocodone polistirex; chlorphenira-mine	Tussionex
Hivid	zalcitabine		
homatropine hydrobromide ophth	Isopto Homatropine		
		hydrocortisone	Cortef Hydrocortone
Humalog	insulin, lispro		
Humatin	paromomycin sulfate	hydrocortisone sodium succinate	Solu-Cortef
Humorsol	demecarium bromide	Hydrocortone	hydrocortisone
Humulin 70/30	isophane insulin suspension 70%, insulin inj 30% (human)	HydroDIURIL	hydrochlorothia-zide
		hydroflumethia-zide	Saluron
		hydromorphone HCl	Dilaudid
Humulin L	insulin zinc suspension (Lente) (human)	Hydromox	quinethazone
		hydroxychloro-quine sulfate	Plaquenil
Humulin N	isophane insulin suspension (NPH) (human)	hydroxyurea	Hydrea
		hydroxyzine HCl	Atarax
		hydroxyzine pamoate	Vistaril
Humulin R	insulin inj (human)	Hygroton	chlorthalidone
		Hylorel	guanadrel sulfate
Humulin U Ultralente	insulin zinc suspension,	hyoscyamine sulfate SR	Cystospaz-M Levbid

Hyper-Tet	tetanus immune globulin (human)	Imodium	loperamide HCl
		Imuran	azathioprine
		Inapsine	droperidol
Hyperstat	diazoxide	indapamide	Lozol
Hytrin	terazosin HCl	Inderal	propranolol HCl
Hyzaar	losartan potassium; hydrochlorothiazide	Inderide	propranolol HCl; hydrochlorothiazide
		indinavir	Crixivan
		Indocin	indomethacin
		indomethacin	Indocin
		INFeD	iron dextran inj
		Innovar	fentanyl citrate; droperidol
		Inocor	amrinone lactate
		insulin inj (human)	Humulin R
			Novolin R
			Velosulin Human

I

		insulin zinc suspension (Lente) (human)	Humulin L
			Novolin L
		insulin zinc suspension, extended (beef)	Ultralente U
ibuprofen	Advil		
	Motrin		
	Nuprin	insulin zinc suspension, extended, (human)	Humulin U
ibutilide fumarate	Corvert		Ultralente
Idamycin	idarubicin	insulin, lispro	Humalog
idarubicin	Idamycin	Intal	cromolyn sodium
idoxuridine	Herplex	interferon alfa-2a	Roferon-A
IFEX	ifosfamide	interferon alfa-2b	Intron A
ifosfamide	IFEX	interferon beta-la	Avonex
Ilosone	erythromycin estolate	interferon beta-1b	Betaseron
imciromab pentetate	Myoscint	Intralipid	fat emulsion
Imdur	isosorbide mononitrate SR	Intron A	interferon alfa-2b
		Intropin	dopamine HCl
		Inversine	mecamylamine HCl
imipenem-cilastatin sodium	Primaxin	Invirase	saquinavir mesylate
imipramine HCl	Tofranil	iodixanol	Visipaque
Imitrex	sumatriptan	iohexol	Omnipaque
immune globulin intravenous	Gamimune N	iopanoic acid	Telepaque
	Gammar-P IV	iopromide	Ultravist
	Sandoglobulin	ioxilan	Oxilan

ipratropium bromide	Atrovent	isoxsuprine HCl	Vasodilan
		isradipine	DynaCirc
irinotecan HCl	Camptosar	Isuprel	isoproterenol HCl
iron dextran inj	INFeD		
	Dexferrum	itraconazole	Sporanox
Ismelin	guanethidine monosulfate		
ISMO	isosorbide mononitrate		
isoetharine HCl aerosol	Bronkometer		

isoetharine HCl soln	Bronkosol		
isoflurane	Forane		
isoflurophate	Floropry l		
isoniazid	Nydrazid	Kadian	morphine sulfate SR
isoniazid; rifampin	Rifamate	kanamycin sulfate	Kantrex
isophane insulin suspension (NPH) (human)	Humulin N Novolin N	Kantrex	kanamycin sulfate
		Kaon	potassium gluconate
isophane insulin suspension (NPH) 70%, insulin inj 30% (human)	Humulin 70/30 Novolin 70/30	Kaon-Cl	potassium chloride SR
		Kayexalate	polystyrene sulfonate sodium
isoproterenol HCl	Isuprel	K-Dur	potassium chloride SR
Isoptin	verapamil HCl	Keflex	cephalexin
Isopto Carbachol	carbachol ophth	Keflin	cephalothin sodium
Isopto Carpine	pilocarpine HCl ophth	Keftab	cephalexin HCl
Isopto Homatropine	homatropine hydrobromide ophth	Kefurox	cefuroxime sodium
Isopto Hyoscine	scopolamine hydrobromide ophth	Kefzol	cefazolin sodium
		Kemadrin	procyclidine HCl
		Kenalog	triamcinolone acetonide
Isordil	isosorbide dinitrate	Kerlone	betaxolol
isosorbide dinitrate	Isordil	Ketalar	ketamine HCl
isosorbide mononitrate	ISMO	ketamine HCl	Ketalar
isosorbide mononitrate SR	Imdur	ketoconazole	Nizoral
		ketoprofen	Orudis
		ketoprofen SR	Oruvail
isotretinoin	Accutane	ketorolac tromethamine	Toradol

ketorolac tromethamine ophth	Acular	*leucovorin calcium*	Wellcovorin
Klonopin	clonazepam	Leukeran	chlorambucil
Klor-Con 10	potassium chloride SR	Leukine	sargramostim
		leuprolide acetate	Lupron
K-Lyte	potassium bicarbonate; potassium citrate effervescent	Leustatin	cladribine
		levamisole HCl	Ergamisol
		Levbid	hyoscyamine sulfate SR
K-Lyte/Cl	potassium chloride potassium bicarbonate effervescent	Levo-Dromoran	levorphanol tartrate
		levobunolol HCl	Betagan
		levocarnitine	Carnitor
		levodopa	Larodopa
Kolyum	potassium chloride; potassium gluconate	levodopa; carbidopa	Sinemet
		levodopa; carbidopa SR	Sinemet CR
Konsyl-D	psyllium	levonorgestrel	Nordette
Kwell	lindane	levonorgestrel implant	Norplant
Kytril	granisetron HCl	levonorgestrel; ethinyl estradiol	Tri-Levlen Triphasil
		Levophed	norepinephrine bitartrate

L

		levorphanol tartrate	Levo-Dromoran
		levothyroxine sodium	Levoxyl Synthroid
labetalol HCl	Normodyne Trandate	Levoxyl	levothyroxine sodium
lactulose	Cephulac Chronulac	Librax	clidinium; chlordiaz-epoxide
Lamictal	lamotrigine	Librium	chlordiazepoxide HCl
Lamisil	terbinafine HCl		
lamivudine	Epivir	Lidex	fluocinonide
lamotrigine	Lamictal	lidocaine HCl	Xylocaine HCl
Lanoxicaps	digoxin capsules	lidocaine; prilocaine cream	EMLA Cream
Lanoxin	digoxin		
lansoprazole	Prevacid	Limbitrol	chlordiazepoxide HCl; amitrip-tyline HCl
Lariam	mefloquine HCl		
Larodopa	levodopa		
Lasix	furosemide	Lincocin	lincomycin HCl
latanoprost	Xalatan	lincomycin HCl	Lincocin
Lescol	fluvastatin sodium	lindane	Kwell

Lioresal	baclofen		bitartrate;
liothyronine sodium	Cytomel		acetaminophen
		losartan potassium	Cozaar
liothyronine sodium inj	Triostat	losartan potassium; hydrochlorothiazide	Hyzaar
liotrix	Euthroid		
Liposyn II and III	fat emulsion		
Liquaemin Sodium	heparin sodium	Lotensin	benazepril HCl
lisinopril	Prinivil	Lotrel	amlodipine besylate; benazepril HCl
	Zestril		
lithium carbonate	Eskalith		
	Lithobid	Lotrimin	clotrimazole
lithium citrate	Cibalith-S	Lotrisone	betamethasone; clotrimazole cream
Lithobid	lithium carbonate		
Lithostat	acetohydroxamic acid		
		lovastatin	Mevacor
Lodine	etodolac	Lovenox	enoxaparin sodium
lodoxamide tromethamine ophth soln	Alomide		
		loxapine succinate	Loxitane
Loestrin	norethindrone acetate; ethinyl estradiol	Loxitane	loxapine succinate
		Lozol	indapamide
		Ludiomil	maprotiline HCl
Lomotil	diphenoxylate HCl; atropine sulfate	Lufyllin	dyphylline
		Lupron	leuprolide acetate
		Luride	sodium fluoride
lomustine	CeeNu	Luvox	fluvoxamine maleate
Loniten	minoxidil tablets		
Lo/Ovral	norgestrel; ethinyl estradiol	lymphocyte immune globulin	Atgam
		lypressin	Diapid
loperamide HCl	Imodium	Lysodren	mitotane
Lopid	gemfibrozil		
Lopressor	metoprolol tartrate		
Lorabid	loracarbef		
loracarbef	Lorabid		
loratadine	Claritin		**M**
loratadine; pseudoephedrine sulfate	Claritin D		
lorazepam	Ativan		
Lorcet	hydrocodone bitartrate; acetaminophen	Maalox	aluminum hydroxide; magnesium hydroxide
Lortab	hydrocodone		

Macrobid	nitrofurantoin macrocrystals and mono-hydrate	medroxyprogesterone acetate	Cycrin Provera
Macrodantin	nitrofurantoin macrocrystals	medroxyprogesterone acetate SR	Depo-Provera
magaldrate	Riopan	mefenamic acid	Ponstel
magnesium chloride SR	Slow-Mag	mefloquine HCl	Lariam
Mandol	cefamandole nafate	Mefoxin	cefoxitin sodium
		Megace	megestrol acetate
maprotiline HCl	Ludiomil	megestrol acetate	Megace
Marcaine HCl	bupivacaine HCl	Mellaril	thioridazine HCl
Marinol	dronabinol	melphalan	Alkeran
Matulane	procarbazine HCl	menadiol sodium diphosphate	Synkayvite
Mavik	trandolapril	menotropins	Pergonal
Maxipime	cefepime HCl	*meperidine HCl*	Demerol
Maxzide	triamterene 75 mg; hydrochlorothiazide 50 mg	mephentermine sulfate	Wyamine
		mephenytoin	Mesantoin
		mephobarbital	Mebaral
Maxzide-25MG	triamterene 37.5 mg; hydrochlorothiazide 25 mg	mepivacaine HCl	Carbocaine
		meprobamate	Equanil Miltown
mazindol	Sanorex	Mepron	atovaquone
measles, mumps, rubella vaccines, combined	M-M-R II	mercaptopurine	Purinethol
		meropenem	Merrem
		Merrem	meropenem
		Meruvax II	rubella virus vaccine live attenuated
Mebaral	mephobarbital	mesalamine	Rowasa
mebendazole	Vermox	Mesantoin	mephenytoin
mecamylamine HCl	Inversine	mesna	Mesnex
		Mesnex	mesna
mechlorethamine HCl	Mustargen	mesoridazine	Serentil
		Mestinon	pyridostigmine bromide
Meclan	meclocycline sulfosalicylate	Metamucil	psyllium
meclizine	Antivert	Metaprel	metaproterenol sulfate
meclocycline sulfosalicylate	Meclan	metaproterenol sulfate	Alupent Metaprel
meclofenamate sodium	Meclomen	metaraminol bitartrate	Aramine
Meclomen	meclofenamate sodium	metformin HCl	Glucophage
		methadone HCl	Dolophine
Medrol	methylprednisolone	methamphetamine HCl	Desoxyn
		methazolamide	Neptazane

methenamine combination	Urised	metoprolol tartrate	Lopressor
methenamine hippurate	Hiprex	*metronidazole*	Flagyl
Methergine	methylergon-ovine maleate	metyrosine	Demser
		Mevacor	lovastatin
methicillin sodium	Staphcillin	Mexate	methotrexate
		mexiletine HCl	Mexitil
methimazole	Tapazole	Mexitil	mexiletine HCl
methocarbamol	Robaxin	Mezlin	mezlocillin
methohexital sodium	Brevital Sodium	mezlocillin	Mezlin
		Miacalcin	calcitonin-salmon
methotrexate	Folex		
	Mexate	Micro K	potassium chloride SR
methotrexate sodium tablets	Rheumatrex		
		miconazole nitrate	Monistat
methoxamine HCl	Vasoxyl		
		Micronase	glyburide
methoxsalen	Oxsoralen	Micronor	norethindrone
methscopamine bromide	Pamine	Midamor	amiloride HCl
		midazolam HCl	Versed
methyclothiazide	Enduron	milrinone lactate	Primacor
methyldopa	Aldomet	Miltown	meprobamate
methyldopa; hydrochlorothi-azide	Aldoril	Minipress	prazosin HCl
		Minocin	minocycline HCl
		minocycline HCl	Minocin
		minoxidil tablets	Loniten
methylergonovine maleate	Methergine	minoxidil topical	Rogaine
		Mintezol	thiabendazole
methylphenidate HCl	Ritalin	Miochol E	acetylcholine ophth
methylpredniso-lone	Medrol	mirtazapine	Remeron
		misoprostol	Cytotec
methylpredniso-lone acetate SR	Depo-Medrol	Mithracin	plicamycin
		mitomycin	Mutamycin
		mitotane	Lysodren
methylpredniso-lone sodium succinate	Solu-Medrol	mitoxantrone HCl	Novantrone
		Mivacron	mivacurium chloride
methyltestoster-one	Oreton Methyl	mivacurium chloride	Mivacron
methysergide maleate	Sansert	M-M-R II	measles, mumps, rubella vaccines, combined
Meticorten	prednisone		
metoclopramide HCl	Reglan		
		Moban	molindone HCl
metolazone	Diulo	Moduretic	amiloride HCl; hydrochlorothi-azide
	Zaroxolyn		
metoprolol succinate SR	Toprol XL		

moexipril HCl	Univasc	Myoscint	imciromab pentetate
molindone HCl	Moban	Mysoline	primidone
mometasone furoate	Elocon		
Monistat	miconazole nitrate		
Monocid	cefonicid sodium		
Monopril	fosinopril sodium	**N**	
moricizine	Ethmozine		
morphine sulfate	Roxanol		
morphine sulfate inj	Duramorph		
morphine sulfate SR	Kadian	nabumetone	Relafen
	MS Contin	nadolol	Corgard
	Oramorph SR	Nafcil	nafcillin sodium
	Roxanol SR	nafcillin sodium	Nafcil
Motrin	ibuprofen		Unipen
MS Contin	morphine sulfate SR	nalbuphine HCl	Nubain
Mucomyst	acetylcysteine	Nalfon	fenoprofen calcium
mupirocin nasal ointment	Bactroban	nalidixic acid	NegGram
muromonab-CD3	Orthoclone OKT3	nalmefene HCl	Revex
		naloxone HCl	Narcan
Mustargen	mechlorethamine HCl	naltrexone	ReVia
		nandrolone phenpropionate	Durabolin
Mutamycin	mitomycin		
M.V.I.-12	vitamin, multiple inj	nandrolone decanoate	Deca-Durabolin
Myambutol	ethambutol HCl	naphazoline ophth soln	Vasocon
Mycelex	clotrimazole	Naprelan	naproxen sodium SR
Mycifradin Sulfate	neomycin sulfate oral soln	Naprosyn	naproxen
Myciguent	neomycin sulfate ointment and cream	naproxen	Naprosyn
		naproxen sodium	Anaprox
		naproxen sodium SR	Naprelan
Mycolog Cream	nystatin; triamcinolone cream	Narcan	naloxone HCl
		Nardil	phenelzine sulfate
mycophenolate mofetil	CellCept	Naropin	ropivacaine HCl
		Nasacort	triamcinolone acetonide nasal inhaler
Mycostatin	nystatin		
Mydriacyl	tropicamide		
Myleran	busulfan	Nasalcrom	cromolyn sodium
Mylicon	simethicone	Navane	thiothixene
Myochrysine	gold sodium thiomalate	Navelbine	vinorelbine tartrate

Nebcin	tobramycin sulfate	Nicorette	nicotine polacrilex
NebuPent	pentamidine isethionate aerosol	nicotine nasal spray	Nicotrol NS
nefazodone HCl	Serzone	nicotine polacrilex	Nicorette
NegGram	nalidixic acid	nicotine transdermal system	Habitrol
Nembutal	pentobarbital sodium		
Neo-Synephrine	phenylephrine HCl	Nicotrol NS	nicotine nasal spray
neomycin sulfate ointment and cream	Myciguent	nifedipine	Adalat Procardia
neomycin sulfate oral soln	Mycifradin Sulfate	nifedipine SR	Adalat CC Procardia XL
Neoral	cyclosporine microemulsion capsules and oral soln	Nimbex	cisatracurium besylate
		nimodipine	Nimotop
Neosar	cyclophospha-mide	Nimotop	nimodipine
		Nipride	nitroprusside sodium
Neosporin Cream	polymyxin; neomycin	nisoldipine SR	Sular
Neosporin Ointment	polymyxin; neomycin; bacitracin	Nitro-Bid	nitroglycerin SR
		Nitro-Dur	nitroglycerin transdermal
Neosporin ophth Ointment	polymyxin; neomycin; bacitracin	nitrofurantoin macrocrystals	Macrodantin
Neosporin ophth soln	polymyxin; neomycin	nitrofurantoin macrocrystals and monohydrate	Macrobid
neostigmine methylsulfate	Prostigmin	nitrofurazone	Furacin
Neptazane	methazolamide	nitroglycerin transdermal	Transderm-Nitro
Nesacaine	chloroprocaine HCl	nitroglycerin inj	Tridil
		nitroglycerin ointment	Nitrol
netilmicin sulfate	Netromycin	nitroglycerin SR	Nitro-Bid
Netromycin	netilmicin sulfate	*nitroglycerin sublingual tablets*	Nitrostat
Neupogen	filgrastim		
Neurontin	gabapentin	nitroglycerin transdermal	Nitro-Dur
Neutrexin	trimetrexate		
nevirapine	Viramune	Nitrol	nitroglycerin ointment
niacin SR	Nicobid		
nicardipine HCl	Cardene	nitroprusside sodium	Nipride
Niclocide	niclosamide		
niclosamide	Niclocide		
Nicobid	niacin SR		

Nitrostat	nitroglycerin sublingual tablets	Novolin L	insulin zinc suspension (Lente) (human)
nizatidine	Axid	Novolin N	isophane insulin suspension (NPH) (human)
Nizoral	ketoconazole		
Nolvadex	tamoxifen citrate		
Norcuron	vecuronium bromide		
Nordette	levonorgestrel	Novolin R	insulin inj (human)
norepinephrine bitartrate	Levophed		
		Nubain	nalbuphine HCl
norethindrone	Micronor	Numorphan	oxymorphone HCl
norethindrone acetate; ethinyl estradiol	Loestrin		
		Nupercainal	dibucaine
		Nuromax	doxacurium chloride
norethindrone; ethinyl estradiol (or mestranol)	Ortho-Novum (products)	Nuprin	ibuprofen
		Nutropin	somatropin for inj
		Nutropin AQ	somatropin inj
Norflex	orphenadrine citrate	Nydrazid	isoniazid
		nylidrin HCl	Arlidin
norfloxacin	Noroxin	*nystatin*	Mycostatin
Norgesic	orphenadrine citrate; aspirin; caffeine	nystatin; triamcinolone cream	Mycolog Cream
norgestrel; ethinyl estradiol	Lo/Ovral		
Normodyne	labetalol HCl		
Noroxin	norfloxacin		
Norpace	disopyramide phosphate		
Norplant	levonorgestrel implant	**O**	
Norpramin	desipramine HCl		
nortriptyline HCl	Aventyl Pamelor		
Norvasc	amlodipine besylate	octreotide acetate	Sandostatin
		ofloxacin	Floxin
Norvir	ritonavir	Ogen	estropipate
Novantrone	mitoxantrone HCl	olanzapine	Zyprexa
		olsalazine sodium	Dipentum
Novocain HCl	procaine HCl		
Novolin 70/30	isophane insulin suspension (NPH) 70%, insulin inj 30% (human)	omeprazole	Prilosec
		Omnipaque	iohexol
		Omnipen	ampicillin
		Omnipen-N	ampicillin sodium

Oncaspar	pegaspargase	Oxsoralen	methoxsalen
Oncovin	vincristine sulfate	oxtriphylline	Choledyl
		oxybutynin chloride	Ditropan
ondansetron	Zofran		
Ophthaine	proparacaine	oxychlorosene sodium	Clorpactin WCS-90
opium; belladonna suppositories	B & O Supprettes	oxycodone HCl	Roxicodone
		oxycodone HCl; acetaminophen	Percocet Roxicet
Opticrom	cromolyn sodium	oxycodone HCl; aspirin	Percodan
Optimine	azatadine maleate	oxymetazoline HCl	Afrin nasal spray Dristan Long Lasting
Oramorph SR	morphine sulfate SR		
Oretic	hydrochlorothiazide	oxymetholone	Anadrol-50
		oxymorphone HCl	Numorphan
Oreton Methyl	methyltestosterone		
Organidin NR	guaifenesin	oxytocin	Pitocin
Orinase	tolbutamide		
Ornade Spansules	phenylpropanolamine HCl; chlorpheniramine maleate SR		
orphenadrine citrate	Norflex		
orphenadrine citrate; aspirin; caffeine	Norgesic	**P**	
Ortho-Cept	desogestrel; ethinyl estradiol		
Ortho-Novum (products)	norethindrone; ethinyl estradiol (or mestranol)	paclitaxel	Taxol
		Pamelor	nortriptyline HCl
		pamidronate disodium	Aredia
Orthoclone OKT3	muromonab-CD3	Pamine	methscopolamine bromide
Orudis	ketoprofen	Pancrease	pancrelipase EC
Oruvail	ketoprofen SR	pancrelipase	Cotazym
Os-Cal 500	calcium carbonate	pancrelipase EC	Cotazym-S Pancrease
Otrivin	xylometazoline	pancuronium bromide	Pavulon
oxacillin sodium	Prostaphlin	papaverine HCl SR	Pavabid
Oxandrin	oxandrolone		
oxandrolone	Oxandrin	Paradione	paramethadione
oxaprozin	Daypro	Paraflex	chlorzoxazone 250 mg
oxazepam	Serax		
Oxilan	ioxilan		

Parafon Forte DSC	chlorzoxazone 500 mg	Pentam 300	pentamidine isethionate inj
paramethadione	Paradione		
Paraplatin	carboplatin	pentamidine isethionate aerosol	NebuPent
paregoric	camphorated tincture of opium	pentamidine isethionate inj	Pentam 300
pargyline HCl	Eutonyl	pentazocine HCl	Talwin
Parlodel	bromocriptine mesylate	pentazocine HCl; naloxone HCl	Talwin Nx
Parnate	tranylcypromine sulfate	pentobarbital sodium	Nembutal
paromomycin sulfate	Humatin	Pentothal	thiopental sodium
paroxetine HCl	Paxil	pentoxifylline	Trental
Parsidol	ethopropazine HCl	Pen Vee K	penicillin V potassium
Pavabid	papaverine HCl SR	Pepcid	famotidine
Pavulon	pancuronium bromide	Peptavlon	pentagastrin
Paxil	paroxetine HCl	Percocet	oxycodone HCl; acetaminophen
PBZ	tripelennamine HCl	Percodan	oxycodone HCl; aspirin
PCE Dispertab	erythromycin base coated particles	Pergonal	menotropins
		Periactin	cyproheptadine HCl
Pediazole	erythromycin ethylsuccinate; sulfisoxazole	Peri-Colace	docusate sodium; casanthranol
PedvaxHIB	haemophilus b vaccine	Peridex	chlorhexidine gluconate mouth rinse
pegaspargase	Oncaspar	Peritrate	pentaerythritol tetranitrate
pemoline	Cylert		
penicillamine	Cuprimine	Permitil	fluphenazine HCl
penicillin G benzathine	Bicillin L-A	perphenazine	Trilafon
penicillin G benzathine; penicillin G procaine	Bicillin C-R	perphenazine; amitriptyline HCl	Etrafon Triavil
penicillin G procaine	Wycillin	Persantine	dipyridamole
		petrolatum, white	Vaseline
penicillin V potassium	Pen Vee K V-Cillin K Veetids	phenazopyridine HCl	Pyridium
pentaerythritol tetranitrate	Peritrate	phendimetrazine tartrate	Plegine
pentagastrin	Peptavlon	phenelzine sulfate	Nardil

Phenergan	promethazine HCl	piperacillin sodium	Pipracil
phenobarbital	phenobarbital	piperacillin sodium; tazobactam sodium	Zosyn
phenobarbital, ergotamine; belladonna	Bellergal-S		
phenolphthalein	Ex-Lax	Pipracil	piperacillin sodium
phenoxybenzamine HCl	Dibenzyline	piroxicam	Feldene
phentermine HCl	Fastin	Pitocin	oxytocin
		Pitressin	vasopressin
phentolamine mesylate	Regitine	Placidyl	ethchlorvynol
phenylbutazone	Butazolidin	Plaquenil	hydroxychloroquine sulfate
phenylbutyrate sodium	Buphenyl	Plasbumin	albumin human
phenylephrine HCl	Neo-Synephrine	plasma protein fraction	Plasma-Plex Plasmanate Plasmatein Protenate
phenylpropanolamine HCl; chlorpheniramine maleate SR	Ornade Spansules		
		Plasma-Plex	plasma protein fraction
phenylpropanolamine HCl; caramiphen edisylate SR	Tuss-Ornade Spansules	Plasmanate	plasma protein fraction
		Plasmatein	plasma protein fraction
		Platinol AQ	cisplatin
phenylpropanolamine HCl; guaifenesin SR	Entex LA	Plegine	phendimetrazine tartrate
		Plendil	felodipine
phenytoin	Dilantin	plicamycin	Mithracin
Pholpholine Iodide	echothiophate iodide	pneumococcal vaccine	Pneumovax
Photofrin	porfimer sodium	Pneumovax	pneumococcal vaccine
physostigmine ophth ointment	Eserine Sulfate		
		Polaramine Repetabs	dexchlorpheniramine maleate SR
physostigmine salicylate	Antilirium	Polycillin	ampicillin
phytonadione	AquaMEPHYTON	Polycillin-N	ampicillin sodium
pilocarpine HCl ophth	Isopto Carpine	polymyxin B sulfate; trimethoprim ophth soln	Polytrim
pilocarpine HCl tablet	Salagen		
pindolol	Visken	polymyxin; neomycin	Neosporin Cream Neosporin ophth soln
pipecuronium bromide	Arduan		

polymyxin; neomycin; bacitracin	Neosporin Ointment	prednisolone syrup	Prelone
	Neosporin ophth Ointment	*prednisone*	Deltasone
polystyrene sulfonate sodium	Kayexalate		Meticorten
		Prelone	prednisolone syrup
polythiazide	Renese	Premarin	estrogens, conjugated
Polytrim	polymyxin B sulfate; trimethoprim ophth soln	Premphase	estrogens, conjugated; medroxyproges-terone acetate
Pondimin	fenfluramine HCl		
Ponstel	mefenamic acid	Prempro	estrogens, conjugated; medroxyproges-terone acetate
Pontocaine	tetracaine HCl		
porfimer sodium	Photofrin		
potassium bicarbonate; potassium citrate effervescent	K-Lyte	Prepidil	dinoprostone gel
		Prevacid	lansoprazole
		Prilosec	omeprazole
		Primacor	milrinone lactate
		Primaxin	imipenemcila-statin sodium
potassium chloride potassium bicarbonate effervescent	K-Lyte/Cl		
		primidone	Mysoline
		Principen	ampicillin
		Prinivil	lisinopril
		Priscoline	tolazoline
		Pro-Banthine	propantheline bromide
potassium chloride SR	Kaon-Cl		
	K-Dur		
	Klor-Con 10	probenecid	Benemid
	Slow-K	probenecid; colchicine	ColBENEMID
	Micro K		
potassium chloride; potassium gluconate	Kolyum	procainamide	Pronestyl
		procainamide HCl SR	Procan SR
			Procanbid
		procaine HCl	Novocain HCl
potassium gluconate	Kaon	Procan SR	procainamide HCl SR
povidone iodine	Betadine	Procanbid	procainamide HCl SR
pralidoxime chloride	Protopam		
		procarbazine HCl	Matulane
pramoxine HCl	Tronothane HCl		
		Procardia	nifedipine
Pravachol	pravastatin sodium	Procardia XL	nifedipine SR
		prochlorperazine	Compazine
		Procrit	epoetin alfa
pravastatin sodium	Pravachol	procyclidine HCl	Kemadrin
prazosin HCl	Minipress	Prograf	tacrolimus
Precose	acarbose	ProHIBiT	haemophilus b vaccine

Prokine	sargramostim
Proleukin	aldesleukin
Prolixin	fluphenazine HCl
Proloid	thyroglobulin
promazine HCl	Sparine
promethazine HCl	Phenergan
Pronestyl	procainamide
Propacet-100	propoxyphene napsylate; acetaminophen
propafenone HCl	Rythmol
propantheline bromide	Pro-Banthine
proparacaine	Ophthaine
Propine	dipivefrin
propofol	Diprivan
propoxyphene HCl	Darvon
propoxyphene HCl; acetaminophen	Wygesic
propoxyphene HCl; aspirin; caffeine	Darvon Compound 65
propoxyphene napsylate; acetaminophen	Darvocet-N 100 Propacet-100
propranolol HCl	Inderal
propranolol HCl; hydrochlorothiazide	Inderide
Propulsid	cisapride
Proscar	finasteride
Prostaphlin	oxacillin sodium
Prostigmin	neostigmine methylsulfate
Prostin E$_2$	dinoprostone vaginal suppositories
Prostin VR	alprostadil
protamine sulfate	protamine sulfate
Protenate	plasma protein fraction
Protopam	pralidoxime chloride
protriptyline HCl	Vivactil
Protropin	somatrem

Protropin II	somatropin for inj
Proventil	albuterol
Provera	medroxyprogesterone acetate
Prozac	fluoxetine HCl
pseudoephedrine HCl	Sudafed
pseudoephedrine HCl; bromphiramine maleate	Drixoral Syrup
psyllium	Konsyl-D Metamucil
Purinethol	mercaptopurine
Pyridium	phenazopyridine HCl
pyridostigmine bromide	Mestinon
pyrimethamine	Daraprim

Q

Quarzan	clidinium bromide
Questran	cholestyramine
Quinaglute	quinidine gluconate SR
quinapril HCl	Accupril
quinethazone	Hydromox
quinidine gluconate SR	Quinaglute
quinidine sulfate	quinidine sulfate

R

ramipril	Altace
ranitidine bismuth citrate	Tritec
ranitidine HCl	Zantac
Recombivax HB	hepatitis B vaccine

Redux	dexfenfluramine HCl	Rifamate	isoniazid; rifampin
Regitine	phentolamine mesylate	rifampin	Rifadin
			Rimactane
Reglan	metoclopramide HCl	Rilutek	riluzole
		riluzole	Rilutek
Regroton	chlorthalidone; reserpine	Rimactane	rifampin
		rimantadine	Flumadine
Relafen	nabumetone	rimexolone	Vexol
Remeron	mirtazapine	Riopan	magaldrate
remifentanil HCl	Ultiva	Risperdal	risperidone
		risperidone	Risperdal
Renese	polythiazide	Ritalin	methylphenidate HCl
Renova	tretinion topical		
ReoPro	abciximab	ritodrine HCl	Yutopar
reserpine	Serpasil	ritonavir	Norvir
RespiGam	respiratory syncytial virus immune globulin intravenous (human)	Robaxin	methocarbamol
		Robinul	glycopyrrolate
		Robitussin	guaifenesin
		Robitussin A-C	guaifenesin; codeine phosphate
respiratory syncytial virus immune globulin intravenous (human)	RespiGam	Robitussin-DM	guaifenesin; dextrometh-orphan
		Rocephin	ceftriaxone sodium
Restoril	temazepam	Roferon-A	interferon alfa-2a
Retin-A	tretinoin topical	Rogaine	minoxidil topical
Retrovir	zidovudine	ropivacaine HCl	Naropin
Revex	nalmefene HCl	Rowasa	mesalamine
ReVia	naltrexone	Roxanol	morphine sulfate
R-Gene	arginine HCl	Roxanol SR	morphine sulfate SR
Rheumatrex	methotrexate sodium tablets	Roxicet	oxycodone HCl; acetaminophen
Rhinocort	budesonide nasal inhaler	Roxicodone	oxycodone HCl
RH_0 (D) immune globulin	RhoGAM	rubella virus vaccine live attenuated	Meruvax II
RH_0 (D) immune globulin intravenous (human)	WinRho SD	Rubex	doxorubicin HCl
		Rythmol	propafenone HCl
RhoGAM	RH_0 (D) immune globulin		
ribavirin	Virazole		**S**
Ridaura	auranofin		
Rifadin	rifampin	Salagen	pilocarpine HCl tablet

salmeterol xinafoate	Serevent	Seromycin	cycloserine
		Serpasil	reserpine
salsalate	Disalcid	Serlect	sertindole
Sal-Tropine	atropine sulfate tablets	sertindole	Serlect
		sertraline HCl	Zoloft
Saluron	hydroflumethi-azide	Serzone	nefazodone HCl
Sandimmune	cyclosporine	sevoflurane	Ultane
Sandoglobulin	immune globulin intravenous	Silvadene	silver sulfadiazine
Sandostatin	octreotide acetate	silver sulfadiazine	Silvadene
Sanorex	mazindol		
Sansert	methysergide maleate	simethicone	Mylicon
		simvastatin	Zocor
Santyl	collagenase	Sinemet	levodopa; carbidopa
saquinavir mesylate	Invirase		
		Sinemet CR	levodopa; carbidopa SR
sargramostim	Leukine Prokine		
		Sinequan	doxepin HCl
Sclerosol	talc, sterile aerosol	Slo-bid	theophylline SR
scopolamine hydrobromide ophth	Isopto Hyoscine	Slo-Phyllin	theophylline SR
		Slow Fe	ferrous sulfate SR
scopolamine transdermal	Transderm Scop	Slow-K	potassium chloride SR
Sectral	acebutolol HCl	Slow-Mag	magnesium chloride SR
Seldane	terfenadine		
Seldane D	terfenadine; pseudoephed-rine HCl	sodium citrate; citric acid	Bicitra
		sodium fluoride	Luride
selegiline HCl	Eldepryl	sodium hyaluronate	Amvisc Healon
selenium sulfide	Selsun Blue		
Selsun Blue	selenium sulfide	sodium tetradecyl sulfate	Sotradecol
senna concentrates	Senokot		
		Solganal	aurothioglucose
Senokot	senna concentrates	Solu-Cortef	hydrocortisone sodium succinate
Septra	sulfamethox-azoletrimeth-oprim		
		Solu-Medrol	methylpredniso-lone sodium succinate
Ser-Ap-Es	hydralazine; hydrochloro-thiazide; reserpine		
		Soma	carisoprodol
		somatrem	Protropin
Serax	oxazepam	somatropin for inj	Nutropin Protropin II
Serentil	mesoridazine		
Serevent	salmeterol xinafoate	somatropin inj	Nutropin AQ
		sotalol	Betapace

Sotradecol	sodium tetradecyl sulfate	sulindac	Clinoril
		Sultrin	triple sulfa vaginal cream
Sparine	promazine HCl		
		sumatriptan	Imitrex
spectinomycin HCl	Trobicin	Sumycin	tetracycline HCl
		Suprane	desflurane
spironolactone	Aldactone	Suprax	cefixime
spironolactone; hydrochlorothi-azide	Aldactazide	Surfak	docusate calcium
		Survanta	beractant
		Symmetrel	amantadine HCl
Sporanox	itraconazole	Synalar	fluocinolone acetonide
Stadol	butorphanol tartrate inj		
		Synkayvite	menadiol sodium diphosphate
Stadol NS	butorphanol tartrate nasal spray		
		Synovir	thalidomide
		Synthroid	levothyroxine sodium
stanozolol	Winstrol		
Staphcillin	methicillin sodium		
Stelazine	trifluoperazine HCl		
Stilphostrol	diethylstilbestrol diphosphate		
		T	
Streptase	streptokinase		
streptokinase	Streptase		
streptomycin sulfate	streptomycin sulfate		
streptozocin	Zanosar	TACE	chlorotrianisene
Sublimaze	fentanyl citrate	tacrine HCl	Cognex
succinylcholine chloride	Anectine	tacrolimus	Prograf
		Tagamet	cimetidine HCl
sucralfate	Carafate	talc, sterile aerosol	Sclerosol
Sudafed	pseudoephedrine HCl		
		Talwin	pentazocine HCl
Sufenta	sufentanil citrate	Talwin Nx	pentazocine HCl; naloxone HCl
sufentanil citrate	Sufenta		
Sulamyd sodium	sulfacetamide sodium ophth	Tambocor	flecainide acetate
		tamoxifen citrate	Nolvadex
Sular	Nisoldipine SR	Tapazole	methimazole
sulfacetamide sodium ophth	Sulamyd sodium	Taractan	chlorprothixene
		Tavist	clemastine fumarate
sulfamethoxazole	Gantanol		
sulfamethoxazole-trimethoprim	Bactrim Cotrim co-trimoxazole Septra	Taxol	paclitaxel
		Taxotere	docetaxel
		Tazicef	ceftazidime
		Tazidime	ceftazidime
sulfasalazine	Azulfidine	Tegopen	cloxacillin sodium
sulfinpyrazone	Anturane		

Tegretol	carbamazepine		Slo-Phyllin
Teldrin	chlorpheniramine maleate SR	theophylline SR	Slo-bid
			Theo-Dur
Telepaque	iopanoic acid	TheraCys	BCG intravesical
temazepam	Restoril	Theragran-M	vitamins; minerals
Tenex	guanfacine HCl		
teniposide	Vumon	thiabendazole	Mintezol
Tenoretic	atenolol; chlorthalidone	thiethylperazine maleate	Torecan
Tenormin	atenolol	thioguanine	thioguanine
Tensilon	edrophonium chloride	thiopental sodium	Pentothal
Tenuate	diethylpropion HCl	Thioplex	thiotepa
		thioridazine HCl	Mellaril
Terazol	terconazole	thiotepa	Thioplex
terazosin HCl	Hytrin	thiothixene	Navane
terbinafine HCl	Lamisil	Thorazine	chlorpromazine
terbutaline sulfate aerosol	Brethaire	thyroglobulin	Proloid
		thyroid	thyroid
terbutaline sulfate tablets and inj	Brethine Bricanyl	thyrotropin	Thytropar
		Thytropar	thyrotropin
		Tiazac	diltiazem HCl SR
terconazole	Terazol		
terfenadine	Seldane	Ticar	ticarcillin disodium
terfenadine; pseudoephedrine HCl	Seldane D	ticarcillin disodium	Ticar
Teslac	testolactone	ticarcillin; clavulanic acid	Timentin
Testoderm	testosterone transdermal system	TICE BCG	BCG intravesical
		Ticlid	ticlopidine
		ticlopidine	Ticlid
testolactone	Teslac	Tigan	trimethobenzamide HCl
testosterone cypionate SR	DEPO-Testosterone		
testosterone transdermal system	Androderm Testoderm	Timentin	ticarcillin; clavulanic acid
		timolol	Timoptic
tetanus immune globulin (human)	Hyper-Tet	timolol maleate	Blocadren
		Timoptic	timolol
		Tinactin	tolnaftate
tetracaine HCl	Pontocaine	tizanidine HCl	Zanaflex
tetracycline HCl	Achromycin Sumycin	TobraDex	tobramycin; dexamethasone
tetrahydrozoline HCl ophth	Collyrium Visine Extra	tobramycin sulfate	Nebcin
thalidomide	Synovir	tobramycin sulfate ophth	Tobrex
Tham	tromethamine		
Theo-Dur	theophylline SR	tobramycin; dexamethasone	TobraDex
theophylline	Elixophyllin		

317

Tobrex	tobramycin sulfate ophth	tretinion topical	Renova Retin-A
tocainide HCl	Tonocard	tretinoin capsules	Vesanoid
Tofranil	imipramine HCl	triamcinolone acetonide	Aristocort Kenalog
tolazamide	Tolinase	triamcinolone acetonide aerosol	Azmacort
tolazoline	Priscoline		
tolbutamide	Orinase	triamcinolone acetonide nasal inhaler	Nasacort
Tolectin	tolmetin sodium		
Tolinase	tolazamide		
tolmetin sodium	Tolectin	triamterene	Dyrenium
tolnaftate	Tinactin	triamterene 37.5 mg; hydro-chlorothiazide 25 mg	Maxzide -25MG Dyazide
Tonocard	tocainide HCl		
Topicort	desoximetasone		
topotecan HCl	Hycamtin		
Toprol XL	metoprolol succinate SR	triamterene 75 mg; hydro-chlorothiazide 50 mg	Maxzide
Toradol	ketorolac tromethamine		
Torecan	thiethylperazine maleate	Triavil	perphenazine; amitriptyline HCl
toremifene citrate	Fareston	triazolam	Halcion
		Tridesilon	desonide
Tornalate	bitolterol mesylate	Tridil	nitroglycerin inj
torsemide	Demadex	Tridione	trimethadione
Totacillin-N	ampicillin sodium	trifluoperazine HCl	Stelazine
Tracrium	atracurium besylate	trifluridine	Viroptic
tramadol HCl	Ultram	trihexyphenidyl HCl	Artane
Trandate	labetalol HCl		
trandolapril	Mavik	Trilafon	perphenazine
Transderm Scop	scopolamine transdermal	Tri-Levlen	levonorgestrel; ethinyl estradiol
Transderm-Nitro	nitroglycerin transdermal	Trilisate	choline magnesium trisalicylate
Tranxene	clorazepate dipotassium		
tranylcypromine sulfate	Parnate	trimethadione	Tridione
		trimethaphan camsylate	Arfonad
Trasylol	aprotinin		
Travasol	amino acid inj	trimethobenza-mide HCl	Tigan
trazodone HCl	Desyrel	trimetrexate	Neutrexin
Trecator-SC	ethionamide	Trimox	amoxicillin
Trental	pentoxifylline	Triostat	liothyronine sodium inj

Tripedia	diphtheria & tetanus toxoids & acellular pertussis vaccine
tripelennamine HCl	PBZ
Triphasil	levonorgestrel; ethinyl estradiol
triple sulfa vaginal cream	Sultrin
triprolidine HCl; pseudoephedrine HCl	Actifed
Tritec	ranitidine bismuth citrate
Tri-Vi-Flor	vitamins A, D, & C; fluoride
Trobicin	spectinomycin HCl
tromethamine	Tham
Tronothane HCl	pramoxine HCl
TrophAmine	amino acid inj
Tropicacyl	tropicamide
tropicamide	Mydriacyl Tropicacyl
Trusopt	dorzolamide HCl
tuberculin skin test	Aplisol
tubocurarine	tubocurarine
Tucks	witch hazel pads
Tums	calcium carbonate
Tuss-Ornade Spansules	phenylpropanolamine HCl; caramiphen edisylate SR
Tussi-Organidin NR	guaifenesin; codeine phosphate
Tussionex	hydrocodone polistirex; chlorpheniramine
Tylenol	acetaminophen

U

Ultane	sevoflurane
Ultiva	remifentanil HCl
Ultralente U	insulin zinc suspension, extended (beef)
Ultram	tramadol HCl
Ultravist	iopromide
Unasyn	ampicillin sodium; sulbactam sodium
Unipen	nafcillin sodium
Univasc	moexipril HCl
Urecholine	bethanechol chloride
Urised	methenamine combination
Urispas	flavoxate HCl
urokinase	Abbokinase
ursodiol	Actigall

V

valacyclovir	Valtrex
Valium	diazepam
valproic acid	Depakene
Valtrex	valacyclovir
Vancenase	beclomethasone dipropionate
Vancenase AQ Nasal	beclomethasone dipropionate
Vanceril	beclomethasone dipropionate

Vancocin	vancomycin HCl	Vermox	mebendazole
vancomycin HCl	Vancocin	Versed	midazolam HCl
Vantin	cefpodoxime proxetil	Vesanoid	tretinoin capsules
		Vexol	rimexolone
Vaponefrin	epinephrine racemic	Vibramycin	doxycycline hyclate
Vaqta	hepatitis A vaccine, inactivated	Vicodin	hydrocodone bitartrate; acetaminophen
varicella virus vaccine	Varivax	vidarabine monohydrate	Vira-A
Varivax	varicella virus vaccine	Videx	didanosine
Vascor	bepridil	vinblastine sulfate	Velban
Vaseline	petrolatum, white	vincristine sulfate	Oncovin
Vaseretic	enalapril maleate; hydrochloro- thiazide	vindesine sulfate	Eldisine
		vinorelbine tartrate	Navelbine
Vasocon	naphazoline ophth soln	Vioform	clioquinol
Vasodilan	isoxsuprine HCl	Vira-A	vidarabine monohydrate
vasopressin	Pitressin	Viramune	nevirapine
Vasotec	enalapril maleate	Virazole	ribavirin
Vasoxyl	methoxamine HCl	Viroptic	trifluridine
V-Cillin K	penicillin V potassium	Visine Extra	tetrahydrozoline HCl ophth
		Visipaque	iodixanol
vecuronium bromide	Norcuron	Visken	pindolol
		Vistaril	hydroxyzine pamoate
Veetids	penicillin V potassium	Vistide	cidofovir
Velban	vinblastine sulfate	vitamin A	Aquasol A
		vitamin B complex; folic acid; vitamin C	Berroca
Velosef	cephradine		
Velosulin Human	insulin inj (human)		
venlafaxine HCl	Effexor	vitamin, multiple inj	M.V.I.-12
Ventolin	albuterol	vitamins A, D, & C; fluoride	Tri-Vi-Flor
VePesid	etoposide		
verapamil HCl	Isoptin		
verapamil HCl SR	Calan SR	vitamins; minerals	Centrum Theragran-M
verapamil HCl SR	Verelan	Vitrasert	ganciclovir ophth implant
verapamil HCl SR bedtime formulation	Covera HS		
		Vivactil	protriptyline HCl
Verelan	verapamil HCl SR		

Vivelle	estradiol transdermal system
Voltaren	diclofenac sodium
Voltaren-XR	diclofenac sodium SR
Vumon	teniposide

W

warfarin sodium	Coumadin
Wellbutrin	bupropion HCl
Wellcovorin	leucovorin calcium
WinRho SD	RH$_O$ (D) immune globulin intravenous (human)
Winstrol	stanozolol
witch hazel pads	Tucks
Wyamine	mephentermine sulfate
Wycillin	penicillin G procaine
Wydase	hyaluronidase
Wygesic	propoxyphene HCl; acetaminophen
Wytensin	guanabenz acetate

XYZ

Xalatan	latanoprost
Xanax	alprazolam
Xylocaine HCl	lidocaine HCl
xylometazoline	Otrivin
Yutopar	ritodrine HCl
zalcitabine	Hivid
Zanaflex	tizanidine HCl
Zanosar	streptozocin
Zantac	ranitidine HCl
Zarontin	ethosuximide
Zaroxolyn	metolazone
Zestril	lisinopril
Zetar	coal tar product
Ziac	bisoprolol fumarate; hydrochloro-thiazide
zidovudine	Retrovir
Zinacef	cefuroxime sodium
Zinecard	dexrazoxane
Zithromax	azithromycin
Zocor	simvastatin
Zofran	ondansetron
Zoladex	goserelin acetate
Zoloft	sertraline HCl
zolpidem tartrate	Ambien
Zosyn	piperacillin so-dium; tazobac-tam sodium
Zovirax	acyclovir
Zyloprim	allopurinol
Zyprexa	olanzapine
Zyrtec	cetirizine HCl

References

1. Olin BR ed. Facts and comparisons. St. Louis: Facts and Comparisons, Inc. (published yearly)

2. Billup NF, Billup SM. American drug index. St. Louis: Facts and Comparisons, Inc. (published yearly)

3. Physicians GenRx. St. Louis: Mosby. (published yearly)

4. Reynolds JEF, ed. Martindale: The extra pharmacopeia. London: 31st edition. The Pharmaceutical Press. 1996

Chapter 6

Normal Laboratory Values*

In the following tables, normal reference values for commonly requested laboratory tests are listed in traditional units and in SI units. The tables are a guideline only. Values are method dependent and "normal values" may vary between laboratories.

	Blood, Plasma or Serum	
	Reference Value	
Determination	**Conventional Units**	**SI Units**
Ammonia (NH₃)	10–80 μg/dl	5–50 μmol/L
Amylase	≤130 units/L	≤130 units/L
Antinuclear antibodies	negative at 1 : 10 dilution of serum	negative a 1 : 10 dilution of serum
Antithrombin III (AT III)	80%–120%	
Bilirubin: conjugated total	≤0.2 mg/dl 0.1–1 mg/dl	≤4 μmol/L 2–18 μmol/L
Calcitonin:	<100 ng/L	<100 ng/L
Calcium: female <50 years old female >50 years old male	8.8–10 mg/dl 8.8–10.2 mg/dl 8.8–10.3 mg/dl	2.2–2.5 mmol/L 2.2–2.56 mmol/L 2.2–2.58 mmol/L
Carbon dioxide content	22–28 mEq/L	22–28 mmol/L
Carcinoembryonic antigen	<3 ng/ml	<3 μg/L
Chloride	95–105 mEq/L	95–105 mmol/L
Coagulation screen: Bleeding time Prothrombin time Partial thromboplastin time (activated) Protein C Protein S	3–9.5 min <2 sec from control 22–37 sec 58%–148% 58%–148%	180–570 sec <2 sec from control 22–37 sec
Copper, total	70–140 μg/dl	11–22 μmol/L
Corticotropin (ACTH)	20–100 pg/mL	4–22 pmol/L
Cortisol: 0800 hr 1800 hr 2400 hr	4–19 μg/dl 2–15 μg/dl <5 μg/dl	110–520 nmol/L 40–410 nmol/L <140 nmol/L
Creatine phosphokinase, total (CK, CPK)	≤150 units/L	≤150 units/L
Creatine phosphokinase isoenzymes, MB fraction	>5% in MI	>0.05 fraction of 1
Creatinine	0.6–1.2 mg/dl	50–110 μmol/L
Fibrinogen (coagulation factor I)	150–350 mg/dl	1.5–3.5 g/L
Follicle stimulating hormone (FSH): female peak production male	2–15 mIU/mL 20–50 mIU/mL 1–10 mIU/mL	2–15 IU/L 20–50 IU/L 1–10 IU/L

*1996 by Facts and Comparisons. Used with permission from *Drug Facts and Comparisons, 1996 ed.* St. Louis: Facts and Comparisons, Inc.

Blood, Plasma or Serum (Cont.)		
	Reference Value	
Determination	**Conventional Units**	**SI Units**
Glucose fasting	70–110 mg/dl	3.9–6.1 mmol/L
Haptoglobin	50–220 mg/dl	0.5–2.2 g/L
Hematologic tests:		
Hematocrit (Hct), female	33%–43%	0.33–0.43 fraction of 1
male	39%–49%	0.39–0.49 fraction of 1
Hemoglobin (Hb), female	11.5–15.5 g/dl	115–155 g/L
male	14–18 g/dl	140–180 g/L
Leukocyte count (WBC)	3200–9800/mm^3	3.2–9.8 × 10^9/L
Erythrocyte count (RBC), female	3.5–5 10^6/mm^3	3.5–5 × 10^{12}/L
male	4.3–5.9 10^6/mm^3	4.3–5.9 × 10^{12}/L
Mean corpuscular volume (MCV)	76–100 μm^3/cell	76–100 fl/cell
Mean corpuscular hemoglobin (MCH)	27–33 pg/RBC	27–33 pg/RBC
Mean corpuscular hemoglobin concentration (MCHC)	33–37 g/dl	330–370 g/L
Erythrocyte sedimentation rate (sedrate, ESR): female	≤30 mm/hr	≤30 mm/hr
male	≤20 mm/hr	≤20 mm/hr
Erythrocyte enzymes:		
Glucose-6-phosphate dehydrogenase (G6PD)	5–15 units/g Hb	5–15 units/g Hb
Pyruvate kinase	13–17 units/g Hb	13–17 units/g Hb
Ferritin	18–300 ng/mL	18–300 μg/L
Folic acid: normal	>3.3 ng/mL	>7.3 nmol/L
borderline	2.5–3.2 ng/mL	5.75–7.39 nmol/L
Platelet count	130–400 × 10^3/mm^3	130–400 × 10^9/L
Vitamin B$_{12}$:	200–1000 pg/mL	150–750 pmol/L
Iron		
female	60–160 μg/dl	11–29 μmol/L
male	80–180 μg/dl	14–32 μmol/L
Iron binding capacity	250–460 μg/dl	45–82 μmol/L
Lactic acid (lactate)	0.5–2 mEq/L	0.5–2.2 mmol/L
Lactic dehydrogenase	50–150 units/L	50–150 units/L
Lead	≤60 μg/dl	≤2.9 μmol/L
Lipids:		
Lipids, total	400–850 mg/dl	4–8.5 g/L
Total cholesterol		
<29 years old	<200 mg/dl	<5.2 mmol/L
30–39 years old	<225 mg/dl	<5.85 mmol/L
40–49 years old	<245 mg/dl	>6.35 mmol/L
>50 years old	<265	<6.85
LDL	50–190 mg/dl	1.3–4.9 mmol/L
HDL		
female	30–90 mg/dl	0.8–2.35 mmol/L
male	30–70 mg/dl	0.8–1.8 mmol/L
Triglycerides	<460 mg/dl	<1.8 g/L
Magnesium	1.6–2.4 mEq/L	0.8–1.2 mmol/L
Osmolality	280–300 mOsm/kg	280–300 mmol/kg
Oxygen saturation (arterial)	96%–100%	0.96–1 fraction of 1

Normal Laboratory Values (Cont.) Blood

	Blood, Plasma or Serum (Cont.)	
	Reference Value	
Determination	**Conventional Units**	**SI Units**
PCO$_2$, Arterial	35–45 mm Hg	4.7–6 kPa
pH, Arterial	7.35–7.45	7.35–7.45
PO$_2$, Arterial: breathing room air[1] on 100% O$_2$	75–100 mm Hg >500 mm Hg	10–13.3 kPa
Phosphatase (acid), total:	≤3 King-Armstrong units/dl ≤3 Bodansky units/dl	≤5.5 units/L ≤16.1 units/L
Phosphatase (alkaline)[2]	30–120 units/L	30–120 units L
Phosphorus, inorganic[3] (phosphate)	2.5–5 mg/dl	0.8–1.6 mmol/L
Potassium	3.5–5 mEq/L	3.5–5 mmol/L
Progesterone: Follicular phase Luteal phase	<2 ng/mL 2–20 ng/mL	<6 nmol/L 6–64 nmol/L
Prolactin	<20 ng/mL	<20 µg/L
Prostate specific antigen	0–4 ng/ml	
Protein: Total Albumin Globulin	6–8 g/dl 4–6 g/dl 2.3–3.5 g/dl	60–80 g/L 40–60 g/L 23–35 g/L
Rheumatoid factor	<80 IU/mL	<80 KIU/L
Sodium	135–147 mEq/L	135–147 mmol/L
Testosterone: female male	<0.6 ng/mL 4–8 ng/mL	<2 nmol/L 14–28 nmol/L
Thyroid Hormone Function Tests: Thyroid-stimulating hormone (TSH) Thyroxine-binding globulin capacity Total triiodothyronine (T$_3$) Total thyroxine by RIA (T$_4$) T$_3$ resin uptake	2–11 µ units/mL 15–28 µg T$_4$/dl 75–220 ng/dl 4–11 µg/dl 25%–35%	2–11 mU/L 150–360 nmol/L 1.2–3.4 nmol/L 52–142 nmol/L 0.25–0.35 fraction of 1
Transaminase, AST (Aspartate aminotransferase, SGOT)	≤35 units/L	≤35 units/L
Transaminase, ALT (Alanine aminotransferase, SGPT)	≤35 units/L	≤35 units/L
Urea nitrogen (BUN)	8–18 mg/dl	3–6.5 mmol/L
Uric acid	2–7 mg/dl	120–420 µmol/L
Vitamin A (retinol)	10–50 µg/dl	0.35–1.75 µmol/L
Zinc	75–120 µg/dl	11.5–18.5 µmol/L

[1]Age dependent.
[2]Infants and adolescents up to 104 units/L.
[3]Infants in the first year up to 6 mg/dl.

Normal Laboratory Values-Drug Levels

Drug Levels†			
		Reference Value	
Drug Determination		**Conventional Units**	**SI Units**
Aminoglycosides (peak levels)	Amikacin	16–32 μg/mL	nd
	Gentamicin	4–8 μg/mL	nd
	Kanamycin	15–40 μg/mL	nd
	Netilmicin	6–10 μg/mL	nd
	Streptomycin	20–30 μg/mL	nd
	Tobramycin	4–8 μg/mL	nd
Anti-arrhythmics	Amiodarone	0.5–2.5 μg/mL	nd
	Bretylium	0.5–1.5 μg/mL	nd
	Digitoxin	9–25 μg/L	11.8–32.8 nmol/L
	Digoxin	0.5–2.2 ng/mL	0.6–2.8 nmol/L
	Disopyramide	2–8 μg/mL	6–18 μmol/L
	Flecainide	0.2–1 μg/mL	nd
	Lidocaine	1.5–6 μg/mL	4.5–21.5 μmol/L
	Mexiletine	0.5–2 μg/mL	nd
	Procainamide	4–8 μg/mL	17–34 μmol/L
	Propranolol	50–200 ng/mL	190–770 nmol/L
	Quinidine	2–6 μg/mL	4.6–9.2 μmol/L
	Tocainide	4–10 μg/mL	nd
	Verapamil	0.08–0.3 μg/mL	nd
Anti-convulsants	Carbamazepine	4–12 μg/mL	17–51 μmol/L
	Phenobarbital	15–40 μg/mL	65–172 μmol/L
	Phenytoin	10–20 μg/mL	40–80 μmol/L
	Primidone	5–12 μg/mL	25–46 μmol/L
	Valproic acid	50–100 μg/mL	350–700 μmol/L
Anti-depressants	Amitriptyline	110–250 ng/mL	nd
	Amoxapine	200–500 ng/mL	nd
	Bupropion	25–100 ng/mL	nd
	Clomipramine	80–100 ng/mL	nd
	Desipramine	125–300 ng/mL	nd
	Doxepin	100–200 ng/mL	nd
	Imipramine	200–350 ng/mL	nd
	Maprotiline	200–300 ng/mL	nd
	Nortriptyline	50–150 ng/mL	nd
	Protriptyline	100–200 ng/mL	nd
	Trazodone	800–1600 ng/mL	nd
Antipsychotics	Chlorpromazine	30–500 ng/mL	nd
	Fluphenazine	0.13–2.8 ng/mL	nd
	Haloperidol	5–20 ng/mL	nd
	Perphenazine	0.8–1.2 ng/mL	nd
	Thiothixene	2–57 ng/mL	nd
Miscellaneous	Amantadine	300 ng/mL	nd
	Amrinone	3.7 μg/mL	nd
	Chloramphenicol	10–20 μg/mL	31–62 μmol/L
	Cyclosporine[1]	250–800 ng/mL (whole blood, RIA)	nd
		50–300 ng/mL (plasma, RIA)	nd
	Ethanol[2]	0 mg/dl	0 mmol/L
	Hydralazine	100 ng/dl	nd
	Lithium	0.5–1.5 mEq/L	0.5–1.5 mmol/L
	Salicylate	100–200 mg/L	724–1448 μmol/L
	Sulfonamide	5–15 mg/dl	nd
	Terbutaline	0.5–4.1 ng/mL	nd
	Theophyline	10–20 μg/mL	55–110 μmol/L
	Vancomycin (peak)	30–40 μg/mL	nd

†The values given are generally accepted as desirable for achieving therapeutic effect without toxicity for most patients. However, exceptions are not uncommon.
[1] 24 hour trough values. [2] Toxic: 50–100 mg/dl (10.9–21.7 mmol/L).
nd—No data available.

Normal Laboratory Values-Urine

URINE		
	Reference Value	
Determination	**Conventional Units**	**SI Units**
Catecholamines: Epinephrine Norepinephrine	<10 µg/day <100 µg/day	<55 nmol/day <590 nmol/day
Creatinine: female male	14–22 mg/kg/24 h 20–26 mg/kg/24 h	0.12–0.19 mmol/kg/day 0.18–0.23 mmol/kg/day
Potassium (diet dependent)	25–100 mEq/day	25–100 mmol/day
Protein, quantitative	<150 mg/day	<0.15 g/day

Steroids:

	Age (yrs)	(mg/day)		(µmol/day)	
		male	female	male	female
17-Ketosteroids	10	1–4	1–4	3–14	3–14
	20	6–21	4–16	21–73	14–56
	30	8–26	4–14	28–90	14–49
	50	5–18	3–9	17–62	10–31
	70	2–10	1–7	7–35	3–24
17-Hydroxycorticosteroids (as cortisol): female male		2–8 mg/day 3–10 mg/day		5–25 µmol/day 10–30 µmol/day	

Please forward additional meanings for these abbreviations, additional abbreviations and their meanings, or corrections to the author so that the list can be updated. Thank you. Dr. Neil M. Davis, 1143 Wright Drive, Huntingdon Valley, PA 19006-2721.
FAX (215) 938 1937. E-mail med@neilmdavis.com

Additions

Additions

Additions

Additions